GALEN AND THE ARABIC RECEPTION OF PLATO'S *TIMAEUS*

This first full-length study of the Arabic reception of Plato's *Timaeus* considers the role of Galen of Pergamum (129–*c.* 216 CE) in shaping medieval perceptions of the text as transgressing disciplinary norms. It argues that Galen appealed to the entangled cosmological scheme of the dialogue, where different relations connect the body, soul, and cosmos, to expand the boundaries of medicine in his pursuit of epistemic authority – the right to define and explain natural reality. Aileen Das situates Galen's work on disciplinary boundaries in the context of medicine's ancient rivalry with philosophy, whose professionals were long seen as possessing superior knowledge of the cosmos vis-à-vis that of doctors. Her case studies show how Galen and four of the most important Christian, Muslim, and Jewish thinkers in the Arabic Middle Ages creatively interpreted key doctrines from the *Timaeus* to reimagine medicine and philosophy as well as their own intellectual identities.

AILEEN R. DAS is an Assistant Professor of Classical Studies and Middle East Studies at the University of Michigan. Her work aims to illuminate the diverse, and often subversive, uses to which medieval Arabic writers put their Graeco-Roman sources in realising their own scientific ambitions. In addition to translating Arabic versions of lost or fragmentary Greek texts, she has published on various topics relating to ancient and medieval medicine and philosophy, including Islamicate receptions of Hippocrates, epitomatory literature, and views on plant life.

GALEN AND THE ARABIC RECEPTION OF PLATO'S *TIMAEUS*

AILEEN R. DAS
University of Michigan, Ann Arbor

CAMBRIDGE
UNIVERSITY PRESS

CAMBRIDGE
UNIVERSITY PRESS

University Printing House, Cambridge CB2 8BS, United Kingdom

One Liberty Plaza, 20th Floor, New York, NY 10006, USA

477 Williamstown Road, Port Melbourne, VIC 3207, Australia

314–321, 3rd Floor, Plot 3, Splendor Forum, Jasola District Centre,
New Delhi – 110025, India

79 Anson Road, #06–04/06, Singapore 079906

Cambridge University Press is part of the University of Cambridge.

It furthers the University's mission by disseminating knowledge in the pursuit of education, learning, and research at the highest international levels of excellence.

www.cambridge.org
Information on this title: www.cambridge.org/9781108499484
DOI: 10.1017/9781108583107

First published 2020

A catalogue record for this publication is available from the British Library.

ISBN 978-1-108-49948-4 Hardback

In memory of Amanda Das (1985–2013)

Contents

Figures

Acknowledgements

This book began around ten years ago as a doctoral thesis at the University of Warwick, which funded my studies through a Warwick Postgraduate Research Fellowship. I am grateful to Peter Pormann and Maude Vanhaelen for their joint supervision; from them, I learned how to navigate my way through medieval Arabic texts without losing sight of the broader historical picture. I also wish to thank Simon Swain, who taught me invaluable lessons during my stay at Warwick, and Uwe Vagelpohl, who read drafts of several chapters. During the preparation of my thesis, I benefited from Gerrit Bos and Rüdiger Arnzen generously making their work available to me pre-publication.

Since the thesis's completion, the project has undergone reconceptualization a few times, prompted in part by the helpful feedback that I received from my Ph.D. examiners, Peter Adamson and Mark Schiefsky. My interest in disciplinarity and knowledge production – issues which inform the conceptual core of the book – was sparked during my time as an Early Career Fellow at the Institute of Advanced Study at the University of Warwick and as a Frances A. Yates Short-Term Fellow at the Warburg Institute, where I found it generative to listen to researchers from diverse disciplinary backgrounds discuss the claims and limitations of their own fields. Special thanks go to Charles Burnett for his warm welcome to the Warburg and to the members of the Arabic philosophy reading group that met weekly at the institute, whose impressive command of medieval Arabic set a model for my own work. During this period, the award of a Leverhulme Small Research Grant to myself and Pauline Koetschet, who has been a supportive interlocutor for some years now, enabled me to write the section on al-Rāzī's Platonic sources in Chapter 3.

My colleagues at the University of Michigan assisted me greatly while I completed this book. My chairs Sara Forsdyke and Artemis Leontis have been very conscientious about protecting my time as a junior faculty member. I am also indebted in particular to Ryan Szpiech, Sara Ahbel-Rappe,

Rafe Neis, and Karla Mallette for their comments on the book during its many stages; their advice both encouraged me to develop further my theoretical arguments and helped me to articulate them clearly. Samer Ali graciously made time to translate with me Arabic passages with which I was having difficulty. My use of the conceptual frame of boundary work to describe the refiguring of medicine and philosophy that is the subject of this book is an outcome of my year of leave at Michigan's Institute for the Humanities, where I profited from intellectual exchanges with the director, Peggy McCracken, and colleagues from sociology, political science, and comparative literature. Off campus, the suggestions of James Uden at Boston University were indispensable for improving the book's introduction. Christina Hoenig also provided valuable observations on a draft version of the monograph.

I wish to express gratitude to my commissioning editor at Cambridge, Michael Sharp, for his interest in and assistance with the project during its various phases of production. Furthermore, this book is a better book because of the considerate responses of the Press's two anonymous readers, from whose reports I learned a lot. In preparing my manuscript for publication, I have received technical aid from a number of individuals and financial support from the Bruce Friar Fund. Salman Elamir Amir and Daniel Davies proofread the Arabic texts, Jonathan Farr copyedited and indexed the entire book, and Molly Schaub compiled the bibliographies. All errors are, of course, my own.

Over the course of the decade during which this book has been taking shape, my family has kept up my spirits when I felt fatigued or uncertain about what I was doing. Finally, words cannot adequately convey my appreciation for the love and support of my colleague and partner Ian Fielding. He has guided me through my grief for the loss of my older sister Amanda, who passed unexpectedly less than a month before my viva, and weathered two transatlantic moves with me. Moreover, I have benefited immensely from watching him approach his own research and receiving feedback from him on my own.

Notes on Texts, Translations, and Transliterations

Editions and Translations

< > Diamond brackets enclose words or letters added by the editor (or by me).

[ ] Square brackets in the edition of a text enclose material an editor or I think should be deleted. In a translation, they indicate words that have been supplied for the sake of clarification.

On an orthographical note, I have kept *tašdīd* (the doubling of consonants) to a minimum – on accusative and preventive particles and where context demands – for typographical reasons.

Transliteration

The following system of transliteration is employed for Arabic:

ا ā; ء ʾ; ب b; ث ṯ; ج ǧ; ح ḥ; خ ḫ; د d; ذ ḏ; ر r; ز z; س s; ش š; ص ṣ; ض ḍ; ط ṭ; ظ ẓ; ع ʿ; غ ġ; ف f; ق q; ل l; م m; ن n; ه h; و w, ū; ي-ية ī, iyya

For Hebrew, I follow the general transliteration rules of the *Encyclopaedia Judaica* (2nd edition), ed. M. Berenbaum and F. Skolnik (Detroit, 2007), vol. I, pp. 197–9. My transliteration of ancient Greek conforms to the American Library Association-Library of Congress romanization scheme. In my bibliography, for Arabic and Hebrew titles, I reproduce the transliterations given in WorldCat.

Abbreviations

All abbreviations of the Galenic corpus follow the system used in the *Cambridge Companion to Galen*. I model my abbreviations of Aristotle's works on the *Oxford Handbook of Aristotle*. The abbreviations of other Graeco-Roman sources follow the usage of the *Oxford Classical Dictionary, 4th edition*. In addition, the following abbreviations are used for reference works, collections, and editions frequently cited:

ANRW	*Aufstieg und Niedergang der römischen Welt*, ed. W. Haase and H. Temporini (Berlin, 1972–).
Com. Tim.	*Galeni Compendium Timaei Platonis*, ed. and trans. P. Kraus and R. Walzer (London, 1951).
EI	*Encyclopaedia of Islam*, 1st edn., 9 vols. (online).
EI^{2}	*Encyclopaedia of Islam*, 2nd edn., 12 vols. (online).
EI^{3}	*Encyclopaedia of Islam, Three* (online).
EIr	*Encyclopaedia Iranica* (electronic resource), ed. E. Yarshater (New York, 1998).
K	*Claudii Galeni Opera Omnia*, ed. K. G. Kühn, 20 vols. (Leipzig, 1821–33).
LG	*L'anima e il dolore: De indolentia-De propriis placitis. Testo greco a fronte*, ed. and trans. A. Lami and I. Garofalo (Milan, 2012).
LSJ	*Greek–English Lexicon*, ed. H. G. Liddell, R. Scott, and H. S. Jones (9th edn., Oxford, 1996).
M–J	*Dalālat al-Ḥā'irīn*, ed. S. Munk and I. Joel (Jerusalem, 1930–1).
NP	*Brill's New Pauly Online Encyclopaedia of the Ancient World* (Leiden, 2005–).

OLD	*Oxford Latin Dictionary*, ed. P. G. W. Glare (2nd edn., Oxford, 2012).
SVF	*Stoicorum Veterum Fragmenta.*, ed. H. von Arnim, 3 vols. (Leipzig, 1903).
WGAÜ	*Wörterbuch zu den griechisch-arabischen Übersetzungen des 9. Jahrhunderts*, Supplement, Band I: A–O, ed. M. Ullmann (Wiesbaden, 2006).

Introduction: Plato's Timaeus *as Universal Text*

ἔδοξεν γὰρ ἡμῖν Τίμαιον μέν, ἅτε ὄντα ἀστρονομικώτατον ἡμῶν καὶ περὶ φύσεως τοῦ παντὸς εἰδέναι μάλιστα ἔργον πεποιημένον, πρῶτον λέγειν ἀρχόμενον ἀπὸ τῆς τοῦ κόσμου γενέσεως, τελευτᾶν δὲ εἰς ἀνθρώπων φύσιν.

We decided that Timaeus shall speak first because he is the most learned of us in astronomy and has especially made it his task to know about the nature of the All. Beginning with the birth of the cosmos, he will finish with the nature of humans. Plato, *Timaeus* 27a3–6

Of Plato's dialogues, the *Timaeus* has had the most constant and pervasive presence in the intellectual cultures of Europe and the Middle East. Its partial translation into Latin by Cicero (106–43 BCE) and Calcidius (*c.* mid. third or early fourth century CE) made it the only Platonic text accessible to medieval readers without Greek before the twelfth century.[1] Owing to its complex transmission into Arabic, it also appears to have been the dialogue with which pre-modern Islamicate thinkers were best acquainted.[2] Modern interpreters have pointed to the 'fluidity' of the language and imagery of the eponymous Timaeus' monologue, which seems to accommodate diverse readings, as one possible reason for the enduring appeal of a work often not ranked among Plato's most

[1] On these Latin translations and their contribution to the medieval reception of Plato in western Europe, see, e.g., Somfai (2002); Lévy (2003); Burnett (2012); Sedley (2013); Hoenig (2018).

[2] On the transmission of the Platonic corpus into Arabic, see below (pp. 22–4). In this book, I use the adjective 'Islamicate', which was coined by Marshall Hodgson (1974: vol. I, 57–60), to designate societies, cultures, and peoples in regions where Muslims are politically and culturally dominant. 'Islamicate' does not refer directly to the religion of Islam but rather to the 'social and cultural complex historically associated with Islam', which is found both among Muslims and non-Muslims (Hodgson 1974: vol. I, 59). This term is especially relevant to my study as Chapter 2 centres on a member of the Church of the East, Ḥunayn ibn Isḥāq, and Chapter 5, a Jew, Moses Maimonides. I give Islamic calendar dates (with the Gregorian calendar equivalents following) for all the Islamicate figures mentioned in this book because it was the official dating system used in the majority-Muslim areas where they were working.

metaphysically important compositions.[3] In particular, the dialogue's depiction of a supreme craftsman god (the Demiurge, *dēmiourgos*), who caused the world to 'become' (*gegonen*, 28b7), invited adherents of Judaism, Christianity, and Islam to draw connections with their monotheistic creation accounts.[4] More recently, physicists and philosophers of science have recognized in the *Timaeus* a cosmology that not only anticipates the Big Bang theory but also wrestles with the same issues at the centre of contemporary speculations about the universe, such as its uniqueness and the contingency of the events occurring in it.[5]

In the passage quoted in the epigraph above, the character Critias draws attention to the extraordinarily ambitious scope of Timaeus' ensuing speech: it aims to cover everything, the world and its contents.[6] The broad range of material that the dialogue encompasses certainly accounts for its rich history of reception outside natural philosophy (namely, 'physics'), which ancient sources list as its subject.[7] Astronomers, musicologists, and mathematicians, among others, found in the text details pertinent to their own interests.[8] The *Timaeus*, however, is 'no mere collection of bits of information'.[9] Plato's narrative links together the parts of the cosmos by sketching out different causal, analogous, or homologous relationships between them: for instance, the composition of the four elements out of triangles explains their transformations (56c8–57d6) as well as why living things age (81b4–d4); the movement of harmonious music is similar to the orbits of the heavens and the soul (47b5–e2); and the metaphysical principle of space has the same function as a uterus or a perfume base (50d2–4, 50e4–8). These

[3] Reydam-Schils (2003), 13. See also Celia and Ulacco (2012), vii. See Owen (1953), 95, who asserts that the *Timaeus* has overshadowed the 'more sophisticated metaphysics' of the 'profoundly important late dialogues' such as the *Philebus*. Sharples and Sheppard (2003: 1) write that the low estimation of the *Timaeus* has ancient precedent.

[4] Niehoff (2007) argues that the dialogue created textual communities among Christian and pagan readers, who respectively championed literal and metaphorical readings of its cosmogony.

[5] See Brisson and Meyerstein (1995) ; Leggett (2010).

[6] As Mohr (2010: 1) observes, this comprehensive narrative unfolds over the course of just sixty-five pages.

[7] The Alexandrian grammarian Aristophanes of Byzantium (*c.* 265–190 or 257–180 BCE) arranged the Platonic dialogues into trilogies, the first of which seems to have contained texts dealing chiefly with physics: *Republic*, *Timaeus*, and *Critias* (Tarrant 1993: 106). See *PHP* 9.9.3 (De Lacy 2005: p. 598 l. 10), where Galen states that the *Timaeus* gives an 'account of the natural world' (*physiologia*). Cf. Albinus (second century CE), *Prol.* 5.25–9, and Proclus (fifth century CE), *In Ti.* I 1.17–20, both of whom relate that the dialogue's enquiry into nature includes theological matters.

[8] On the use of Plato's *Timaeus* by pre-modern and early modern astronomers, mathematicians, and musicologists, see Gregory (2003); Barker (2003); Allen (2003); Prins (2014).

[9] Reydam-Schils (2003), 4.

connections appear to signify that the domains of knowledge concerned with the aforementioned phenomena – geometry, physics, biology, etc. – are not self-sufficient but 'entangled'.[10] Moreover, as I will mention below, the dialogue's own reflection on the epistemological status of its narrative, which it famously calls an *eikōs logos* or *mythos* ('a likely account or myth'), suggests that these very domains are not fixed but alterable.

Among the many ancient readers of the *Timaeus* who responded to the text's fluidity, Galen of Pergamum (129–*c.* 216 CE), after Hippocrates the most famous doctor of Graeco-Roman antiquity, was one of the most significant and provocative. This book is about Galen's reading of the *Timaeus,* and about the reception of that reading in the Middle Ages, mainly in the Islamicate world. It makes two key arguments: first, that Galen was the first to seize on the potential in the *Timaeus* to reimagine the discipline of medicine.[11] While doctors before Galen engaged with Plato's *Timaeus,* he is unprecedented in his use of the dialogue to conceptualize not only aspects of human physiology but also the boundaries of medical knowledge, which he shows a distinctive concern to define.[12] I situate Galen's anxiety about the epistemic topography of this discipline in the context of the broader rivalry between medicine and philosophy that had been ongoing since Plato but whose stakes were raised in the agonistic climate of the Second Sophistic. At the root of the competitive displays of learning (*paideia*) characteristic of the period of the Second Sophistic (*c.* 60–230 CE) were struggles for power – including wealth, political office, and socio-cultural prestige – that resulted in the re-creation or reinscription of group identities (ethnic and professional, for example).[13] Besides rewards such as increased patronage, Galen, this book maintains, turned to

[10] I adopt Barad's (2007) concept of 'entanglement', which denies an inherent separation between entities in the world. For Barad, entanglement does not 'mean just any old kind of connection, interweaving, or enmeshment in a complicated situation' (160), but rather speaks to a relational ontology, in which boundaries and properties become determinate when 'cuts' are made between what is included or excluded from consideration during acts of observation (or any way of knowing). While Barad is primarily interested in the relations between material bodies, her framework (or as she calls it, 'onto-epistem-ology') does not assume an intrinsic difference between 'human and nonhuman, subject and object, mind and body, matter and discourse' (185).

[11] On my use of 'discipline', see pp. 10–12 below.

[12] For example, Polito (2013) discusses how the doctor Asclepiades of Bithynia (first century BCE) developed his atomistic theory of matter in response to the Platonist Heraclides of Pontus' (fourth century BCE) interpretation of the dialogue's account of the geometrical shapes of the four elements.

[13] On the Second Sophistic, see Bowersock (1969); Anderson (1993); Gleason (1995); Swain (1996); Whitmarsh (2001, 2005). Cf. Eshleman (2012) and Dench (2017), who encourage a new approach to the Second Sophistic that does not see Greekness but rather profession as the foundational concern of its identity dynamics.

the *Timaeus* to invest medicine with epistemic authority – the right, long enjoyed by philosophy, to define, describe, and explain the different domains of reality – and thus to enhance the standing of his own profession. Galen's youthful training in philosophy made him uniquely qualified to leverage the dialogue's model of knowledge to redraw the boundaries of medicine; his education also equipped him to anticipate the critiques of philosophers, for whom the text was a visible site for working out sectarian doctrine and identity.[14]

Galen does not comment on whether his disciplinary project gained traction among his contemporaries, perhaps because the degree of its success is irrelevant to his self-presentation, which he crafts through a rhetoric of exceptionalism. The further entrenchment of medicine's lowly position in late antique and medieval hierarchies of knowledge appears to testify to Galen's failure to revise the epistemic landscape. The second argument developed in this book is that Galen's project and its significance cannot fully be understood without considering its medieval reception in Arabic writings. The Islamicate receptions studied in the second part of this book will reveal, in fact, that his disciplinary boundary work – a phrase that I borrow from science and technology studies (STS), to be explained more fully below – with the *Timaeus* was productive of new ways of thinking about knowledge categories and professional identities.[15] A similar story to the one that will unfold over the bulk of this book (Chapters 2–5) could perhaps be told about the late antique Mediterranean or medieval Latin West, in which Galen was an important presence.[16] I have historical and ideological reasons, however, for foregrounding medieval Islamicate responses to Galen's use of the *Timaeus*.

First, the medieval Islamicate world lends itself to a study of shifts in disciplinary thinking because the large-scale translation of scientific texts from the Graeco-Roman Mediterranean and other pre-modern societies into Arabic encouraged reflection from those living both during and after this activity on their own cultural boundaries of knowledge vis-à-vis this assimilated past. Second, in giving full attention to Islamicate actors, my aim is to redress their marginalization in medical and intellectual histories

[14] For the *Timaeus*' presence in contemporary philosophical debate, see Fowler (2017) *passim* and pp. 36–8 below.

[15] See pp. 11–12 below.

[16] For Galen's reception in the Graeco-Roman Mediterranean during the centuries immediately following his death and in the medieval West, I refer the reader to the relevant chapters in the recent *Brill's Companion to the Reception of Galen* (Bouras-Vallianatos and Zipser 2019).

that define their historical value in terms of their preservation and transmission of a (largely) Greek past to the West.[17] The point of my analysis of the four Islamicate thinkers treated in the latter half of this book – Ḥunayn ibn Isḥāq (d. 260/873 or 264/877), Abū Bakr al-Rāzī (d. *c.* 313/925), Avicenna (d. 428/1037), and Maimonides (d. 600/1204) – is to demonstrate that they continually refigure, rather than adopt, Galen's map of medical and philosophical knowledge when seeking to establish their own authority. My examination also calls into question the adequacy of terms such as 'synthesis' and 'adaptation' for describing medieval knowledge projects such as those that form the core of this book, for, while more agentive, they still imply that the 'synthesizer' or 'adaptor' is confined by the prior system(s) in which they are working. This book hopes to stimulate a new approach to pre-modern knowledge that denies a significant disjunct between ancient and medieval 'scientific' categories and their modern counterparts, whose rhetorical nature STS research over the past thirty years has underscored.[18]

Although medicine wields significant cultural authority today, I argue in this introduction that the impetus behind Galen's boundary work was the discipline's inferior ranking in the epistemic hierarchies of antiquity. The first section will connect these ancient claims about medicine's inferiority to earlier, often polemically charged, observations on the contingent nature of its knowledge, as well as the social status of the majority of its practitioners. After outlining my methodological approach to 'science' as a discursive and iterative practice, I will consider how the *Timaeus* itself recognizes the dynamism of knowledge: its potential to be divided and bounded differently by each knower. Galen's philosophical training may have brought him into initial contact with Plato's dialogue, but, as I will next discuss, he exploits the text's epistemic possibilities to promote his professional identity as a doctor in contests with philosophers (both dead and living) for credibility. Finally, to preface the second part of this book, I propose that Galen's own role in interfacing Arabic readers with the *Timaeus* called for Islamicate doctors and philosophers to re-evaluate their own categories and taxonomies of knowledge, which had been shaped by late antique epistemologies.

[17] Cf. Brentjes' (2012: 154–6) call for more agential histories of science in Islamic societies that give serious consideration to local contexts, individuality, and identity.

[18] For now-classic studies of the rhetorical constitution of science, which are overwhelmingly centred on the modern and contemporary periods, see Gieryn (1983); Latour and Woolgar (1986); Shapin (1992); Gross (1996); Taylor (1996).

Ancient Hierarchies of Knowledge: Medicine as a *Technē*

Most ancient, and subsequently medieval Islamicate, epistemologies put forward a pyramidal vision of knowledge, which recognizes different forms of knowing and gives some of these forms priority over others. Although medicine's classification and position in these epistemological schemes may be at the root of the struggle of doctors such as Galen to endow their expertise with prestige, it is important to note that there is no absolute consensus regarding how this unit of knowledge should be categorized. The inconsistency in the labelling of medicine across ancient and medieval writings, and even within individual authors, is one of the reasons why I find it more productive to refer to this area of knowledge as a 'discipline' – a term with ancient roots but especially modern associations, as I will explain in more detail below.[19] Traditionally rendered as 'art' or 'craft', *technē* (Lat. *ars*; Arab. *ṣināʿa*) is the designation most commonly applied to medicine in Greek; as a category of knowledge, it is often distinguished from *empeiria* ('knack', 'routine') and *epistēmē* ('science', 'theoretical knowledge': Lat. *scientia*; Arab. *ʿilm*), which philosophy is usually called. The Hippocratic Corpus, in particular the tracts *On Ancient Medicine* (Περὶ ἀρχαίης ἰητρικῆς) and *On the Art* (Περὶ τέχνης), offers the earliest surviving comments on the defining characteristics of a *technē* when responding to critics who deny that medicine warrants the identification or that this kind of knowledge exists at all.[20] The Hippocratic idea that a *technē* utilizes a rational, teachable method to achieve a goal, and in so doing asserts control over luck (*tychē*) and nature (*physis*), anticipates – and might even have informed – Plato and Aristotle's understandings of the concept.[21] For an activity to qualify as a *technē*, both philosophers require it to have a goal (*telos*), which determines the domain of the action, and that its practitioners be able to explain what and why they do what they do.[22]

19 *OLD*, s.v. 'disciplina 2a'.

20 See Schiefsky (2005), 5–25, and Mann (2012), 1–20, who review how these two texts respectively define the concept of *technē* and defend medicine's classification as such. See also Lloyd's (1991) discussion of the polemical targets of the two aforementioned Hippocratic treatises, *On Regimen in Acute Diseases* (Περὶ διαίτης ὀξέων), and *On the Sacred Disease* (Περὶ ἱερῆς νούσου). Craik (2015: 40, 285) dates *On the Art* and *On Ancient Medicine* to the late fifth century BCE. This dating suggests that these Hippocratic authors may be drawing on earlier sixth- and fifth-century conceptions of *technē*.

21 See Schiefsky (2005), 5, who states that Plato and Aristotle adopted the same notion of *technē* at the basis of *On Ancient Medicine*. Cf. Mann (2012), 1, who is more cautious about linking the Hippocratic, Platonic, and Aristotelian theories of *technē*. For the opposition between *technē* and *tychē*, see Nussbaum (2001), 89–106; on the sometimes adversarial relationship between *technē* and *physis*, see von Staden (2007).

22 There is a large amount of secondary scholarship on the meaning of *technē* in Plato and Aristotle; for good overviews of their definitions of the term, see, e.g., Isnardi Parente (1966); Roochnik (1996); Balansard (2001); Löbl (2003), 61–150, 178–264.

The ability of a *technē* to provide an account of its goal and methods is the feature that differentiates it from an *empeiria* – which, according to Plato, is unable to give a reason for each of the things that it does – but it also blurs the distinction between this form of knowledge and *epistēmē*.[23] Among the different relations that Plato sketches out between *technē* and *epistēmē*, he seems in certain dialogues to make the latter a component of the former by calling the reasoning of *technai* '*epistēmai*'.[24] Furthermore, the definition of the medical art as 'the science of health' (ἐπιστήμη . . . τοῦ ὑγιεινοῦ) at *Chrm.* 165c8 indicates a more radical elision of the two knowledge types in that this passage views *technē* as nothing other than an *epistēmē*.[25] The contrast introduced elsewhere in Plato's writings between practical and theoretical knowledge, which does not produce anything, may have stimulated Aristotle's own separation and evaluation of the categories of *technē* and *epistēmē*.[26] Pointing to the productive nature of *technē*, Aristotle assigns it an inferior ontological and epistemological value vis-à-vis *epistēmē* because it deals with things that change (not always systematically); thus, the instability of their subject compels practitioners to depend at times on conjecture.[27] The superiority of *epistēmē*, then, follows from its concern with invariable and eternal objects, which can be known with certainty through demonstration (*apodeixis*, proof by deduction).[28] At *Met.* 981b13–25 Aristotle also interprets the unproductivity, or uselessness (τὸ μὴ πρὸς χρῆσιν εἶναι), of *epistēmē* as a marker of its elite social status, for those who pursue it have the leisure to think about issues that will bring them little to no financial gain.[29]

To upgrade the *technē* of medicine in the hierarchy of the arts and sciences, Galen has to confront the idea that the ontological inferiority of the body, which is a realm of change, disqualifies it from being a source of

[23] At *Grg.* 501a4–b1, Plato describes the *empeiria* of cooking as acting 'without reason' (*alogōs*). On the distinction between *technē* and *empeiria* in the *Gorgias* and other dialogues, see Schiefsky (2005), 346–50; Levin (2014), 7–20.

[24] E.g., *Euthyd.* 281a4–5: 'Furthermore, I presume that in the working connected with furniture it is theoretical knowledge that effects the right work' (ἀλλὰ μήν που καὶ ἐν τῇ περὶ τὰ σκεύη ἐργασίᾳ τὸ ὀρθῶς ἐπιστήμη ἐστὶν ἡ ἀπεργαζομένη: Lamb 1924: 413 [slightly modified]).

[25] Isnardi Parente (1966) charts a progressive separation of the concept of *technē* from *epistēmē* in the Academy and Aristotle that eventually collapses in the Hellenistic period. For a critique of Isnardi Parente's methodology, especially with reference to her analysis of Aristotle, see Natali (2007), 5.

[26] See *Plt.* 258d–260a. In this text, Plato seems to use *technē* and *epistēmē* interchangeably; his concern is not to establish *technē* as being inherently more practical than *epistēmē* but to assert the existence of a kind of knowledge that is unproductive.

[27] See *EN* 1140a. On Aristotle's recognition of the imprecision of *technē*, see Schiefsky (2005), 366–70.

[28] See *EN* 1139b. For Aristotle's notion of 'demonstration', see, e.g., *APo* 71b20–5 and Barnes (1969); Lloyd (1992); Mendell (1998); Allen (2011).

[29] In this passage, Aristotle seems to conflate *epistēmē* with a subset of *technai* that concentrate on theoretical questions, such as mathematics.

demonstrative knowledge. Notwithstanding Galen's efforts to rehabilitate utility as a desirable quality of *technē*, the social stigma associated with doctors' and other craftpersons' receipt of pay for their services was hard to erase. In antiquity, work for wages was regarded as akin to slavery and therefore beneath the elite, who ideally were to draw on inherited wealth to fund their careers in politics.[30] Additionally, the participation of slaves, freedpersons, and foreigners in medicine, at least in the Roman world, contributed to the low esteem of the *technē*, and may account for why it was never regarded as one of the canonical *artes liberales* – 'the arts worthy of a free person'.[31] Banned from Athens and Rome for brief intervals, philosophy had its own problems with its reputation during antiquity, but philosophers' education of the elite and, in many cases, their own elite backgrounds meant that the field did not have the same social baggage as medicine.[32]

A Roman citizen with landed property, Galen is conspicuous proof that medicine was not just an occupation of the non-elite.[33] It has been argued that, long before Galen, doctors from more well-to-do families or with

30 Kudlien (1976), 448; Horstmanshoff (1990), 193. As Horstmanshoff (1990: 180–1) observes, it was not until the nineteenth century that medicine was viewed as a profession of high social status.

31 Nutton (2004: 165) reports that three-quarters of the doctors recorded in inscriptions in the western part of the Roman Empire in the first century CE were slaves (either born into slavery or captured in war) and ex-slaves. See also Kobayashi (1988); Pleket (1995). On medicine's place among the 'liberal arts', see Kudlien (1976), 450–1; Horstmanshoff (1990), 195. The Greek precursor of the *artes liberales* was the ἐγκύκλιος παιδεία, a general education for elite youths that did not usually include medicine (see *NP*, s.v. 'enkyklios paideia'). While some elite women such as Minicia Marcella, the second daughter of the younger Pliny's friend Minicius Fundanus, were permitted by their male relatives to study the *artes liberales*, this education was intended for freeborn men (see Hemelrijk 1999: 60–1). On ancient education as an 'essentially masculine process', see Morgan (1998), 48.

32 For the social standing of philosophers in the classical and Hellenistic periods, see Korhonen (1997) and Chang (2008). The decree of Sophocles of Sounion in 307–306 BCE, which was repealed within a year, forbade philosophers to hold seminars and classes in Athens (Korhonen 1997: 75–85). In Rome, the Senate approved the expulsion of philosophers and rhetors from the city in 161 BCE; in 173 or 154 BCE two Epicurean philosophers were banished; and the emperors Vespasian and Domitian exiled philosophers in 71 (or 74), 85, and 90 CE (see Gell. *NA* 15.11 and Gruen 1990: 171–9). As Striker (1995: 54) observes, when attempting to show the respectability of philosophy to his elite Roman readers, Cicero, like Plato before him, had to address their suspicions that it was politically disruptive. Hine (2016: 15) adds that republican and early imperial Romans such as Cicero and Seneca the Younger were hesitant to apply the label *philosophus* to themselves on account of its ethnic connotations – at this time it usually described Greek professional teachers of philosophy. Because they received pay from their aristocratic clientele, philosophers were not immune from accusations of greed and chicanery; for example, they were lampooned in Greek comedy for their mercenary behaviour (see Korhonen 1997: 86–96).

33 On the social status and wealth of Galen's family, see Nutton (2004), 216–17; Mattern (2013), 28–35. According to ancient bibliographies (on which, see Pinault 1992: 5–34), Hippocrates claimed noble descent from the Asclepiads, who traced their lineage back to the healing god Asclepius. At *Opt.Med. Cogn.* 1.3–4 (Iskandar 1988: p. 40 l. 11–p. 42 l. 6), which is extant only in Arabic, Galen alludes to medicine's divine origins to attest to the discipline's former prestige.

social ambitions in the fifth and fourth centuries BCE set out to distance themselves from their non-elite colleagues by adopting theories from philosophy.[34] Thus, medicine had its own internal hierarchy, which prioritized doctors who possessed the theoretical training to investigate the nature and cause of disease over those focused on identifying and subsequently treating their patients' complaints.[35] Galen's invocation of Plato's *Timaeus* should be viewed as a continuation of this strategy to increase the social and intellectual profile of medicine through a connection with philosophy. The ways in which this relationship was typically framed in antiquity subordinated medicine to philosophy: medicine borrows from philosophy because of a lack in its conceptual resources, or is a part of philosophy and thus not completely autonomous.[36] This book maintains, however, that Galen interprets the link between medicine and philosophy to imply neither a one-sided dependence nor a conflation of the two areas of knowledge. His aim is to prove that medicine can offer an equally valid – and sometimes superior – method for accessing truths about the cosmos.

Although Galen's defence of medicine starts from its assumed inferiority, philosophy did not enjoy its position as the highest form of knowledge without contest even prior to him. As Levin reveals, Plato himself treats medicine as a serious challenger for philosophy's claim to authority on nature and human flourishing (*eudaimonia*).[37] In response to this threat, Plato cites the primacy of the soul over the body as grounds for demoting medicine, whose domain he restricts to bodily health.[38] Furthermore, the doctor Eryximachus' incompetent foray into cosmology and ethics at *Symp.* 185e6–188e5, where this character not only gets previous physical theories wrong but also allows for the indulgence of unhealthy desires, calls into question medicine's right to comment on these subjects, which should fall under philosophy's jurisdiction.[39] Considering Plato's rivalry with

[34] Horstmanshoff (1990); Chang (2008).

[35] Plato, *Leg.* 720a–c, and Aristotle, *Pol.* 1282a4–8, famously distinguish between types of physicians: elite, non-elite, and lay. In the Platonic text the contrast is specifically between free and slave doctors. Because of the latter's inability to give a rational account (*logos*) of their activities, they practise the *empeiria* rather than the *technē* of medicine.

[36] Cf. Philo, *De congressu erud. gratia* §§ 141–57, which alleges that the *technai* have stolen ideas from philosophy and passed them off as their own. Cf. also Celsus, *De Medicina* pr.6–8: 'At first, the science of healing was considered a part of philosophy . . . the pupil Hippocrates of Cos, the first [doctor] worthy of mention, separated this discipline from the study of wisdom, a man marked by both his skill and eloquence' (*Primoque medendi scientia sapientiae pars habebatur . . . discipulus Hippocrates Cous, primus ex omnibus memoria dignus, a studio sapientiae disciplinam hanc separavit, vir et arte et facundia insignis*). On the philosophical origins of medicine in Celsus' history, see Mudry (1982), 63–5.

[37] Levin (2014) tracks this rivalry across the *Gorgias*, *Symposium*, *Republic*, and *Laws*.

[38] Levin (2014), 20–40, 122–8. [39] Levin (2014), 73–109.

medicine, it seems especially subversive that Galen has recourse to one of his dialogues to justify his own more expansive notion of the *technē*'s epistemic reach.[40] Galen never addresses the tension between medicine and philosophy in the Platonic corpus, but this silence may have more to do with his rhetorical strategy, which seeks to cast Plato as a prototype for his own blend of medical and philosophical expertise, than obliviousness on his part. Before delving into why the *Timaeus* lends itself to Galen's reworking of medicine, it will be helpful to clarify my use of the term 'discipline' to refer to medicine and philosophy.

The foregoing discussion has reviewed the ancient structuring of knowledge into categories that were assigned different epistemological, ontological, and social values. While the continued presence of terms such as *technē* and *epistēmē* in ancient discourses of knowledge gives the impression of a certain constancy in their meaning, it is important to observe that they are subject to considerable slippage, even in an author who is concerned to maintain a distinction between them, such as Aristotle. Although Aristotle regularly calls medicine a *technē* (for example, at *Met.* 1070a29, *Pol.* 1279a1, *Poet.* 1460b20, and *EN* 1097a9), in the *Prior Analytics* (26a10–13, 64a40–b28) he takes it for granted that the proposition 'medicine (*iatrikē*) is a science (*epistēmē*)' is true, and he uses it to check the validity of certain argumentative forms. Less consistent authors such as Galen contribute to this 'terminological promiscuity' (as Isnardi Parente puts it) by defining *technē* and *epistēmē* to suit their ideological purposes.[41] In including philosophy in the same rank of *technai* as medicine, Galen's *Exhortation to the Arts*, for instance, makes the ability to produce demonstrative knowledge a characteristic of *technē* and therefore deprives *epistēmē* of its monopoly on this way of knowing.[42] For this reason, I am not going to insist on strict definitions of the two terms when ancient and medieval authors do not actually adhere to their own. Instead, I want to emphasize that what these words express is a power relationship: they are devices that can be

[40] Levin (2014) does not include the *Timaeus* in her analysis. Her reading of *Laws* proposes that Plato has resolved his rivalry with medicine by acknowledging its contribution to *eudaimonia* at this late stage of his career (Levin 2014: 177–211). One of his mature dialogues, the *Timaeus* also seems to be sympathetic to medicine in that it recognizes the pertinence of the body to the study of the cosmos; however, the fact that an expert in astronomy and physics, rather than a doctor, is the source of the medical information may represent a move to subsume medicine into natural philosophy. For Plato's subordination of medicine to philosophy in the *Timaeus*, see Chapter 1 (pp. 54–6 below).

[41] Isnardi Parente (1966), 1.

[42] See *Protr.* 5.2 (Boudon-Millot 2002a: p. 88 l. 23–p. 89 l. 2), where medicine and philosophy occupy the highest level of the hierarchy of *technai*. Cf. Levin (2014), 110–41, who discusses how Plato redefines *technē* in the *Republic* to exclude medicine from this category of knowledge.

reformulated to exclude or legitimize contenders for intellectual and social authority. The purpose of the above terminological survey is to show that medicine did not occupy a dominant position in the epistemological schemes before (and, as I will show, even after) Galen, so this study's broader examination of his and his Islamicate successors' reconfiguration of medical knowledge should be viewed as part of a play for power.

In my translations of primary source passages, I render *epistēmē* and its Arabic equivalent *ʿilm* as 'science' and *technē* and its Arabic equivalent *ṣināʿa* as 'art', but I employ the word 'discipline', a term more attuned to an analysis of power relations, to describe the fields of philosophical and medical knowledge captured by these pre-modern terms. Similar to the ancient and medieval categories, 'discipline' is not without its problems, and the term may seem anachronistic because it is commonly invoked with reference to modern institutional contexts – for example, research universities, professional societies, and governmental agencies.[43] The concept, nonetheless, has been generative in both knowledge studies and STS in the investigation of how types of knowledge are related to one another and the power dynamics involved.[44] My book pursues this line of enquiry by looking into the discursive practice of discipline construction with regard to 'medicine' and 'philosophy', and the struggles for legitimacy and influence behind it.[45] I do not consider disciplines to be historically transcendent categories but fields of possibilities, some of which are put forward over others in conflicts for what Bourdieu calls symbolic capital – that is, intellectual and socio-cultural prestige.[46] The following study focuses on disciplines in theory rather than in practice, for how

[43] Cf., e.g., the definitions of 'discipline' or 'disciplinarity' given by Messer-Davidow, Shumway, and Sylvan (1993: 3): 'disciplinarity is about the coherence of a set of otherwise disparate elements, objects of study, methods of analysis, scholars, students, journals, and grants, to name a few'; and Jacobs (2013: 35): 'discipline is a self-regulating body of researchers and scholars based in a university'. Foucault famously associated disciplinarity with power in *Discipline and Punish: The Birth of the Prison* (*Surveiller et punir: Naissance de la prison*, 1975), which builds on *The Archaeology of Knowledge* (*L'archéologie du savoir*, 1969). This work is not specifically concerned with the formation of knowledge categories but with social power-wielding activities. Be that as it may, as Goldstein (1984: 178) notes, Foucault draws implicit connections between the two practices throughout the text. See, e.g., Foucault's (1975: 187–8) discussion of the well-ordered hospital and the discipline of medicine.

[44] See, e.g., Messer-Davidow, Shumway, and Sylvan (1993); Klein (1996), 57–84.

[45] Cf. Lloyd (2009), who surveys the role of elite cadres in the development of disciplines such as medicine, philosophy, and law in pre-modern Greece and China.

[46] In this conceptualization of discipline, I draw on Bourdieu's (1993) field theory, which argues that social agents transform intellectual spaces such as 'science' and 'art' by redefining the terms of entry

Graeco-Roman and Islamicate practitioners wrote about their expertise could differ significantly from how they taught it in the classroom.[47] As a result, the discourses that I will highlight are pointedly elite and masculine; non-elite and women rivals are shut out from these struggles for disciplinary control and authority.

The theoretical framework of this book is indebted to Gieryn's sociological approach to science (in the modern understanding of the word) as a 'cultural map' that is drawn and redrawn according to context.[48] He proposes that science maintains its cultural authority through a process called 'boundary work': the attribution of certain qualities to scientists, their methods, and claims with the purpose of establishing a rhetorical boundary between science and other less 'credible' non-sciences.[49] What is at stake in this mapping out of science is 'epistemic authority' – the power to act as a believed and trusted interpreter of natural reality, and the symbolic and economic capital that goes with it.[50] In pursuit of this prize, rival authorities variously constrict or expand 'scientific' knowledge to include themselves or deny access to the privileged space of science.[51] The instances of boundary work explored in the ensuing five chapters will highlight how the contours of philosophy and medicine in premodernity were shaped by a similar competition for epistemic authority, which encompasses mastery over the sublunary world ('nature' in the pre-modern sense) but also the wider cosmos. By Galen's time, philosophy had mapped itself out as a space of epistemic authority by placing demonstrative knowledge, the soul, and macrocosm within its terrain, so the boundary work of philosophers mostly consists in policing its borders to protect its claim to these subjects. As the 'poser-science', however, medicine sought to allocate epistemic authority to itself by challenging philosophy's exclusive jurisdictional control over the body, soul, and cosmos. For Galen, the *Timaeus* was a resource in this contest for epistemic authority because, as I will now argue, it showed that

(who can be called a 'scientist' or 'artist' and what they need to know) in their pursuit of symbolic capital.

47 For educational theories and practices in Graeco-Roman antiquity and the medieval Islamicate world, see, e.g., Cribiore (2001); Xenophontos (2016); Makdisi (1981); Brentjes (2018).

48 It should be stressed that his approach does not reduce science to a mere social construct: 'The problem is not that there is no "real science" behind the cartographic representations, but that there are too many "real sciences". And even when all those sciences are added up, they still together do not allow either the sociologist or the players themselves to know a priori what science will look like on the next occasion for its mapping. But neither does it make much sense to think of science-on-the-map as just made up any old way' (Gieryn 1999: 19).

49 Gieryn (1999), 4. Cf. also Gieryn (1983).

50 Gieryn (1999), 1.

51 Gieryn (1999), 15–18.

knowledge was not fixed, and accordingly individual domains could be redrawn – and even done so more expansively.

Mapping Knowledge with the *Timaeus*

In contrast to ancient epistemological hierarchies, which impose stability on knowledge through their division and ranking of its domains, the *Timaeus* seems to accept that human knowledge of the world is provisional. Timaeus has cause to reflect on the nature of knowledge when addressing the epistemological status of his own cosmic account in the so-called methodological passage at the beginning of his monologue.[52] After positing that an account derives its epistemological status from the ontological status of its subject matter, Timaeus identifies two types of discourse on the basis of there being two orders of existence, being and becoming:

> τοῦ μὲν οὖν μονίμου καὶ βεβαίου καὶ μετὰ νοῦ καταφανοῦς μονίμους καὶ ἀμεταπτώτους [. . .] τοὺς δὲ τοῦ πρὸς μὲν ἐκεῖνο ἀπεικασθέντος, ὄντος δὲ εἰκόνος εἰκότας ἀνὰ λόγον τε ἐκείνων ὄντας (29b5–7, 29c1–2).

> An account of that which is abiding and stable and discoverable by the aid of reason will itself be abiding and unchangeable . . . while an account of what is made in the image of that other, but is only a likeness, will itself be but likely.[53]

In view of his previous assertion that the world has come into existence by being created after an eternal model (27d6–29b2), Timaeus associates his cosmology, which he describes as both an *eikōs mythos* (29d2) and an *eikōs logos* (30b7), with the second discourse type. While the meaning of the designation *eikōs mythos* or *logos* remains controversial, it appears to signal that a firm grasp of the world is unachievable because the cosmos is a copy (albeit of something stable) caught up in a realm of unceasing change.[54] Furthermore, Timaeus remarks that his own cognitive distance (as a human) from the gods contributes to his inability to produce

[52] See *Ti.* 27d–29d. [53] Cornford (1937), 23.

[54] See Cornford (1937), 23–30; Zeyl (2000), xxxii; Betegh (2010). Johansen (2004: 59) alleges that the difficulty in achieving certain knowledge about the world is not connected to its changeability per se; rather, because the likeness and model belong to different ontological categories, we cannot know for certain how accurately the former represents the latter. Cf. Burnyeat (2005), who claims that *eikōs* does not indicate an epistemological limitation but a positive norm – an *eikōs* account successfully reveals something to be an *eikōn*. Against Burnyeat, Mourelatos (2010) shows that it is not anachronistic to see the *Timaeus* as treating human knowledge as provisional. For the interpretation of *mythos* as a 'myth' (i.e. an account of the divine), see, e.g., Betegh (2010), 221, and Brisson (2012); for it meaning a 'narrative story', see Vlastos (1939), 71–3; according to Johansen (2004: 64–8), the word calls attention to the teleological nature of the account.

'self-consistent' (ἑαυτοῖς ὁμολογουμένους) and 'exact' (ἀπηκριβωμένους) accounts of their creation (29c4–d1). The dialogue seems to leave room for multiple interpretations of the material world in acknowledging that apodeictic certainty about it cannot be reached on account of its instability and the human nature of its investigators. Timaeus goes so far as to invite the reader to revise his own explanation, if they can improve on it: 'if anyone can tell us about a better kind that he [the Demiurge] has chosen for the construction of these bodies [that is, the elements], his will be the victory, not of an enemy, but of a friend' (ἂν οὖν τις ἔχῃ κάλλιον ἐκλεξάμενος εἰπεῖν εἰς τὴν τούτων σύστασιν, ἐκεῖνος οὐκ ἐχθρὸς ὢν ἀλλὰ φίλος κρατεῖ, 54a4–5).[55]

In his commentary on the dialogue, the Neoplatonist Proclus (*c.* 411–85) concludes from Timaeus' preface that there are as many understandings of the perceptible cosmos as there are 'knowers' of it.[56] He attributes this diversity in understanding to the kind of knowledge available in physics (*physiologia*), which the *Timaeus* articulates, in addition to the cognitive limitations of humans.[57] Building on Timaeus' declaration at 29b4–5 that accounts should be akin (*syngeneis*) to the realities they explain, Proclus asserts that multiplicity is inherent to physics as its objects – copies of the eternal, intelligible realm – are plural and neither stable nor clear.[58] Whereas intelligible realities can be grasped by intuitive knowledge all at once, even the highest form of knowing in physics – 'science' (*epistēmē*), which ranks above sensation, imagination, and opinion – involves division and fragmentation.[59] Perhaps in the light of the kinship that *Ti.* 29b4–5 forges between accounts and their subjects, Proclus alleges just prior to his exegesis of these lines that the *Timaeus* imitates (*mimeitai*) the Demiurge's act of creation.[60] Thus, according to Proclus, readers of the *Timaeus* are presented with a textual cosmos, which, in Gersh's words, 'functions as a map of the real world with a point by point correspondence between its

[55] Cornford (1937), 214. Cf. 54b1–2: 'But if anyone should put the matter [i.e. the construction of the elements out of triangles] to the test and discover that it is not so, the prize is theirs with all good will' (ἀλλὰ τῷ τοῦτο ἐλέγξαντι καὶ ἀνευρόντι δὴ οὕτως ἔχον κεῖται φίλια τὰ ἆθλα; Cornford 1937: 214).

[56] See *In Ti.* II 352.15–20; Runia and Share (2008), 210.

[57] See *In Ti.* I 1.5–20 (Tarrant 2007: 91) and II 352.5 (Runia and Share 2008: 210).

[58] See *In Ti.* II 340.10, 351.5; Runia and Share (2008), 197, 208. However, at II 348.25 (Runia and Share 2008: 205), Proclus states that, as nature is the product of the 'intellective light beam' of the Demiurge, accounts of it will necessarily include both things that change (i.e. sensibles) and things that are stable and unaltering (i.e. intelligibles).

[59] *In Ti.* II 342.5–343.15; Runia and Share (2008), 198, 200.

[60] *In Ti.* II 339.20–25; Runia and Share (2008), 196. Cf. Johansen's (2004: 190) description of Timaeus as a 'creator of the cosmos in words' rather than 'in deeds'.

own constituent elements and those of its counterpart'.[61] In 'knowing' the dialogue, they divide up the cosmos.

Although Proclus' interpretation elaborates a distinctively Neoplatonic theory of knowledge, it brings out the epistemological offerings of the *Timaeus*: an entire world of knowledge that can be mapped out differently because of the fundamental instability of its objects.[62] The *Timaeus*' reluctance to draw hard boundaries between 'landmarks' such as the body of the cosmos, the human body, and the soul seems to encourage various mappers to introduce their own demarcations on to this world. At the end of his monologue (92c4–9), Timaeus places emphasis on the oneness (*heis*) and singularity (*monogenēs*) of the cosmos (*kosmos, ouranos*) that has come into being – here, he appears to refer to his own (literary) creation, as well as that of the Demiurge.[63] The passage verbally recalls Timaeus' rejection of a plurality of worlds at 31a8–b3, but it also serves to underscore the unity, or entanglement, of each component of the cosmos and his speech.[64] On a structural level, Timaeus constructs this unity through narrative links that establish causal relations between the parts of his discourse, and thus the parts of the cosmos. For example, with the statement 'this being premissed, we must state what follows next' (τούτου δ' ὑπάρχοντος αὖ τὰ τούτοις ἐφεξῆς ἡμῖν λεκτέον, 30c2), Timaeus transitions from his description of the Demiurge's benevolence to his discussion of the divinity's choice of cosmic models, for he wishes to portray the latter as being determined by the former. Moreover, he implicitly invokes the teleological nature of creation, which is itself a unifying theme of the dialogue, to justify his digression on plants (77a3–c5): as the digestive tract exists for the purpose of breaking down nutriment, what these organs were designed to deal with must necessarily be recounted first.[65]

Timaeus' narrative progresses in a downward direction from the Demiurge's crafting of the outer realms of the cosmos to the generation of the various creatures populating the earth. Through analogy and homology, Timaeus seems to deny a strict separation of these remote ends. Shaped in imitation (*apomimēsamenoi*) of the spherical body of

[61] Gersh (1973), 88. See also Martijn (2010), 276–85.

[62] In my use of the phrase 'world of knowledge', I am influenced by Gill, Whitmarsh, and Wilkins (2009: 8–9), whose edited collection *Galen and the World of Knowledge* aims to capture Galen's (and his culture's) aspiration to construct a universal, orderly, all-encompassing system of knowledge.

[63] See Johansen (2004), 188–90.

[64] At 31b3, Timaeus calls the universe (*ouranos*) 'one' (*heis*) and 'singular' (*monogenēs*).

[65] Cf. 59d2–3.

the world, in order to be capable of the same cognitive activities as the World Soul, the human head is paradigmatic of the connections that Timaeus makes between the heavens and earth.[66] As Chapters 1–3 will highlight, Galen, Ḥunayn, and al-Rāzī interpret these entangled relations to signify that the human body can be studied to understand the cosmos – or that it cannot be understood without fully comprehending its broader cosmic context. On their reading, Plato's text authorizes their expansion of medicine's boundaries beyond the limits of the human body. Its famous doctrine of a tripartite soul housed in the brain, heart, and lower belly (69c5–71e2), which appears in *Republic* 4 (435e1–439e4) too, is also cited to bring psychology within the domain of their expertise. Therefore, while the *Timaeus* resists the division and bounding of knowledge of other ancient epistemological schemes, thinkers such as Galen, who remain committed to these hierarchical epistemologies without being entirely happy with them, approach it as an amorphous map that can be carved up to further their disciplinary visions.

Galen, the Philosopher-Doctor

Galen's boundary work with the *Timaeus* appears to have two interconnected purposes – one of which is to improve medicine's socio-intellectual standing, as I have already suggested, and the other to defend his unusual expertise by remaking the discipline in his own image. Compared to the education of most ancient doctors, which routinely revolved around an apprenticeship, Galen's was long, wide-ranging, and expensive.[67] Galen credits his atypical training to his architect father Nicon, who taught him mathematics, arithmetic, and grammar and encouraged him to become a philosopher.[68] In Pergamum and later in Smyrna (modern İzmir in Turkey), the young Galen attended lectures from two students of the Platonist Gaius (early second century) – only one of whom he names, Albinus (second century) – and received tuition as well from Peripatetic, Stoic,

[66] 44d3–6. Cornford (1937: 295n4) observes that the varied movement of the lower parts of the body reflects the irregularity of the 'wandering cause' (τῆς πλανωμένης . . . αἰτίας, 48a6–7), or Necessity. Cf. 73e1–4, where Timaeus uses the same mixing-bowl imagery as in his account of the Demiurge's creation of the rational part of the human soul (41d4–7) to describe the deity's construction of bone.

[67] For Galen's training in Pergamum, Smyrna, and Alexandria, see Mattern (2013), 36–80.

[68] See *Ord.Lib.Prop.* 4.2–4; Boudon-Millot (2007), p. 99 l. 13–p. 100 l. 4. The inheritance that Galen received after his father's death in 148 helped him to fund his studies outside Pergamum.

and Epicurean instructors.[69] Notwithstanding his claim at *Aff.Dig.* 8.3 that he did not derive much benefit from his time with his Platonist teachers (that is, the one he does not care to name), Galen was probably introduced then to the *Timaeus*, its commentary tradition, and current, 'Middle Platonic' approaches to exegesis, which can be seen in his own utilization of Peripatetic and Stoic doctrine to illuminate the Platonic text.[70] Perhaps as an apology for his abandonment of the more prestigious career of a philosopher, Galen relates on several occasions that the divine intervened through his father's dreams to steer him towards medicine.[71]

Depicting his medical occupation as a divine calling, Galen presents himself foremost as a doctor, even if he boasts about being mistaken for a philosopher with a sideline in medicine and not vice versa.[72] Despite the financial and social success that his medical career in Rome brought him, culminating in his appointment as personal physician to the imperial family, Galen still had to contend with biases against medicine's, and therefore his own, intellectual capacities, as one contemporary response to his work reveals.[73] The chair of Aristotelian philosophy at Athens, Alexander of Aphrodisias (late second–early third century), cited Euripides' *Orest.* 258–9 ('Wretched man, keep still in your bed! / For, you see nothing of which you think you see well'; μέν', ὦ ταλαίπωρ', ἀτρέμα σοῖς ἐν δεμνίοις | ὁρᾷς γὰρ οὐδὲν ὧν δοκεῖς σάφ' εἰδέναι) to reprimand Galen for treating philosophical topics beyond his medical

[69] Mattern (2013: 37) observes that Galen does not identify by name most of his philosophical teachers because they were not well known and therefore would not add much to his intellectual pedigree.

[70] See de Boer (1937), p. 28 ll. 12–15. The modern term 'Middle Platonism' designates a stage in the development of Platonism from the time of Antiochus of Ascalon (*c.* 130–68 BCE) to Plotinus (205–70 CE). On Galen's syncretic Platonism, see Hankinson (1992), 3507. A citation in Proclus' commentary on the *Timaeus* (II 290.5) indicates that Galen's teacher Albinus wrote some kind of exegesis of the dialogue (see also Dillon 1996: 270). Moreover, parallels between Galen's *Synopsis of Plato's Timaeus* (*Com.Tim.*), which is mostly extant in Arabic (on this text, see pp. 22–3), and Alcinous' *Primer on Plato's Doctrines* (Διδασκαλικὸς τῶν Πλάτωνος δογμάτων), which was once attributed to Albinus, demonstrate Galen's familiarity with Middle Platonic readings of the dialogue (see Festugière 1952). Dörrie and Baltes (2002: 312) also note that Galen's explanation of the dialogue's account of the soul in *Com.Tim.* shares similarities with Plutarch's and Atticus' (*c.* 176) interpretations.

[71] See *Ord.Lib.Prop.* 4.4 (Boudon-Millot 2007: p. 100 ll. 2–4); *Praen.* 2.12 (Nutton 1979: p. 76 l. 29–p. 78 l. 2; and *MM* 9 10.609K.

[72] See *Praen.* 2.5.11–12 (Nutton 1979: p. 76 ll. 26–9), where Galen recounts how his patient the Peripatetic philosopher Eudemus mistook him for a philosopher because he accurately predicted his fever's crisis. On Galen's self-identification as a doctor as opposed to a *professional* philosopher, see Singer (2014) and pp. 36–7 below.

[73] In 169 Galen was appointed to the post of personal physician to Marcus Aurelius' (r. 161–80) heir Commodus (r. 177–92).

expertise.[74] Alexander's authorship of two refutations of Galen's views on the philosophical themes of potentiality and the prime mover shows, however, a polemical recognition that he thought them serious enough to warrant an attack.[75]

My analysis in Chapter 1 will be concerned with Galen's struggle to convince philosophers of the investigative promise of medicine, but it is worth mentioning that he had to advertise his more expansive conception of the discipline to doctors too. In imperial Rome Galen was part of a larger medical marketplace, where not only patients but also would-be doctors could choose from a variety of practical and doctrinal options. As Galen observes with contempt, one popular alternative, Methodism, held that logic and theoretical knowledge of the natural world is irrelevant to medicine.[76] Galen performs his disciplinary boundary work in texts written with a medical reader in mind, such as *The Best Doctor is Also a Philosopher*, to persuade them to accept his vision of medicine as more authentically Hippocratic and thus authoritative. In its criticism of 'doctors nowadays' (οἱ νῦν ἰατροί), *Opt.Med.* fashions Hippocrates into a philosophical figure to bring logic, physics, and ethics within medicine's purview.[77] Galen takes Hippocrates' attribution of therapeutic failure to an inability to distinguish diseases by species and genus as a protreptic to study logic; Hippocrates' emphasis on acquiring accurate knowledge of the body before venturing into medicine directs doctors to preface their training with physics; and his prioritization of public benefit over personal gain signals that ethics should underpin a medical education.[78] Compared to the treatises surveyed in Chapter 1, *Opt.Med.* does not recommend the study of these parts of philosophy for theoretical ends but rather for their potential to assist the

[74] See Olympiodorus, *Commentary on the First Alcibiades of Plato* § 170 (Westerink 1956: p. 108 ll. 11–12) and Nutton (1984), 319.

[75] Alexander's treatises *A refutation of Galen 'On the possible'* and *A refutation of Galen 'On the first mover'* are extant in Arabic; for these texts, see Rescher and Marmura (1965). Alexander of Aphrodisias may have met and argued with Galen in person. At *Praen.* 5.9–15 (Nutton 1979: p. 9 l. 5–p. 98 l. 8), Galen relates that an Alexander of Damascus, who was the chair of Aristotelian philosophy at Athens, interrupted one of his anatomical demonstrations. It is unclear whether Alexander of Aphrodisias and Alexander of Damascus are the same person, because their professorships at Athens do not seem to line up (see Nutton 1984: 318–19; Mattern 2013: 148).

[76] For Galen's criticism of the Methodist medical education, see *MM* 1.5. On the Methodist sect in general, see Meyer-Steineg (1916); Pigeaud (1993); Nutton (2004), 187–201; Tecusan (2004).

[77] See Boudon-Millot (2007), p. 284, l. 4–p. 285, l. 12. Here, Galen also refers to Hippocrates' interest in astronomy to argue that it and its preliminary, geometry, should also form part of the doctor's knowledge. On Galen's portrayal of Hippocrates as a link between medicine and philosophy, see Vegetti (1994), 1694. Cf. *Protr.* 5.4 (Boudon-Millot 2002a: p. 89, ll. 18–19), where Galen groups Hippocrates with Socrates, Plato, and Homer.

[78] See respectively Boudon-Millot (2007), p. 285 ll. 5–9, p. 284 l. 13–p. 285 l. 2, and p. 288 ll. 3–8.

doctor in selecting the appropriate remedies. This purpose led Temkin to label the ideal physician of *Opt.Med.* a 'limited philosopher'.[79]

New Epistemic Terrains

As his books attained canonical status in the late antique medical schools at Alexandria and Ravenna, Galen the philosopher-doctor became the career model to which elite doctors aspired.[80] Even so, this philosophical–medical paradigm represented an epistemic problem for the powerfully essentializing hierarchies of knowledge outlined in philosophical prolegomena of the period. The introductory texts of, for instance, the Neoplatonists Olympiodorus (b. *c.* 505), pseudo-Elias (sixth century), and David of Armenia (second half of the sixth century) equated the Aristotelian corpus with philosophy itself; they matched individual treatises with the different parts of philosophy and arranged them to reflect their notion of ontological reality.[81] Their classifications, which were not merely dialectical but purported to uncover things as they are, segregated the philosophical sciences (*epistēmai*) according to their degree of abstraction from the material world. On this scheme, metaphysics ranks highest because it deals with things beyond matter and substance, whereas physics' treatment of the sublunary world makes it inferior.[82] As David explains, the ontological rift between the domains of knowledge entails certain restrictions on what 'lesser' disciplines such as medicine can learn about the areas above them:

> καὶ γὰρ τῇ ἰατρικῇ ὑπόκεινται τὰ ἀνθρώπεια σώματα, τῇ δὲ φιλοσοφίᾳ αὐτὴ ἡ ἰατρικὴ ὑπόκειται . . . ἔτι δὲ διὰ τοῦτο εἶπε τὴν φιλοσοφίαν τέχνην τεχνῶν καὶ ἐπιστήμην ἐπιστημῶν, ἐπειδὴ αὕτη μὲν τὴν φύσιν τῶν πραγμάτων γινώσκει, τὰ δὲ παρεπόμενα δίδωσι γινώσκειν ταῖς τέχναις καὶ ἐπιστήμαις· καὶ γὰρ αὕτη λαμβάνουσα κατὰ τὴν γνῶσιν τὸ εἶδος καὶ τὴν ὕλην ἀποτελεῖ τὰ τέσσαρα στοιχεῖα καὶ ἐκ τούτων ἀποτελεῖ τὰ ὁμοιομερῆ καὶ ἐκ τῶν ὁμοιομερῶν τὰ ὀργανικὰ καὶ ἐκ τούτων τὸ ἀνθρώπειον σῶμα, καὶ λοιπὸν τὰ ἄλλα δίδωσι γινώσκειν τῇ ἰατρικῇ,

[79] Temkin (1953), 224.

[80] On Galen's late antique reception, see Temkin (1973), 51–69. Based on the commentary of Agnellus of Ravena (*c.* 600) on Galen's *SI* and evidence from the Arabic writings of the Egyptian doctor ʿAlī ibn Riḍwān (388–453/998–1061), Roueché (1999) concludes that certain late antique medical professors in Alexandria lectured on both medicine and dialectic.

[81] See Olympiodorus, *Prolegomena to Aristotle's Logic and Commentary on Aristotle's Categories*; pseudo-Elias, *Commentaries on Porphyry's Introduction and Aristotle's Categories*; and David, *Prolegomena and Commentary on Porphyry's Introduction.* For a survey of late antique divisions of philosophy, see Hein (1985).

[82] On the normative force of these hierarchies, see Gutas (1983), 247–8.

> φημὶ δὲ τὴν νόσον καὶ τὴν ὑγίειαν, οὐχ ὡς ἀγνοοῦσα αὐτά (γινώσκει γὰρ καὶ ταῦτα), ἀλλ᾽ ὡς μὴ βουλομένη καταρρυποῦν ἑαυτὴν καὶ ἐπὶ τὰ ἔσχατα ἔρχεσθαι.[83]
>
> Human bodies are subordinate to [lit. lie under] medicine, and medicine is itself subordinate to philosophy . . . For this reason also he [i.e. Aristotle] said that philosophy is the art of arts and the science of sciences, because it knows the nature of things, while it leaves it to the arts and sciences to know their consequences. For it takes matter and form and, according to knowledge, produces the four elements, and from these, it produces similar [lit. homoiomerous] parts and from similar parts, organic things and from these, human bodies. But it leaves medicine the rest to know – I mean illness and health – not because it does not know these things (for it knows them), but because it does not wish to dirty itself by coming down to these lowest things.

While the theoretical basis of medicine derives from philosophy (or physics, as David goes on to specify), the relationship does not permit medicine to work back from its subject matter to get at the nature of the philosophical concepts underlying it.[84] The explanatory direction in this epistemological scheme goes only one way: an investigator can move from a higher to a lower science because they understand the latter's principles – however, there is a limit to how far down they should go owing to the ontological differences between the ranks of knowledge.

Through the efforts of the translators participating in the 'Graeco-Arabic translation movement' (second–fourth/eighth–tenth centuries), which was sponsored by elite officials at the ʿAbbāsid court in Baghdad, scholars first in Iraq and then throughout the diverse regions of the Islamicate world became acquainted with late antique Greek (and Syriac) epistemologies such as the above.[85] A mass of taxonomic literature,

[83] Busse (1904), p. 40 ll. 10–21.

[84] See Busse (1904), p. 40 ll. 29–30: 'The doctor also knows that human bodies are composed of the four elements, but he sends along the reason why to natural philosophy' (καὶ πάλιν ὁ ἰατρὸς οἶδεν ὅτι ἐκ τῶν τεσσάρων στοιχείων τὰ ἀνθρώπεια συνίστανται σώματα, τὴν δὲ αἰτίαν παραπέμπει τῇ φυσικῇ φιλοσοφίᾳ). Cf. the Armenian translation in Kendall and Thomson (1983), 97, which appears to be based on an older tradition than the Greek manuscripts.

[85] While it is now standard to refer to the period of translation activity that took place in the second–fourth/eighth–tenth centuries in Baghdad as the 'Graeco-Arabic translation movement', this appellation obscures not only the role of Syriac in the transmission of Greek learning but also the fact that texts in other languages (e.g., Middle Persian and Sanskrit) were rendered into Arabic at this time. See Le Coz (2006), who highlights the substantial contribution that Syriac-literate Christians made to this translation enterprise. For the interest in Sanskrit texts at the ʿAbbāsid court, see van Bladel (2011). On the possible motivations for the ʿAbbāsids' sponsorship of this translation activity, see Gutas (1998), 28–74. Gutas (1983) highlights the contribution of the theologian of the Church of the East Paul the Persian (*fl.* 567–80 CE) to the transmission of these late antique epistemologies into Arabic.

produced from the beginning of ʿAbbāsid rule to the Ottoman period (ninth–fourteenth/fifteenth–nineteenth centuries), responded to these prior hierarchical classifications by introducing additional divisions to accommodate 'local' sciences – for example, Arabic grammar, Qurʾānic exegesis, and knowledge of Islamic law (*fiqh*).[86] At a macroscopic level, these writings in Arabic, Persian, and Hebrew, among other languages, encapsulate the imperial ambitions of the regimes under which they were composed, governments seeking to impose order on the various peoples now under their domain.[87] While certain changes to the ancient epistemological schemes in these medieval taxonomies of knowledge may reflect the cultural preferences of the new hegemonies, their authors also formulated different relations between the fields of learning to better their own position in the epistemic and political landscapes, where, as in Galen's day, intellectual prestige as well as material rewards through patronage were on offer.[88]

Notwithstanding these restructurings, medicine (Arab. *ṭibb*) generally still ranked lower than philosophy (Arab. *falsafa*).[89] The stories circulating in biographical literature about the financial success of various doctors – among whom the Islamicate figures covered in this book are usually counted – occlude the social reality of the average practitioner, who was often no better off than a shopkeeper.[90] Philosophy, on the other hand, was, as Rosenthal puts it, 'the slogan of the elite', at least during the first two centuries of the ʿAbbāsids' reign.[91] The involvement of individuals at the top of the social hierarchy, such as the caliph, may have helped to raise the socio-cultural profile of philosophy, but it is important to stress that, as in Graeco-Roman antiquity, this warm reception was not universal – although its critics frequently utilized the idiom of philosophy to express their objections.[92]

86 Many Islamicate intellectuals, starting with al-Kindī (*c.* 185–252/801–66) and including famous figures such as the philosopher al-Fārābī (*c.* 259–339/872–950), the polymath al-Balḫī (d. 322/934), the religious scholar al-Ġazālī (d. 505/1111), and the 'sociologist' Ibn Ḫaldūn (d. 808/1406), composed their own classifications of the sciences and arts. For an introduction to this substantial body of literature, see Vesel (1986), Heinrichs (1995), and Biesterfeldt (2000, 2002).

87 Cf. König and Whitmarsh (2007: 7), who, with regard to the Roman Empire, forcefully argue for a connection between knowledge and imperial ordering projects: 'The world of knowledge – comprising both the institutions defining it and the texts embodying it – is never neutral, detached, objective. The assumption that the textual compilation of knowledge is a practice distinct from political power will not stand.'

88 See Rosenthal (1992), 52–3.

89 See the texts surveyed by Rosenthal (1992: 54–63), Biesterfeldt (2000, 2002), and Gutas (2003).

90 See Rosenthal (1978) and Chapter 2 (p. 80n47) for further references.

91 Rosenthal (1978), 491.

92 See Brentjes (2014) for the role of the ruling class in sanctioning the pursuit of a range of ancient sciences (e.g., philosophy, mathematics, and geography). See also Druart (2003) for a helpful sketch of the differing attitudes towards philosophy's compatibility with Islam in the medieval period.

As I argue in Chapters 2 and 3, whose respective subjects are Ḥunayn ibn Isḥāq and Abū Bakr al-Rāzī, Galen's boundary work with Plato's *Timaeus* showed Islamicate doctors wishing to improve the cachet of their profession how their discipline, and thus epistemic landscapes, could be redrawn to give themselves a greater share in cosmic knowledge and authority. My studies of Avicenna and Maimonides in Chapters 4 and 5 contend, on the other hand, that, for critics of the Platonic elements of Galen's and his followers' (namely, al-Rāzī's) thought, the dominant epistemologies furnished them with a discourse that could be weaponized to neutralize this doctrinal threat. These philosophical reactionaries have recourse to the notion that each discipline is a self-contained unit to circumscribe their medical adversaries' expertise and, in so doing, deprive them of the right to engage in psychological and cosmic debates. A thread running through these two pairs of chapters is that Galen is more than a model for the four Islamicate authors in this book: he is a point of departure for their own projects of self-fashioning, the stakes of which seem to be their pre-eminence over both (near) contemporaries and the remote past. While the entanglement of body, soul, and cosmos in the *Timaeus* meant that the dialogue did not map exactly on to the hierarchical epistemologies described above, I want to conclude this introduction by considering how the text's disciplinary subversiveness may also have to do with Galen's own formative role in bringing Arabic readers into contact with it.

Islamicate Receptions

Despite the reports of Arabic translations of the Platonic corpus in medieval bibliographies such as Ibn al-Nadīm's (d. *c.* 385/995) *Catalogue* (*al-Fihrist*), it does not appear that the *Timaeus* or any other dialogue was rendered completely into Arabic in the pre-modern period.[93] Arnzen concludes from his analysis of the bibliographical evidence that medieval Islamicate writers refer to three separate works by the title '*Timaeus*', all of which are secondary treatments of the Platonic text: (1) a tripartite paraphrase or epitome that was sometimes entitled 'Spiritual Timaeus' (*Ṭīmāwus al-rūḥānī*) and was translated into Arabic by Yaḥyā ibn al-Biṭrīq (*fl. c.* 200/815), who was connected to the circle of the philosopher al-Kindī; (2) Galen's *Com.Tim.*, which occasionally circulated as the 'Physical Timaeus'

[93] Arnzen (2012). For a review of the Platonic material available to medieval Arabic readers, see Gutas (2012). See also Moseley (2018a, 2018b, 2019), whose philological study of certain Arabic quotations of the *Phaedo*, *Laws*, and *Symposium* considers the role of different (including Galenic) indirect traditions in the transmission of these texts.

(*Ṭīmāwus al-ṭabīʿī*) and was translated into Arabic by Ḥunayn ibn Isḥāq and his associate ʿĪsā ibn Yaḥyā; and (3) Galen's commentary on the *Medical Statements in Plato's Timaeus*, which was frequently called the 'Medical Timaeus' (*Ṭīmāwus al-ṭibbī*) and was rendered into Arabic by Ḥunayn and his son Isḥāq.[94] None of the surviving Timaean material in Arabic has been identified definitively as coming from Ibn al-Biṭrīq's 'Spiritual Timaeus', so this version remains shadowy.[95] Its supposed explanation of the 'hierarchy of the worlds' (*tartīb al-ʿawālim*) – the spiritual, noetic, and psychic – indicates, however, that it was probably based on a Neoplatonic source as this structuring of reality reflects the Plotinian hypostases the One, Intellect, and Soul.[96]

Individual doctrines from Plato's *Timaeus* also made their way into Arabic through translations of Aristotle, his commentators, and treatises ascribed to him.[97] This Aristotelian corpus offered Islamicate authors contrasting lenses through which to view the relationship between Aristotle and Plato. *On the Soul* and *On the Heavens*, for example, emphasized the two philosophers' theoretical opposition, specifically on the origin of the world and the nature of the soul, whereas the pseudonymous *Theology of Aristotle* (*Kitāb Uṯūlūǧiya Arisṭāṭālīs*) – a creative reworking of Plotinus' *Enneads* 4–6 – fostered the idea of a fundamental harmony between them.[98] Nonetheless, the bulk of Arabic citations with explicit attributions to the *Timaeus* appear to derive from Galen's two exegeses and other treatments of the dialogue. These references imply that for many Islamicate thinkers there was no clear distinction between Plato's *Timaeus* and Galen's interpretation of it.[99]

94 Arnzen (2012). On Ibn al-Biṭrīq, see Dunlop (1959) and Endress (1997), 55–8. On Ḥunayn's translations of Galen's two exegeses of the *Timaeus*, see Bergsträsser (1925), p. 50 ll. 3–7=Lamoreaux (2016), p. 125 l. 6; and Bergsträsser (1925), p. 50 l. 14–p. 51 l. 2, with corrections from Bergsträsser (1932), p. 23 ll. 10–11=Lamoreaux (2016), p. 125 l. 9–p. 127 l. 2.

95 Arnzen (2012: 212, 227) speculates that ʿAlī ibn Sahl ibn Rabban al-Ṭabarī (third/ninth century) in his medical compilation *Paradise of Wisdom* (*Firdaws al-ḥikma*) and al-Bīrūnī (362–*c.* 442/973–*c.* 1050) in *The Book Confirming What Pertains to India, Whether Rational or Despicable* (*Kitāb Taḥqīq mā li-l-Hind min maqūla maqbūla fī l-ʿaql aw marḏūla*) may have drawn on al-Biṭrīq's summary of the *Timaeus*.

96 As Arnzen (2012: 206) notes, this ontological scheme is prefigured in Middle Platonic sources.

97 For a list of the Aristotelian texts that were translated into Arabic during the medieval period, see Peters (1968).

98 On the *Theology of Aristotle* and other Plotinian materials in Arabic, see Zimmermann (1986); Aouad (1989); D'Ancona (2003a, 2003b); Gutas (2007); Hansberger (2011). For the Aristotelianizing tendencies of these texts, see Adamson (2002). See also Endress (1991) and D'Ancona (2006), who examine the topos of the harmony between Plato and Aristotle in medieval Arabic philosophy.

99 Arnzen (2013) demonstrates that Ḥunayn rendered a small section of Proclus' commentary on the *Timaeus* (89e3–90e7) into Arabic for the purpose of clarifying Platonic ideas in Galen's *On Character Traits* (Περὶ ἐθῶν).

The fact that these quotations are almost always ascribed to Plato (Aflāṭūn) instead of Galen (Ǧālīnūs) further testifies to the conflation of the Platonic and Galenic *Timaeus*.[100] Arabic readers encountered a Plato with apparent interests in pharmacology, anatomy, and fevers, among other medical topics.[101] Moreover, this Plato seems to sanction the broadening of medicine's boundaries because Galen plays down aspects of his thought, such as his dualism, that do not align with his conception of the body as an access point to the soul and cosmos.

The work of cataloguing references to the *Timaeus* in Arabic is not undertaken in this book merely to corroborate Arnzen's conclusion about the absence of a medieval translation of the Platonic original, nor even to determine how widely Galen was read as a source for Plato in the pre-modern Islamicate world (although these secondary points do indeed emerge from the chapters that follow). Rather, this book approaches the reception history of the *Timaeus* in Arabic through a series of case studies in order to emphasize what the dialogue was doing for medieval thinkers – or, to be more precise, what medieval thinkers were doing with the dialogue, and how they used it to shape their epistemic landscapes. Although my analysis privileges Galenic over, for instance, Aristotelian and Neoplatonic readings of the dialogue, I show in several places how closely implicated these strands of reception are. It might be possible to write a book that takes into full account the reception histories of the Aristotelian, Galenic, and Plotinian *Timaeus* in Arabic – but in writing this history I have decided to pursue thickness rather than breadth. Even then, there are simply too many leads to follow. While my main goal is to demonstrate how deeply some of the most important thinkers of the Islamicate world engaged with Galen's thought, I also want to represent the diverse intellectual contexts of which he was a part. The four Islamicate cases in the second part of this book deal with authors who all claimed expertise in both medicine and philosophy, came from the three prophetic monotheisms, and lived in different areas under Muslim rule (now in Iraq, Iran, Uzbekistan, Spain, and Egypt). These episodes all highlight how the Galenic *Timaeus* provoked reflection on disciplinary identities and the boundaries of knowledge itself.

Chapter 1 sets the scene for the reception history that ensues by examining Galen's attempts to appropriate Plato's *Timaeus* for medicine in a group of works aimed (although not exclusively) at a philosophical

[100] See Arnzen (2012), 220; Das (2019). [101] See Das (2019).

readership. During the first two centuries of the imperial period, the dialogue was the object of considerable exegetical interest in the different philosophical schools. In view of this attention, I argue that Galen's proposal in *On the Medical Statements in Plato's Timaeus* (Περὶ τῶν ἐν τῷ Πλάτωνος Τιμαίῳ ἰατρικῶς εἰρημένων) and the Arabo-Latin prologue to the *Synopsis of Plato's Timaeus* that the *Timaeus* contains 'medical' information serves to compel philosophical insiders to accept his right as a doctor to the epistemic contents of the dialogue over which they had long asserted authority. In denying the exteriority of the soul, among other subjects that receive treatment in Plato's text, to medicine, Galen refigures more expansively this field of knowledge. I next establish that a similar form of boundary work can be seen in *On the Doctrines of Hippocrates and Plato* (Περὶ τῶν Ἱπποκράτους καὶ Πλάτωνος δογμάτων) and *The Faculties of the Soul Follow the Mixture of the Body* (Ὅτι ταῖς τοῦ σώματος κράσεσιν αἱ τῆς ψυχῆς δυνάμεις ἕπονται), in which Galen advances more monopolistic claims on the soul for medicine. The first text refers to Galen's anatomical expertise, which he honed through study, experimentation, and clinical practice, to position doctors as best able to resolve a psychological controversy with roots in the *Timaeus* – the corporeal location of the ruling part of the soul. The second text, on the other hand, subversively interprets *Ti.* 86b–87b, which links bodily and psychic diseases, to leave room for doctors in character formation, when the dialogue itself appears to refuse them this space. Finally, I turn back to *On the Medical Statements in Plato's Timaeus* to demonstrate how Galen exploits the dialogue's homology between human and plant in his account of vegetative sensation to extend medicine's boundaries beyond the world of the body.

The second chapter studies the efforts of the Christian Ḥunayn ibn Isḥāq (d. 260/873 or 264/877), whose workshop in ʿAbbāsid Baghdad translated the Galenic sources considered in this book, to enhance the respectability of the specialism of ophthalmology in his *Ten Treatises on the Eye* (*Kitāb al-ʿAšr al-maqālāt fī l-ʿayn*). Even more than medicine, ophthalmology was at a disadvantage in its pursuit of epistemic authority because Galen himself had attacked the sub-field as an exemplar of the worrying tendency among doctors in Rome and other cities towards specialization, which threatened the unity of the discipline and the health of patients. I maintain that Ḥunayn, concerned with his own intellectual standing at the ʿAbbāsid court, constructs an ophthalmology that recognizes the eyes' connection with the body and cosmos, perhaps in reply to Galen's criticisms. The characterization in the *Timaeus* of the eye and its function as paradigms of the joint work of the two cosmic forces of Reason and Necessity, to which Ḥunayn has access through Galen, provides him with a framework with which to express his disciplinary vision. My examination of treatises one through three of *Ten Treatises on the Eye* reveals how Ḥunayn builds on Galen's explanation of the dialogue's description of the eyes' service to the rational soul to perform his own boundary work, which aims to give ophthalmologists a stake in the controversial subject of sensation. I also expose how Ḥunayn modifies Galen's interpretation of Plato's teleological ocular anatomy and visual theory in order to privilege the eye over all other organs as a window to cosmic knowledge. As I conclude, Ḥunayn's ophthalmology assumes that its students have a grounding in physics and 'generalist' medicine – a requirement that helps to distance the sub-field from its non-elite associations; nonetheless, he subordinates these disciplines to his own expertise by making specialist knowledge the *telos* of his idealized education.

Chapter 3 shifts eastward to Iran and centres on the 'Arab Galen', the Muslim doctor Abū Bakr al-Rāzī (251–*c.* 313/865–*c.* 925), who was attacked by later Islamicate thinkers for his attempts to replace Galenism with his own more theologically informed system of medicine and philosophy. In particular, it claims that al-Rāzī seeks to weaken the epistemic authority of Galenism through his critiques of Galen's readings of certain doctrines from Plato's *Timaeus*. Calling attention to al-Rāzī's discussions of creation, pleasure, and the materialism of the soul in the *Doubts about Galen* (*al-Šukūk ʿalā Ǧālīnūs*), my analysis shows that he undermines Galen's Platonic credentials by suggesting that his predecessor's interpretations of the *Timaeus* play down, and perhaps even neglect, God's role in the cosmos. To preface this fight over the title of Plato's successor and the authority that it bestows, the first section of the chapter reviews the Middle Platonic and Neoplatonic sources on which al-Rāzī may have drawn to elaborate his 'anti-Platonism' – his Platonism in response to Galen's Platonism. In reformulating the boundaries of medicine to include theological knowledge, which belonged in ancient epistemological schemes to metaphysics, al-Rāzī, I conclude, promotes the doctor-metaphysician in opposition to Galen's more limited philosopher-doctor as the most reliable investigator of the cosmos.

The fourth chapter moves on to Central Asia and Avicenna (Ibn Sīnā, *c.* 370–428/980–1037), arguably the most famous medical and philosophical writer of the medieval Islamicate world. I demonstrate that

Avicenna's widely read compilation, the *Canon of Medicine* (*al-Qānūn fī l-ṭibb*), tries to reassert the epistemic authority of philosophy by restoring the 'proper' boundaries of medicine, which Galen had obscured in particular through his engagements with Plato's *Timaeus*. My contention is that Avicenna shows his commitment to the restrictive epistemic hierarchies of his intellectual milieu because of the polemical work that they can do for him. In the eyes of Avicenna, a student of Aristotle, Galen's defence of the dialogue's brain-centred psycho-physiology, which elevated the organ as the seat of the rational soul and thus principal contributor to sensation, put the credibility of Aristotelian cardiocentrism on the line. Thus, Avicenna invokes Galen's professional identity as a doctor, who – according to the prevailing epistemologies, should keep to subjects only relevant to the production or preservation of bodily health – to delegitimize his contributions to natural philosophy. The rhetorical, as opposed to normalizing, force of Avicenna's disciplinary prescriptions will, however, become evident from my examination of the chapters on the hegemonic organ and pleasure in the *Canon of Medicine*, *Cardiac Drugs* (*Maqāla fī Aḥkām al-adwiya al-qalbiyya*), and the *Metaphysics* (*al-Ilāhiyyāt*) of *The Cure* (*Kitāb al-Šifāʾ*). There, Avicenna can be seen to transgress his own 'laws' when disputing or even adopting Galen's Timaean positions on these issues.

Ending in Egypt via southern Iberia, the last chapter concentrates on the reformist efforts of Rabbi Moses Maimonides (Mūsā ibn Maymūn or Moshe ben Maimon, 532–600/1138–1204) to rid Galenism of its Timaean elements. While, as in Avicenna's case, Maimonides' affiliation with Aristotelianism put him in conflict with Galen, the Platonic lines in Galenism also generated problems for his conception of Jewish belief. My discussion of Maimonides' *The Guide for the Perplexed* (*Dalālat al-ḥāʾirīn*) and *Medical Aphorisms* (*Kitāb al-Fuṣūl fī l-ṭibb*) will uncover that he rejected Galen's interpretation of the dialogue's cosmogony as heterodox on account of its denial of creation *ex nihilo* and the omnipotence of God. To curtail Galen's philosophical, and therefore theological, reach, Maimonides sets out to limit the relevance of his predecessor's thought to the domain of the body. I survey Maimonides' medical corpus, with special attention given to the *Medical Aphorisms*, which purports to cover the essentials of medicine, to illustrate that he performs his boundary work, or 'de-philosophization' of Galenism, by giving more restricted senses to Galen's philosophically loaded terminology. I close the chapter with a study of Maimonides' criticism of Galen's Timaean psycho-physiology in the *Medical Aphorisms*, in which he mobilizes evidence from his own anatomical observations and perhaps experiments to dispute the theory's claim to truth.

I have framed this book as a study of receptions rather than transmission, influence, or (in particular) tradition. As my readings make clear, in line with current theorizations, I understand reception to be dialogic in the sense that each participant's response not only shows an active renegotiation of a text's meaning but also betrays what in the text or artefact may have been generative of the response.[102] On the other hand, while recent scholarship may envision 'the classical tradition' as a succession of creative responses to ancient materials (for example, texts, monuments, and art), the core meaning of tradition – 'a passing on' – essentializes the classical past by giving it a single point of origin, often in Athens or Rome.[103] This idea of descent encourages the localization of the classical tradition in western Europe, with which Greece and Rome have often been equated in light of the modern geopolitical landscape. It seems to give grounds for the further identification of classical culture with Western culture.

As a result, histories of the classical tradition often reduce Islamicate thinkers to vehicles of Graeco-Roman science and philosophy that serve Western readers: they made classical ideas accessible to those in western Europe before the Renaissance, which saw the 'return' of Greek manuscripts after the Ottoman conquest of Constantinople (1453), or furnish modern philologists with sources to mine to recover lost texts or improve extant ones. In terms of their religious, linguistic, political, and other cultural affiliations, Ḥunayn, al-Rāzī, Avicenna, and Maimonides were not focused on western Europe – the supposed 'heartland' of the classical tradition.[104] Moreover, the construction of European identity, in which the classical tradition is implicated, has long been oppositional to Islam: notably, the Latin noun *Europenses* ('Europeans') was first used to distinguish Christian from Muslim forces at the Battle of Poitiers-Tours (732).[105] Plato is often claimed as one of the founding figures of western civilization, but this book will make clear that he and Galen and other Graeco-Roman authors are also an

102 I am using 'text' in the broadest sense possible. See Martindale (1993), Hardwick (2003), 12, and Porter (2008), 474.

103 On the diverse responses constituting the 'classical tradition', see, e.g., Grafton, Most, and Settis (2010) and the essays in Silk, Gildenhard, and Barrow (2014) .

104 Cf. Silk, Gildenhard, and Barrow (2014) , 7.

105 See *The Spanish Continuation of Isidore. The Mozarab Chronicle of 754* (*Continuatio Isidoriana Hispana. Cronica Mozarabe de 754*): Lopez Pereira (2009), p. 258 l. 19. See also Appiah (2012), 427.

important presence in the Islamicate world. Although the cultures of Europe and the Middle East have these classical figures in common, I am not seeking to highlight the latter's intellectual value by subsuming it within some hegemonic western tradition: these Islamicate receptions are worth studying in their own right. As I aim to show in what follows, the *Timaeus* is a text that calls all boundaries – including the putative boundaries between 'East' and 'West' – into question.

CHAPTER I

Galen and the 'Medical' Timaeus

In the final years of his life, Galen wrote *On my Own Opinions* (*Prop.Plac.*) to clarify the subjects of which he had either certain (βεβαίως), probable (πιθανόν), or no (μηδεμία) knowledge.[1] He explains his motivation for composing this 'auto-doxography' by recounting an anecdote about Parthenius of Nicaea (or Myrlea, *c.* 70–30 BCE) that describes the poet's encounter with two schoolteachers (γραμματικοί) quarrelling about the meaning of one of his poems.[2] Parthenius intercedes on behalf of the schoolteacher who has correctly interpreted the poem to show the fallaciousness of his opponent's reading. The latter, however, dismisses the interpretation, which prompts Parthenius to deplore the necessity of having one of his friends verify his identity. Galen alleges that he has found himself in a situation similar to Parthenius', as certain doctors and philosophers, who lack preliminary training in grammar and rhetoric, have misinterpreted his views.[3] He uses the story to cast himself as the reluctant author, who is compelled to write *Prop.Plac.* not out of self-interest but for didactic reasons: to correct the mistakes of the poorly educated.[4] Nonetheless, it is part of a strategy of self-promotion, for, in comparing

[1] See *Prop.Plac.* 1.4;Lami and Garofalo (2012), p. 60 ll. 6–8. I refer here and below to Lami and Garofalo's edition [=LG], which improves on the *editio princeps* of Boudon-Millot and Pietrobelli (2005). For the textual divergences between the two editions, see Lami (2010). Prior to the publication of Boudon-Millot and Pietrobelli's Greek edition, the text of *Prop.Plac.* was only accessible through a medieval Arabo-Latin translation, which Nutton (1999) edited and translated into English. Dating to as late as the second decade of the third century (*c.* 209–16), *Prop.Plac.* is probably Galen's last work (Pietrobelli 2013: 107).

[2] *Prop.Plac.* 1.1–2; LG, p. 56 l. 1–p. 58 l. 10. On Parthenius' life, see Lightfoot (1999), 9–16. On *Prop. Plac.* as an 'auto-doxography', see Hankinson (2009), 133.

[3] *Prop.Plac.* 1.3; LG, p. 58 ll. 11–16. Cf. *Lib.Prop.* pr. (Boudon-Millot 2007: p. 134 l. 1–p. 136 l. 22), where Galen relates how he saw in Rome two men arguing about the authenticity of a tract ascribed to him. On the similarities between the prefaces of *Prop.Plac.* and *Lib.Prop.*, see Nutton (1999), 126. Pietrobelli (2013: 129) argues that a concern to resolve authenticity issues surrounding his corpus underlies Galen's composition of both *Prop.Plac.* and *Lib.Prop.*

[4] On Galen's exploitation of this motif, see König (2009), 44, 50–8.

himself to Parthenius, Galen suggests that he, too, is a Greek intellectual celebrity in Roman society.

Galen seems to have his own scholarly credibility – if not his posthumous legacy – in mind when composing this tract. As in Parthenius' case, Galen's patrons were among the intelligentsia (πεπαιδευμένοι) of Rome, so he may have viewed any charge of epistemological inconsistency as a threat to his authority in this circle.[5] The duelling schoolteachers in the Parthenius anecdote, who are debating out in the open, recall Galen's own participation in public disputes on learned subjects, which were a defining feature of the intellectual culture of the Second Sophistic.[6] In contrast to Galen's earlier anatomical performances, which established his superiority over rivals through displays of technical proficiency, *Prop.Plac.* upholds his status as an elite intellectual by denying any wavering in his opinions.[7] This text appears to be as concerned with demarcating the boundaries of Galen's knowledge as with staking out the epistemic topography of medicine, so it serves to defend and advertise his conception of the medical discipline as well.

Prop.Plac. situates Galen's knowledge in relation to five disciplinary categories: 'medicine', 'practical philosophy', 'political philosophy', 'ethical philosophy', and 'theoretical philosophy'.[8] To the apparent exclusion of the latter category, Galen's knowledge seems to encompass what is 'useful' (χρήσιμον) to or 'necessary' (ἀναγκαῖον) for the other four. Because Galen himself determines what is 'useful' to these four fields of learning, the treatise collapses their epistemology with his own. For example, without access to demonstrative proof about the immortality and substance of the soul, Galen professes to have no certain knowledge of these topics, which he characterizes as not 'useful' (χρήσιμον) to the doctor in their treatment of diseases.[9] While *Prop.Plac.* sets up a binary between 'useful' and 'useless' knowledge, which seems to map onto its distinction between 'practical'

[5] Parthenius counted among his patrons the poet and statesman Cornelius Gallus, to whom he dedicated the surviving Ἐρωτικὰ Παθήματα (a collection of love stories), and possibly Helvius Cinna, the author of the lost epyllion *Zmyrna*. See Lightfoot (1999), 11–12, 74–6. For a list of Galen's patrons, which included members of the imperial family, ex-proconsuls, and philosophers, see von Staden (1997), 47–51.

[6] On the Second Sophistic, see p. 3n13 above. For Galen as a Second Sophistic author, see Eichholz (1951); Bowersock (1969); 59–75, von Staden (1995, 1997); Swain (1996), 357–79.

[7] On Galen's anatomical experiments as displays of power and cultural elitism, see Gleason (2009).

[8] See *Prop.Plac.* 8.4, 13.7, 14.5, 15.2, 15.5, 15.7, 15.9; LG, p. 94 l. 14–p. 96 l. 3, p. 126 ll. 14–16, p. 134 l. 13, p. 138 l. 6, p. 140 ll. 4–5, p. 142 ll. 20–1 (on this passage, see p. 35 below), and p. 144 ll. 1, 3.

[9] See, e.g., *Prop.Plac.* 7.3–4; LG, p. 86 l. 19–p. 88 l. 11. He also labels as irrelevant to medicine the issues of empsychosis ('ensoulment') and metempsychosis (LG, p. 138 ll. 6–8) and the nature of vegetative sensation (LG, p. 142 ll. 19–26). For Galen's engagement with the latter subject, see pp. 56–66 below.

and 'theoretical' as well as 'demonstrated' and 'undemonstrated' knowledge, it attenuates this dichotomy by recognizing a third epistemological category that mediates the opposing pair: 'things whose knowledge is not necessary for the health of the body or for the ethical virtues of the soul, but which would – if securely known – be an additional adornment to the things accomplished by medicine and ethical philosophy'.[10] Through the mutual participation of medicine and ethics in this intermediate category, which allows them both to lay claim to a more theoretical (albeit less certain) kind of knowledge, *Prop.Plac.* questions the disjunction between the two fields themselves as well as theoretical philosophy.[11]

Thus, compared to Galen's prior writings on medical disciplinarity (*Ars Med.*, *Protr.*, *Thras.*, *CAM*, *PAM*, and *Opt.Med.*), *Prop.Plac.* seems to advance a more expansive medicine. Whereas these earlier texts are nearly silent about the soul, Galen comes close to giving a materialist (or physicalist) account of the soul at *Prop.Plac.* 7.1–2, notwithstanding his aporia about its substance.[12] He also reiterates throughout the tract his certainty about the soul being the 'source' (ἀρχή) of three movements in the body.[13] Unlike works such as *The Faculties of the Soul Follow the Mixture of the Body* (*QAM*) and *On the Doctrines of Hippocrates and Plato* (*PHP*), which will be discussed below, *Prop.Plac.* does not tease out the medical significance of this 'psychological' information; moreover, after introducing his inference about the soul's material generation from the elements, Galen is quick to qualify that he has only demonstrated what is 'useful' for the doctor to know.[14] Galen's certain knowledge about the soul's involvement in the body as the source of three movements works, however, to undercut the separability of the soul and body. By making the soul a concern of medicine and ethics in addition to theoretical philosophy, Galen, at the very least, softens the edges between these disciplines. In her study of embodiment in classical Greece, Holmes argues that Greek philosophers promoted body–soul dualism to secure a monopoly on psychological expertise.[15] Galen's rejection of this sharp division of body and soul in *Prop.Plac.* may represent an attempt to break down the boundary between

[10] *Prop.Plac.* 14.5; LG, p. 134 ll. 10–13; the translation is from Singer (2014), 17. See also Gill (2010), 150.

[11] For Galen's coupling of ethics and medicine in *Prop.Plac.*, see the reference in the note above and *Prop.Plac.* 15.5; LG, p. 140 ll. 1–5.

[12] See LG, p. 86 ll. 1–18; on this passage, see Gill (2010), 151–2.

[13] *Prop.Plac.* 3.3, 8.2; LG, p. 66 ll. 1–4, p. 92 l. 14–p. 94 l. 2. At *Ars Med.* 23.8 (Boudon-Millot 2002a: p. 347 l. 1), Galen lists 'psychic affections' (ψυχικὰ πάθη) as one of the six non-naturals that alter the condition of the body. Nonetheless, this text does not explain how psychic affections arise in and influence the body, but merely warns against their excess.

[14] See LG, p. 86 ll. 19–21.

[15] See especially Holmes (2010), 192–227.

medicine and philosophy with the aim of challenging philosophers' dominion over the soul. The reference in the text to 'medical philosophy' (ἰατρικὴ φιλοσοφία) – a phrase unprecedented in this sense – suggests that Galen counts his enmeshment of the two disciplines among the greatest achievements of his career.[16]

The notion of the soul's governance of three movements of the body, with which Galen asserts his claim to psychological knowledge, goes back to Plato's theory of a tripartite soul in the *Republic* and *Timaeus*. *Prop.Plac.* presents the *Timaeus* in particular as a foundational text for Galen's own linking of medicine and philosophy – this is the dialogue from which he takes the subjects that determine the boundaries of his own (and thus medicine's) knowledge.[17] While Galen puts the *Timaeus*' cosmological questions about the createdness of the world (28b2–29b1) and the corporeality of the Demiurge (29d7–30c1) beyond the knowledge of doctors, he indicates that they should learn about Plato's tripartite soul (69c5–71e20) and have a rough familiarity with his account of plant life (76e7–77c5).[18] This chapter proposes that, with its vision of the human body as entangled with the soul and macrocosm, the *Timaeus* appealed to Galen because it enabled him to connect medicine to other fields of knowledge.[19] Specifically, I will look at Galen's efforts to define the dialogue, a work on 'physical theory' (τὴν φυσικὴν θεωρίαν) according to *Prop.Plac.*, as a medically relevant resource to extend medicine's jurisdiction to include areas that traditionally fell under philosophy's domain: the 'physical', 'biological', 'psychological', and 'ethical'.[20] As I will show, Galen's

16 While the MS Vlatadon 14 (which preserves *Prop.Plac.*) reads ἰατρικὴ φιλοσοφία (see Boudon-Millot and Pietrobelli 2005: p. 190 l. 5), Lami and Garofalo emend this *hapax* to τὴν ἠθικὴν ('ethics'). Lami (2010: 125) points to the pairing of medicine and ethics at section 14.5 (LG, p. 134 l. 13), among other passages, for support for this emendation. Pietrobelli (2013: 125), on the other hand, defends the manuscript reading on conceptual grounds and on the basis of *variatio*. In *Who is the Heir of Divine Things* (59, § 297), Philo uses ἰατρικὴ φιλοσοφία to designate a form of philosophy that can heal the errors of the soul. Elias (sixth century) uses the phrase similarly in *On Porphyry's Introduction*: Busse (1900), p. 9 l. 9. For a later author who refers to ἰατρικὴ φιλοσοφία in the sense of 'medical philosophy', see John Malalas (*c.* 491–578), *Chronographia* 14.15.

17 Galen refers to the *Timaeus* by name at *Prop.Plac.* 8.3 and 13.4 (LG, p. 94 l. 8, p. 124 l. 2). If one excludes references to book titles, Galen also cites Plato more than Hippocrates – nine times opposed to eight.

18 These are the topics of *Prop.Plac.* 2, 3, 8, 10, 13, and 15.

19 Cf. Gill (2010), 64–84, who attributes Galen and the Stoics' attraction to the dialogue to the text's 'high naturalism'. Gill defines 'high naturalism' as a teleological view of nature, where natural entities possess an innate source of life and capacities that are responsible for their character and structure (66).

20 See *Prop.Plac.* 13.4; LG, p. 124 l. 2. As I mentioned in the Introduction (p. 2n7), Galen also identifies the subject matter of the *Timaeus* as 'physics' in *PHP*. Notwithstanding its Greek etymology, 'biology' is not an ancient category of knowledge – the *Oxford English Dictionary, 2nd Edition*

disciplinary boundary work with the *Timaeus* ranges from denying physics and ethics' exteriority to medicine to undermining philosophy's hegemony over the health of the soul and the world beyond the body. Through this questioning of philosophy's autonomy and 'invasion' of its territory, Galen draws more expansive boundaries for medicine to advance the discipline's epistemic authority.

The first half of the chapter situates Galen's exegetical activity on the *Timaeus* in the context of his rivalry with philosophy. I focus on three related texts: *On the Medical Statements in Plato's Timaeus* (*Plat. Tim.*), *On the Doctrines of Hippocrates and Plato* (*PHP*), and *The Faculties of the Soul Follow the Mixtures of the Body* (*QAM*). These writings, I maintain, engage in a positive polemic with philosophy in the sense that they are not concerned with demolishing this rival claimant to epistemic authority but with illustrating the equal, if not superior, explanatory power of medicine. Galen, however, has to confront medicine's own credibility problems, which supposedly stem from contemporary practitioners' greed and incompetence.[21] My analysis first examines how *Plat. Tim.*, a commentary often neglected in modern scholarship on account of its textual state, represents a move by Galen to further medicine's epistemic standing by arguing for its capacity to investigate some of the same questions as philosophy. I demonstrate that, in purporting to uncover 'medical' (ἰατρικῶς) passages in the *Timaeus*, the exegesis makes medicine a requirement for comprehending the dialogue's cosmological narrative, and therefore contests philosophy's monopolistic command of the body, soul, and cosmos.[22]

I next turn to *PHP* and *QAM*, both of which utilize the embodied soul of the *Timaeus* (and, to a lesser extent, the *Republic*) to perform their disciplinary boundary work. Famously, Galen dedicates the bulk of *PHP*, books one through seven, to defending Plato's tripartition of the soul and location of its rational part in the brain (*Ti.* 69d6–e4, 73c6–d2).

credits the German naturalist Gottfried Reinhold with the coinage of the term in 1802. As Aristotle's writings on animal anatomy and physiology (e.g., *HA*, *PA*, and *GA*) indicate, subjects now considered 'biological' (e.g., physiology and anatomy) were often subsumed under 'physics'.

21 *On Recognizing the Best Physician* (*Opt.Med.Cogn.*), which survives in an Arabic translation by Ḥunayn ibn Isḥāq (see Iskandar 1988), contains Galen's fullest discussion of the supposed decline of medicine.

22 Of the four books of *Plat. Tim.*, only fragments from book three and possibly one and two survive in Greek; however, we have citations from all four books in Arabic. For the Greek and Arabic fragments, see Schröder (1934); Moraux (1977), 44, 49–50; Larrain (1991, 1992); Lorusso (2005), 51, 55–6; Das (2019). Nickel (2002) has dismissed the Greek fragments from books one and two as spurious, whereas I (Das 2014) have defended their authenticity by drawing on evidence from medieval Arabic witnesses.

Concentrating on the issue of the corporeal seat of the rational soul, I call attention to the ways in which this work 'medicalizes' the controversy to position the doctor with clinical experience in addition to logical and anatomical training as better able to settle it than the philosopher. My study also touches on book eight of *PHP*, where Galen invokes the dialogue's aetiology of bodily disease (81e–86a) to legitimize his interest, qua doctor, in the elements. Here, I show that, while Galen's interpretation of the *Timaeus* may license him to broach a subject 'belonging' to physics, he highlights errors in Plato's nosological account to discredit philosophers as reliable producers of knowledge about the body.

Characterized as a 'propagandizing manifesto, devoted principally to promoting the image and the office of the doctor', *QAM* reveals a similarly subversive appropriation of the *Timaeus*.[23] I will review how the tract's materialist theory of the soul serves Galen's expansionist agenda in that it allows medicine to stake out a greater role in character formation vis-à-vis ethics, the established authority on the practice. *Ti.* 86b–87b, which attributes all psychic diseases to bodily causes, is a key passage for Galen's allocation of a share in the soul's health to doctors.[24] Nonetheless, as I will observe, Galen's reading of this section of the dialogue suppresses Plato's criticism of doctors' intervention in psychic illnesses to construct a textual ally for his disciplinary boundary work.

Whereas the first half of the chapter deals with debates centred on the human body, the final part examines Galen's reformulation of the boundaries of medicine to include the non-human: plants. I noted above that *Prop.Plac.* emphasizes the practical orientation of medicine but still leaves room for a more speculative kind of medical knowledge. The philosophical controversy regarding the sensitive ability of plants – an 'unnecessary' (μηδὲ [. . .] ἀναγκαίας) subject according to *Prop.Plac.* – provides Galen with a pretext to display the theoretical potential as well as universal applicability of his theory of the natural faculties, which he presents as a product of his medical learning and experience.[25] Returning to *Plat.Tim.*, I explore how Galen exploits the homologous relationship that the *Timaeus* forges between the micro- and macrocosms to justify his departure from the confines of the human body. Through his contribution to this

[23] Donini (2008), 200.

[24] As I will explain (p. 53), I follow Gill's (2000: 60–1) strong reading of *Ti.* 86b1–2 ('the diseases of the psyche arise because of the condition of the body in the following way', καὶ τὰ μὲν περὶ τὸ σῶμα νοσήματα ταύτῃ συμβαίνει γιγνόμενα, τὰ δὲ περὶ ψυχὴν διὰ σώματος ἕξιν τῇδε), which proposes that *all* psychic defects have a bodily basis.

[25] *Prop.Plac.* 15.8; LG, p. 142 ll. 19–20.

long-standing dispute about vegetative sensation, Galen puts forward doctors such as himself as credible examiners of the cosmos. I then conclude by considering how the 'Galenic *Timaeus*' came to be associated with the destabilization of disciplinary boundaries in the medieval Islamicate world.

Inter-Disciplinary Polemics: Galen and 'Plato Medicus'

Galen famously recounts in *On the Order of my Own Books* (*Ord.Lib.Prop.*) that, as a youth, he was on course to become a philosopher before divine intervention steered him towards medicine.[26] While this story serves to highlight his dual expertise in medicine and philosophy, Singer has argued that Galen did not want to be seen as a philosopher, in spite of his philosophical interests and involvement with elites at Rome whose intellectual koine was philosophy.[27] Galen's rejection of the philosophical profession is predicated on his refusal to commit himself to any philosophical sect, which the career demanded at this point in time.[28] This 'anti-philosophical' stance, however, does not entail an absolute disavowal of philosophy but rather its current dogmatic instantiation.[29] The following discussion will show that, as with the relationship that he constructs between himself and Hippocrates, Galen presents himself as having an unmediated connection to Plato by claiming to recover the original meaning of his work.[30] Nonetheless, the fact that Galen employs many of the same interpretive strategies – for example, the use of Aristotelian and Stoic concepts to explain Platonic theories – as his Middle Platonic peers reveals his own embeddedness in contemporary philosophical culture.[31] Because the *Timaeus* was a focal point of interest for philosophical schools in the first and second centuries CE, the dialogue provided Galen with

[26] His father Nicon was moved by 'vivid dreams' (ὄνειρα ἐναργῆ) to make him study medicine (Boudon-Millot 2007: p. 99 l. 23–p. 100 l. 4). This same story is mentioned in *On Prognosis* (*Praen.*): Nutton (1979), p. 76 l. 29–p. 78 l. 2.

[27] Singer (2014), 1–20.

[28] Singer (2014), 18. At *PHP* 4.4.38 and 9.7.5–6 Galen criticizes the follower of any philosophical or medical sect who disregards the truth in order to defend their master's doctrines. Hankinson (1992: 3507) emphasizes Galen's intellectual independence and contends that he should be viewed as an eclectic who chooses from the 'intellectual *smørgasbord*' offered by rival philosophical (and medical) traditions'.

[29] Singer (2014), 17.

[30] On Galen's attempts to distance himself from Hellenistic and post-Hellenistic Hippocratic commentators, to whom his own Hippocratic exegeses are enormously indebted, see von Staden (2009).

[31] See pp. 56–66. below. Chiaradonna (2009a) maintains that Galen should not be considered a Middle Platonic author, as he is not interested in the hot topics of the period (e.g. the createdness of the cosmos). This lack of interest, however, does not mean that Galen's approach to Plato is not informed by Middle Platonic exegetical trends, on which see Karamanolis (2006).

a conspicuous platform from which he could demonstrate the strength of medicine as a conceptual apparatus for resolving theoretical controversies.[32] Galen's entry into Timaean exegesis presupposes a familiarity with the philosophical disputes surrounding the text, so he admits only the idealized doctor of *Opt.Med.*, who has training in logic, physics, and ethics, into these debates.[33]

Galen composed a number of works on Platonic philosophy, but four of them take theories from the *Timaeus* as their central concern: *PHP*, *QAM*, *Plat.Tim.*, and the *Synopsis of Plato's Timaeus* (*Com.Tim.*), which forms part of an eight-volume set of summaries of Plato's dialogues.[34] The first two texts give considerable attention to Plato's notion of a tripartite soul, which is expounded at *Ti.* 69a–72d and *Republic* 4, 8–9 (419a–445e; 543a–592b). While fragments from the first book of *PHP* indicate that Galen intended to discuss all points of agreement between Hippocrates and Plato, seven of its nine books focus on demonstrating how the two authorities hold similar views on the number and location of the parts of the soul.[35] *QAM* appeals to Plato's location of the rational and irrational parts of the soul in the brain, heart, and liver to develop a link between corporeal and psychic health. *Plat.Tim.* and *Com.Tim.*, the latter of which is almost fully extant in a ninth-century Arabic translation from Ḥunayn ibn Iṣḥāq and his associate ʿĪsā ibn Yaḥyā ibn Ibrāhīm, treat the dialogue's cosmological, physiological, and psychological passages.[36]

The overlapping dates of these writings reveal that Galen may have conceived of them as a unified project. As I will now explain, the internal references which help to date this group of works and the preface of *Com. Tim.* suggest that they constitute a polemic against philosophy. All these

32 There survives from this period a rich body of exegetical material on the *Timaeus*: commentaries from the Peripatetic philosopher Adrastus of Aphrodisias (first half of the second century CE) and the Platonists Calvenus Taurus (mid-second century CE) and Atticus (*c.* 176 CE); a more thematic summary of the dialogue is provided by Alcinous' (second century CE) *Primer on Plato's Doctrines* (Διδασκαλικὸς τῶν Πλάτωνος δογμάτων); and Plutarch (*c.* 45–*c.* 125 CE) treats particular sections of the text in *On the Birth of the Soul in the Timaeus* (Περὶ τῆς ἐν τῷ Τιμαίῳ ψυχογονίας) and *On the World's Having Come into Being According to Plato* (Περὶ τοῦ γεγονέναι κατὰ Πλάτωνα τὸν κόσμον). On these authors, see Dillon (1993, 1996); on their commentaries on the *Timaeus*, see Dörrie and Baltes (1993), 48–54.

33 On Galen's 'intra-disciplinary' polemics, see the Introduction (p. 18 above.).

34 For Galen's other Platonic works, see *Lib.Prop.* 16; Boudon-Millot (2007), p. 170 l. 14–p. 171 l. 5. As Ḥunayn reports in his *Epistle*, his manuscript of Galen's Platonic synopses contained only four of the eight volumes. See Bergsträsser (1925), p. 50 l. 14–p. 51 l. 2, with corrections from Bergsträsser (1932), p. 23 ll. 10–11=Lamoreaux (2016), p. 125 l. 14–p. 127 l. 2.

35 See De Lacy (2005), p. 64 ll. 5–14. Books eight and nine deal with the elements (on which, see pp. 50–1 below) and logical methods of enquiry.

36 On the Arabic translation of *Com.Tim.*, see Kraus and Walzer (1951), 18–19.

texts appear to have been published after 169 CE, during or following Galen's second stay in Rome. Traditionally dated to about 192 CE, *QAM* seems to post-date the other works by almost twenty years, but there is a clear thematic link with Galen's earlier explanations of the *Timaeus*' psychology.[37] Although Galen finished the first six books of *PHP* during his initial stay in Rome (162–6 CE), the last three books were completed around the same time as *Plat. Tim.* and *Com. Tim.* – that is, in the interval between his return to Rome (169 CE) and the emperor Marcus Aurelius' homecoming from the German front (176 CE). In book eight of *PHP* (8.5.13–14; 8.6.57), Galen mentions his plans to write a commentary on the *Timaeus* after he is done with the present work. He relates that some unnamed friends of his have requested that he expound the 'medical statements' (ἰατρικῶς εἰρημένων) in the dialogue because 'few have written on this subject, and they not well' (εἰς ταῦτα δ' ὀλίγοι τε καὶ οὐδ' οὗτοι καλῶς ἔγραψαν).[38] This dearth of exegetical activity is contrasted with the numerous commentaries on 'the rest' (τἆλλα) of the *Timaeus*, some of which are 'longer than what is seemly' (μακρότερον τοῦ προσήκοντος).

Galen divides the dialogue into two sections: 'medical' and 'philosophical' (to which 'the rest' probably refers). He does not identify a line of demarcation in the text, however. The passages in *PHP* promise a full commentary on the *Timaeus* to excuse their cursory examination of Plato's humoural pathology at *Ti.* 84c8–86a8, so by 'medical statements' Galen may mean here the dialogue's description of disease (81e6–86a8) at the very minimum. He is able to leverage doctors' uncontested expertise in the diagnosis and treatment of disease to devise a role for himself in Timaean exegesis and thus assert medicine's right to the dialogue's knowledge. The criticism in *PHP* of the near neglect and incompetent handling of the 'medical' material functions as a further justification for Galen's exegetical interest in the *Timaeus* by establishing a need for his medical learning. While Galen does not name the authors of the few 'not good' commentaries on the dialogue's medical sections, the lack of any prior systematic analysis of the text by a doctor and later evidence of philosophical engagements with these passages suggest that these offenders are philosophers.[39]

[37] Cf. Singer (2013b), 40, who questions the tract's dating based on the tenuous evidence cited in support of it: an apparent reference in the text (4.768K) to *On Character Traits*, which was composed after 192 CE.

[38] De Lacy (2005), p. 508 ll. 5–9.

[39] Presumably following his predecessors' lead, Proclus covered the entire dialogue, including the 'medical' passages, in his commentary. Although the extant text of Proclus' commentary on the *Timaeus* only goes up to *Ti.* 44d, fragments in Arabic (for which, see Arnzen 2013) demonstrate the comprehensiveness of his explanation.

In targeting philosophers for their disregard for and misunderstanding of parts of the *Timaeus*, Galen alleges that the purpose of his future exegetical endeavour is to rescue a lost side of Plato's thought.

Galen offers similar reasons for writing *Plat. Tim.* in the preface to *Com. Tim.* but credits himself with discovering that the *Timaeus* contains 'medical' information. Remarks in *Com. Tim.* regarding his intentions to compose an eighth book of *PHP* and *Plat. Tim.* give the impression that the synopsis was the first of his Timaean expositions to be completed.[40] Nonetheless, according to the prologue to *Com. Tim.*, which survives in a Latin version of a medieval Arabic treatise on magic entitled *The Book of Laws* (*Liber aneguemis*, or *Kitāb al-Nawāmīs*), Galen finished the synopsis after at least *Plat. Tim.*, for he interrupted his work on it to give his full attention to the commentary.[41] He discloses:

> Declinavi ergo secundum id quod visum est michi ad expositionem et cognovi quia ipse est medicus et quod ipse est modus rectitudinis ut faciam cognitionem meam et fatigem animam meam in huius libri expositione.[42]
>
> Therefore, in accordance with my decision, I abandoned [this summary] and started writing a commentary. I realized that Plato is a doctor and the correct method was that I put this realization into practice and make every effort to produce a commentary on this book.

The prologue establishes not only a close chronological connection but also a hermeneutic relationship between *Com. Tim.* and *Plat. Tim.* by adding after the above that the latter is supposed to facilitate comprehension of the former. The Arabic author of *The Book of Laws*, who has in all likelihood adapted Galen's comments, uses an allegory to articulate how the two exegeses should be read, where the synopsis is a sword locked in its sheath (*ensis . . . est in concavitate vagine et est desuper clausum*) and the commentary is an incision (*incidit ex eo portionem parvam in concavitatem vagine*) above the lock that can be enlarged to release the sword.[43] *Plat. Tim.* provides a shortcut to the contents of *Com. Tim.*, but exactly how it helps

[40] See Kraus and Walzer (1951), p. 29 ll. 12–15, where Galen reveals his intention to discuss the dialogue's aetiology of diseases in *PHP* and *Plat. Tim.* Galen appears to have begun writing *Com. Tim.* after book seven of *PHP*, for he refers the reader to his explanation of Plato's theory of vision in the seventh 'chapter' (*maqāla*) (Kraus and Walzer 1951: p. 12 l. 5).

[41] See Rashed (2009). [42] Rashed (2009), 92.

[43] Rashed (2009), 93. Scopelliti and Chaouech (2006: 12–14) reject the manuscripts' ascription of *The Book of Laws* to Ḥunayn ibn Isḥāq and argue for a Muslim author with possible connections to the philosopher al-Šahrastānī (sixth/twelfth century). Pingree (2014: 468–9), on the other hand, maintains that the Arabic author of *The Book of Laws* must have published their work some time between 850 and 900 CE, as the figure(s) writing under the name of the alchemist Ǧābir ibn Ḥayyān (*fl.* end of the ninth or beginning of the tenth century) attacks this treatise. Whatever their identity, the

the reader to understand the shorter text is left unexplained: the commentary may supply the requisite background for grasping the brief analysis of the synopsis by providing line-by-line examinations of a large portion of Timaeus' narrative.

The Arabo-Latin translation's reworking of the Galenic original also raises questions about the significance of the prologue's claim that Plato is a 'doctor' (*medicus*). Nowhere in Galen's extant Greek corpus is Plato called a 'doctor' (ἰατρός); in fact, in book eight of *PHP* Galen ascribes certain omissions in the *Timaeus* to the philosopher's lack of practical medical experience.[44] Perhaps, in line with the references in *PHP* to the future composition of *Plat. Tim.*, the Greek prologue to *Com. Tim.* may have relayed how Galen discovered that medical training is a hermeneutic necessity in the interpretation of the *Timaeus*.[45] Therefore, although Galen may wish to stress the medical content of the *Timaeus* to create an entry point into the dialogue for himself qua doctor, the Arabo-Latin text's characterization of Plato as a *medicus* is probably more reflective of Galen's formative role in shaping Plato's reception in the medieval Islamicate world than his own perception of the philosopher.

Rashed views *Plat. Tim.* as part of a larger Galenic project of shifting focus away from the *Timaeus*' cosmogony, which was the subject of considerable debate among contemporary Platonists, to the less examined 'third part', which contains more practical theories.[46] It is not necessary to assume that Galen would have perceived the same divisions in the structure of the dialogue that have been proposed by modern commentators, who traditionally order it into three sections on 'the craftsmanship of Intellect' (29d7–47e2), 'the effects of Necessity' (47e3–69a5), and 'the cooperation of Intellect and Necessity' (69a6–92c9).[47] While the undisputed Greek fragments of *Plat. Tim.* discuss aspects of human physiology such as the formation of the nails (76d3–e6) and respiration (77c6–81e5), a citation in Abū l-Rayḥān al-Bīrūnī's (362–*c.* 442/973–*c.* 1050) ethnographic *The Book Confirming What Pertains to India, Whether Rational or Despicable* (*Kitāb Taḥqīq mā li-l-Hind min maqūla maqbūla fī l-ʿaql aw marḏūla*) indicates that the commentary may have started around *Ti.* 41a3–41d3, where the Demiurge commands the lesser gods to fashion the mortal creatures of the cosmos.[48] Al-Bīrūnī does not identify from which book of the 'Medical Timaeus' (*Ṭīmāwus al-ṭibbī*) the citation derives, but it has

writer appears to have incorporated part of Ḥunayn and ʿĪsā's translation of Galen's *Com. Tim.* into their text (Rashed 2009: 95–7).

44 See p. 51n100 below.

45 Cf. Rashed (2009), 96.

46 Rashed (2009), 98–9.

47 See, e.g., Cornford (1937), xi–xiv; Zeyl (2000), xci–v.

48 See Sachau (1887), p. 17 ll. 6–9.

been attributed to book one of *Plat. Tim.*[49] Galen appears to have taken Plato's description of the creation and incarnation of individual souls, which belongs in modern schemes to the cosmogonic 'first part' of the *Timaeus*, to represent the initial 'medical statement' (ἰατρικῶς εἰρημένον) of the dialogue.

Galen brings subjects such as form and matter, the elements, and the composition of the human soul as well as the body within medicine's boundaries by designating the passages in the *Timaeus* where they receive treatment as 'medical'. This reconceptualization of the 'medical' finds parallels in Galen's non-Timaean outputs such as *On Semen* and *On the Elements according to Hippocrates*, whose investigations of the interaction of form and matter and elemental change similarly deny the exteriority of these philosophical topics to medicine.[50] Therefore, Galen points to the medical aspects of the *Timaeus* to justify not only his own pertinence to the tradition of Platonic exegesis but also his expansion of the medical discipline. In addition to drawing broader parameters for medicine, Galen's boundary work in the prologue to *Com. Tim.* and *Plat. Tim.* also works to undermine philosophy's autonomy. His suggestion that philosophers lack the expertise to comprehend fully Plato's text implies philosophy's dependence on medicine. Galen contests the exclusivity of philosophy's authority on the *Timaeus* – and the domains of knowledge that the dialogue encompasses in its cosmic account – to enhance medicine's epistemic standing.

As I proposed in the Introduction, Galen's polemic with philosophy may be motivated by an anxiety about medicine's credibility in Roman society. Although Galen's blanket characterization of Roman doctors as cheats and butchers in *On Recognizing the Best Physician* serves his rhetoric of exceptionalism, the tract's complaint about these individuals' inadequate educations reflects the reality that most practitioners could not afford the lengthy training extolled in *Lib.Ord.Prop.* and *Opt.Med.*[51] Galen is by no means the first well-educated and well-to-do doctor in Rome or the wider Graeco-Roman world, but, despite his elite predecessors' efforts to increase medicine's prestige by distancing their practice from that of their sub-elite peers (for example, slaves, freed- and freepersons, and women), the discipline still occupied an inferior status in

49 Larrain (1992), 9–11. Unaware of the reference in al-Bīrūnī, Schröder (1934: 34) placed the beginning of *Plat. Tim.* somewhere between *Ti.* 41d4 and 42e5.

50 See, e.g., *Sem.* 2.1.45–2.24 and *Hipp.Elem.* 3.2.1–22.

51 On the social status of doctors in the Graeco-Roman world, see Pleket (1995) and p. 8 above. For Galen's criticism of the proliferation of medical specialists in Rome and other large cities, see Chapter 2 (pp. 77–80.).

relation to philosophy.[52] Whereas medicine continued to have commercial associations in Rome, the preoccupation of the emperor Marcus Aurelius and other figures at the highest social levels with philosophy certainly contributed to its eminence during Galen's lifetime.[53] Texts such as *Plat. Tim.* and *Com.Tim.* show that the *Timaeus* allowed Galen to question the separation of medicine and philosophy and to establish, through this weakening of disciplinary boundaries, a link between them. Medicine improves its standing by its association with philosophy. The following sections highlight an arguably stronger form of boundary work that aims to install medicine in a position of epistemic authority by edging philosophy out of domains that its expertise had long comprised: psychological health and the question of the location of the 'ruling part' (ἡγεμονικόν) of the soul. Targeting philosophical readers, the two texts that are the focus of my investigation, *PHP* and *QAM*, dispute not only philosophy's monopoly on these subjects but also its very ability to handle them.

Anatomizing the Ruling Part of the Soul

Galen wrote the first six books of *PHP* at the behest of a student of Aristotelian philosophy, the senator and ex-consul Flavius Boethus.[54] The way in which the text builds its arguments on anatomical observations and logical reasoning would have resonated with an Aristotelian, who might see Galen as following in the methodological footsteps of Aristotle. Nonetheless, while *PHP* aims to discuss all points of agreement between Hippocrates and Plato, seven of its nine books defend Plato's tripartite division of the soul and location of its rational, or 'ruling' (ἡγεμονικόν), part in the brain (*Ti.* 44d3–8, 69d6–e3) against the Stoic Chrysippus' (third century BCE), and with less vehemence Aristotle's, idea of a unitary soul whose command

[52] See p. 17 above and the notes for the relevant bibliography. On the diverse social backgrounds of the doctors (both male and female) practising in republican and imperial Rome, see, e.g., Parker (1997), 142–4; Israelowich (2015), 11–44.

[53] Israelowich (2015: 43) emphasizes the precariousness of most Roman doctors' economic situation in that, as 'artisans', their livelihoods depended on their ability to attract and retain clients. Cf. *Opt. Med.Cogn.* 1.3 (Iskandar 1988: p. 40 l. 11–p. 42 l. 2), where Galen recounts how ancient kings used to teach their sons medicine. On philosophy's mixed reception in Rome, see p. 8 above. Marcus Aurelius' *Meditations*, a private notebook written on the German front, shows that he was a formidable student of Stoic philosophy (see Gill 2013).

[54] At *Lib.Prop.* 1.17 (Boudon-Millot 2007: p. 139, l. 27–p. 140, l. 5), Galen recounts that Boethus took the first six books of *PHP* to the province of Syria-Palestine, where he was to be governor, and died shortly thereafter. Singer (2014: 13n14) notes that many of Galen's elite contacts in Rome were Aristotelian philosophers or individuals interested in Aristotelianism.

centre is in the heart.[55] Moreover, the harmony that *PHP* establishes between Hippocrates and Plato may suggest an equivalence between medicine and philosophy, which the two authorities represent metonymically, but these initial seven books give preference to medicine owing to its capacity to resolve the aforementioned psychological controversies with demonstrative proof. At the risk of simplifying a complex concept, 'demonstration' (ἀπόδειξις), according to Galen, is a logically valid argument that proceeds from premises universally agreed upon because they are evident to the senses and reason.[56] Concentrating on Galen's attack on Aristotle and Chrysippus' cardiocentrism in support of Plato's encephalocentric ('brain-centred') thesis, I will now show how he allocates authority in this dispute to the field best able to uncover the phenomena that are the starting points of a demonstration of the issue.[57] Galen frames the debate about the identity of the hegemonic organ, which is responsible for sensation and voluntary motion, as a search for the 'origin' (ἀρχή) of the nerves.[58] In so doing, he underscores the anatomical dimension of the controversy, and thus positions doctors, whose training and clinical experience produce a superior grasp of anatomy, as the most credible contributors to it.

Medicine did not have exclusive jurisdiction over anatomy in Graeco-Roman antiquity. Aristotle's 'biological' works reveal that philosophers from at least the early period of the Lyceum were interested in anatomy and dissected animals.[59] As I remarked above, Galen's own anatomical approach to the question of the hegemonic organ is an Aristotelian inheritance, for Aristotle appears to have been among the first to argue for the physiological significance of the heart in the light of dissection.[60] While the

[55] I will concentrate below on Galen's arguments rather than Chrysippus', for which see the detailed studies of Tieleman (1996, 2003).

[56] For Galen's understanding of demonstration, see Lloyd (1996); Morison (2008), 70–5. See Tieleman (1996) on Galen's method of argumentation and demonstration in *PHP* 2–3.

[57] Galen also draws on the *Timaeus* to refute Chrysippus' theory of the soul's unitary structure: see, e.g., *PHP* 6.8.72, which quotes *Ti.* 70a7–c1 to explain how reason directs the irascible soul to grow angry when the desiderative soul attempts to do something unjust.

[58] See *PHP* 1, testimonium 3 (De Lacy 2005: p. 66 ll. 19–20): 'where the beginning of the nerves is, there is also the governing part of the soul' (ὅπουν τῶν νεύρων ἡ ἀρχή, ἐνταῦθα καὶ τὸ τῆς ψυχῆς ἡγεμονικόν). Rocca (2003: 54) points out that, despite Galen's statements to the contrary, this assertion is not axiomatic. For Havrda (2015: 271), this proposition is 'the most complete example of the demonstrative method in Galen's writings'.

[59] See Lloyd (1987) for an important qualification to Aristotle's empiricism in his biological research.

[60] As Rocca (2003: 29) observes, Aristotle does not frame his investigation as a search for the hegemonic organ, but he contends that the heart is important because it is the source of vital heat, which is the embodiment of the soul, and the blood vessels, which play a key role in sensation. Moreover, as the term ἡγεμονικόν is of Stoic origin (see Long and Sedley 1987: vol. II, 313n5), it would be anachronistic to say that Aristotle identified the heart as the 'ruling part'.

Alexandrian anatomists Herophilus (330/20–260/50 BCE) and Erasistratus (*fl.* 280 BCE) had proved against Aristotle that the nerves originate in the brain through their dissection and vivisection of human, rather than animal, bodies, Galen appears to have felt that the anatomical cachet of cardiocentrism was still significant enough to warrant addressing.[61] To undermine his opponents' cardiocentric position, Galen's tactic in *PHP* is to call attention to either their neglect or imperfect knowledge of anatomy. He weaponizes Chrysippus' own admission of his ignorance of anatomy against the philosopher's depiction of the heart as the source of the nerves and psychic pneuma (ψυχικὸν πνεῦμα) – an invisible substance that is the principal instrument of sensation.[62] Aristotle's competence in anatomy is harder to dismiss, but Galen attributes his erroneous conclusion that the heart is the source of the nerves to a possibly wilful disregard of evidence.[63] This passage from *PHP* 1 also accuses the physician Praxagoras of Cos (late fourth or early third century BCE), another cardiocentrist, of making the same anatomical mistakes as Aristotle.[64] The disproportionate amount of energy that Galen expends in refuting Praxagoras instead of Aristotle gives the impression that the former is the greater threat on account of his medical background.[65] *PHP* deprives philosophers, even those with anatomical experience such as Aristotle, of epistemic authority in the dispute over the hegemonic organ by devaluing their knowledge of anatomy, because it is not based on first-hand contact with the human body.[66]

Galen's defence of Plato's encephalocentrism interweaves episodes from his clinical practice, anatomical demonstrations, and observations of animal sacrifices to imply that the evidence for this position is not only ample but also more convincing – it derives from his experience as a doctor with human anatomy. His refutation, in book one, of Chrysippus' notion that the heart contains psychic pneuma is paradigmatic in this respect. Notwithstanding the fragmentary state of the text, Galen's argumentative

[61] For Herophilus and Erasistratus' experiments on the brain, see von Staden (1989), 155–60, 247–59. These fragments show that both men do not explicitly support encephalocentrism, but the physiological importance which they attribute to the brain suggests that they were sympathetic to this view. Erasistratus locates the origin of the nerves in the meningeal layer of the brain (Rocca 2003: 50).

[62] See *PHP* 1.6.13: De Lacy (2005), p. 80 ll. 21–4. For Galen's identification of pneuma as the instrument of sensation, see *PHP* 7.43.21, 7.3.30: De Lacy (2005), p. 444 ll. 7–10, p. 446 ll. 11–17.

[63] *PHP* 1.6.14–15: De Lacy (2005), p. 80 ll. 24–9.

[64] On Praxagoras' understanding of the heart's role in sensation, see Lewis (2017), 252–87.

[65] See *PHP* 1.6.17–7.55: De Lacy (2005), p. 80 l. 33–p. 90 l. 25.

[66] While Herophilus and Erasistratus championed the 'correct' position in the controversy, Galen also highlights mistakes in their anatomical descriptions (see *PHP* 1.10.3–5, 1.6.1–4: De Lacy 2005: p. 96 ll. 18–20, p. 78 ll. 16–26). In mentioning these errors, Galen indicates that he offers a more perfect anatomy.

strategy consists in showing that damage to the heart does not lead to the cessation of sensation because the organ is full of blood instead of pneuma.[67] Galen describes his examination of a living patient's heart in anticipation of opponents who assign no weight to post-mortem dissections owing to their belief that the organ is deprived of its sensory powers when pneuma escapes at the time of death.[68] This case, with further details about the patient, his injury, and eventual treatment, also appears in *On Anatomical Procedures* (7.13), where it is put to different rhetorical use by Galen.[69] Preserved in Arabic, the pertinent section of *PHP* 1 recounts how Galen removed part of the sternum of a *ġulām* ('slave' or, in De Lacy's translation, 'young boy') afflicted by a pectoral fistula, which had caused the pericardium (the membrane encasing the heart) to mortify. *On Anatomical Procedures* gives the backstory to Galen's surgical intervention: the patient, a slave (παιδάριον) owned by the mime actor Maryllus, developed a fistula on his sternum after a wrestling accident; left untreated for about four months, the injury began to fester and damage the pericardium. Additionally, *PHP* omits that Galen was one of several doctors summoned to treat the slave following a failed first attempt to heal the wound. In *On Anatomical Procedures*, the case both serves to illustrate the work's didactic message that anatomical expertise results in surgical skill and functions as self-promotion for Galen (he alone has the courage and know-how to cure the slave), whereas in *PHP* it disproves the heart's hegemonic role.[70] Galen reasons that the power of sensation and voluntary motion must lie elsewhere, because the patient did not suffer any impairment of function (οὔτε . . . ἐβέβλαπτο τὴν ἐνέργειαν) when he exposed his heart while extracting the corrupted pieces of sternum.[71]

Besides militating against cardiocentrism, this case compels the reader of *PHP* 1 to recognize how Galen's surgical proficiency, acquired through anatomical study and medical practice, gives him access to evidence hidden from view – and from philosophers. Galen has to do more work, however,

[67] *PHP* 1, testimonium 7: De Lacy (2005), p. 70 l. 13–p. 76 l. 13. Here, Galen uses the general term pneuma, but only later qualifies (p. 78 l. 25) that he is arguing against Chrysippus' location of psychic pneuma in the left ventricle.

[68] De Lacy (2005), p. 72 l. 1–p. 76 l. 13.

[69] See Garofalo (2000), 458, 460 [Arabic], 459, 461 [Greek]; Singer (1956), 192–3. See also Mattern (2008), 74, 222n146.

[70] As a counterpoint to his expert treatment of the slave, Galen relates in *AA* how a contemporary physician dealing with gangrene in a less vital part of the body – the arm – severed an artery and caused his patient to bleed to death because of his ignorance of anatomy (see Garofalo 2000: p. 460 ll. 13–18 [Arabic], p. 461 ll. 18–24 [Greek]; Singer 1956: 193).

[71] De Lacy (2005), p. 76 ll. 11–12.

to establish that the absence of psychic pneuma in the heart accounts for the slave's unimpeded use of his sensory and motor faculties during the course of the injury, so he appeals to his vivisection of animal hearts and brains for clarification.[72] Based on his manipulation of the two organs, Galen concludes that the brain must be replete with pneuma, for, when pierced, it does not emit blood, as opposed to the heart. As an exception, he mentions that blood sometimes can be seen in the anterior ventricles of the brains of sacrificed cattle, but the clotting arises from the death blow's severing of various arteries and veins at the base of the neck.[73] Galen never circles back to the case history after listing these various experiments and observations; thus, the text leaves the reader to infer that the slave's injury did not interrupt perception or movement because both ventricles of the heart contain blood.

To deny the heart any role in sensation, Galen sets up a rigid dichotomy between the heart and brain as receptacles of blood and pneuma that does not reflect his conception of the pneumatic system developed elsewhere in *PHP*. In book seven he explains that inhaled air and vaporized humours are transformed into vital pneuma (ζωτικὸν πνεῦμα) in the arteries and heart; when this pneuma is carried via the arteries through the retiform and choroid plexuses of the brain, it changes into psychic pneuma.[74] Moreover, in *PHP* 6 Galen connects blood and pneuma in writing that the left ventricle produces a yellow, warm, 'pneuma-like' (πνευματώδους) blood.[75] He appears to downplay the heart's pneumatic contribution in the aforementioned section of book one because it weakens the value of his 'argument from dissection'. As the presence of blood in the heart does not necessarily entail the absence of pneuma, his anatomical experiments do not refute the organ's hegemonic status.[76] Galen actually has the harder task of demonstrating that Chrysippus' cardiocentric thesis is incorrect due to his misidentification of the *type* of pneuma in the heart.

The passage of book seven that outlines the transformation of pneuma also highlights the limits of what anatomy can reveal about the exact location of the rational soul in the brain.[77] It recounts Galen's attempts to pinpoint the rational soul by determining where in the brain injury

[72] De Lacy (2005), p. 76 ll. 14–26.

[73] De Lacy (2005), p. 76 ll. 26–8. Galen does not specify that these cattle are sacrificial victims; nonetheless, at sacrifices larger animals were similarly stunned by a blow to the neck before their throats were cut (see Ekroth 2014: 325–30).

[74] *PHP* 7.3.28–9: De Lacy (2005), p. 444 l. 33–p. 446 l. 10. See also Rocca (2003), 64–5.

[75] *PHP* 6.8.36: De Lacy (2005), p. 414 ll. 31–2. On this passage, see Rocca (2012), 637.

[76] I borrow the phrase 'argument from dissection' from Rocca (2003), 33.

[77] *PHP* 7.3.14–22: De Lacy (2005), p. 442 l. 19–p. 444 l. 11.

brings about a complete loss of sensation and movement. Through his vivisections, Galen found that cutting the posterior ventricle disrupted sensory and motor functions the most; the animals recovered these activities, however, as soon as he closed the incision. In view of the fact that the animals did not die when pneuma escaped from the posterior ventricle, Galen speculates that the rational soul neither is psychic pneuma nor resident in the ventricular system.[78] His anatomical investigation has reached an impasse: it has demonstrated against cardiocentrists that the rational soul is in the brain but cannot ascertain how it abides there – whether as a material substance or as an incorporeal power.[79] This aporia about the soul's substance shows that Galen does not make any totalizing claim on the soul for medicine as part of his boundary work in *PHP*, but rather has the more restricted aim of redefining the issue of the hegemonic organ as a medical question. The foregoing text of *PHP* has stressed that even to arrive at this point of perplexity requires a mastery of anatomy honed by not only research but also clinical experience. Nonetheless, Galen's larger purpose in reallocating this controversy to medicine may be to grant doctors such as himself a share in psychological expertise and thus to weaken philosophers' monopoly on knowledge of the soul.

Book nine of *PHP* takes a different tack to appropriating the dispute for medicine by suggesting that it has only medical relevance. Galen alleges that the subject is 'useful' (χρήσιμον) to doctors because they need to know where to apply remedies to cure the 'reasoning power' (λογισμός) when injured, whereas it will not help philosophers to acquire the virtues.[80] He mobilizes a rhetoric of utility to close this debate off from ethical philosophers, whom he regards as having a stake in the problem because of their involvement in psychic health. Galen's conceptualization of ethical therapy – conversation directed at getting patients to recognize the affections and errors of their soul with the goal of restoring harmony between its parts – underlies his assertion that the location of the hegemonic organ has no bearing on ethics.[81]

Here, *PHP* 9 does not go so far as to say that doctors have the same capacity as ethical philosophers to treat the soul itself – rather, they treat the soul's physical medium, the nervous system. Even so, the link between

78 See Rocca (2003), 197.

79 Cf. *Ut.Resp.* 4.509K. As will be explained below (pp. 51–2), *QAM* seems to argue for the soul's materiality.

80 *PHP* 9.7.7–8: De Lacy (2005), p. 586 l. 33–p. 588 l. 6.

81 On Galen's 'ethical–philosophical' notion of psychic therapy, as expounded in treatises such as *Aff. Dig.*, *Pecc.Dig.*, and *Mor.*, see Singer (2018), 383–7.

bodily trauma and cognitive damage speaks against the idea of the soul as a separable entity.[82] Thus, although Galen is unclear in this text about how doctors interact with the soul, he still presents them as agents of psychic well-being because their care of the brain affects the soul's exercise of its rational faculties, and presumably its ability to distinguish between error and virtue.[83] This intervention for the soul's benefit, however mediated, allows Galen to insert doctors back into a realm that he may feel was unduly ceded to philosophy in the classical period, when philosophers 'isolated the soul as a discrete target of therapy' to maintain exclusive dominion over it.[84] In *PHP*, the body of the *Timaeus*, bound and fused (43a2–6) with a soul seated in the brain, heart, and lower belly, enables Galen to complicate the dichotomous distribution of psychic and bodily welfare to philosophers and doctors. As will be shown in the next section, the dialogue's troubling of the body–soul division furthers a more hegemonic agenda in *QAM*, which seeks to deflate philosophers' assertion that they alone can doctor the soul.[85]

In the boundary work examined above, the psychology of the *Timaeus* features as a positive point of reference that gives Galen grounds for expanding medical knowledge. Other passages of *PHP* approach the dialogue as a tool that can be used oppositionally to the same end. For instance, immediately following his dismissal of the pertinence of the hegemonic organ debate to ethical philosophers, Galen enumerates a range of 'theoretical' (θεωρητικήν) questions that are also irrelevant to them: whether there is anything outside the cosmos; whether there are multiple worlds; whether the cosmos had a beginning or not; and whether a certain god was the 'artisan' (δημιουργός) of it.[86] These issues are addressed in the *Timaeus*' cosmogony and, as I noted at the start of the chapter, appear in *Prop.Plac.*, where Galen puts them beyond his own

[82] Havrda (2017), 83–4. Cf. Singer (2018), 403.

[83] Donini (2008: 195) summarizes that, in Galen's ethical writings, an 'affection' or 'passion' (πάθος) deals with the irrational parts of the soul, whereas an 'error' (ἁμάρτημα), which consists in incorrect reasoning, involves the rational part of the soul. Accordingly, the ability to identify an error in one's own soul presumes the use of an operational 'reasoning power' (λογισμός). For Galen's depiction of doctors as an 'essential node' in a network of corporeal and psychic health, see Holmes (2013), 172.

[84] Holmes (2010), 322.

[85] Nussbaum (2009: 48–101) traces the motif of philosophers as 'doctors of the soul' back to Aristotle. As Tieleman (2003: 142–57) shows, Chrysippus drew an analogy between medicine and philosophy, because he held that the body and soul are interrelated entities – both are composed of the four elements. Therefore, Galen may also be attacking Chrysippus' recommendation that philosophers should be involved in treating the body to cure the soul. For Chrysippus' interest in regimen, see Tieleman (2003), 162–6.

[86] For the complete list of questions, see *PHP* 9.7.9: De Lacy (2005), p. 588 ll. 7–15.

understanding, and that of medicine as a whole, because they are not empirically verifiable.[87] This section of *PHP* 9 seems to invoke the standard division of philosophy into practical and theoretical parts to create an antithesis – familiar to readers of the later *Prop.Plac.* – between practical and theoretical knowledge, with the former represented by medicine, ethics, and politics. The text, however, goes on to suggest that all of philosophy is intrinsically 'practical', which does not mean 'verifiable' here but what is 'useful' to individuals and communities. Galen refers to an unnamed group (ἔνιοι, 'some people') who believes that philosophy has a 'practical end' (πρακτικὸν . . . τέλος) in the light of its contribution to the management of households and public affairs (πρὸς τὸ καλῶς οἰκεῖν τὸ ἴδιον οἶκον ἢ τῶν τῆς πόλεως πραγμάτων).[88] Their venture into theoretical matters is the result of a logical error – a failure to distinguish between similar queries with different practical values.[89]

Galen reinforces the idea that theory, meaning speculative knowledge, is extraneous to philosophy in his explanation of why Plato made Timaeus the mouthpiece of his dialogue. Because Socrates and his pupils (including Xenophon and Plato) were interested in subjects relating to ethical and political virtues and actions, Galen asserts that Plato, when 'he appended a theory of nature to his philosophy' (τὴν φυσικὴν θεωρίαν τῇ φιλοσοφίᾳ προσθείς), gave the account to Timaeus.[90] Accordingly, physical theory (θεωρία) is something that is added on to Plato's philosophy. Galen cites the cosmological concerns of the *Timaeus* to accentuate the dialogue's difference from Plato's other works and thus distance 'useless' (ἄχρηστα), abstract theories from the body of philosophical knowledge.[91] The functionality of this more circumscribed philosophy supports Galen's linkage of the philosophical discipline to medicine, whose own utility he has stressed in the preceding remarks about the hegemonic organ.

The diverse subjects covered in the *Timaeus*, as well as their interconnectedness, invite Galen to formulate different relations between medicine

[87] See *Ti.* 28b2–33a3 and p. 33 above. [88] *PHP* 9.7.9–10: De Lacy (2005), p. 588 ll. 15–19.

[89] *PHP* 9.7.11–14: De Lacy (2005), p. 588 ll. 18–25. As examples of these queries, Galen remarks that it is 'better' (βέλτιον) to investigate whether there is something more powerful and wiser than humans in the cosmos, whereas it is 'unnecessary' (οὐ . . . ἀναγκαῖον) to ask whether these entities (i.e. the gods) have a body. This discussion is part of a larger argument regarding the importance of logical training (see 9.1.2–3: De Lacy 2005: p. 540 ll. 7–13).

[90] *PHP* 9.7.14–16: De Lacy (2005), p. 588 ll. 25–32. Galen also refers to the *Parmenides*, where Zeno and Parmenides mount several challenges to Socrates'/Plato's theory of Forms.

[91] Forms and derivatives of χρήσιμος ('useful') and ἄχρηστος ('useless') appear seven times in *PHP* 9.7.9–18 (De Lacy 2005: p. 588 l. 7–p. 590 l. 2).

and the areas of knowledge that they represent. While Galen appeals to these epistemological relations to reconfigure medicine's boundaries, the relations themselves are not static. *PHP* 9 may situate theory (θεωρία) outside medicine, but my analysis of the discussion of vegetative sensation in *Plat. Tim.* will illustrate how the dialogue's homology between plant and human appears to permit Galen to redefine as 'medical' (ἰατρικῶς) a theoretical issue which, if not 'useless', at best 'acts as an adornment' (ἐπεκόσμησε) to the discipline.[92] I would like to close this section by looking at how these relations are variable not only across Galen's corpus but also within *PHP* itself.

Composed of an assortment of topics stemming from the *Timaeus*, book eight of *PHP* first investigates the nature and number of the elements.[93] In addition to citing the Hippocratic *On the Nature of the Human*, Galen quotes *Ti.* 82a1–7, which attributes disease to an unnatural excess or deficiency of the body's elemental components (fire, air, water, and earth), to justify his own interest, as a doctor, in these questions.[94] He interprets the causal relation in this Platonic passage to imply an epistemological connection between 'physical theory' – which, after Aristotle, normally involved discussion of the elements – and medicine. Following this attempt to construct a link between the two fields of knowledge, Galen attenuates it by asserting the exteriority of fundamental information about the elements to medicine. He writes:

> ὁ δὲ Πλάτων ὡς ἂν τὴν θεωρητικὴν φιλοσοφίαν ἡγούμενος εἶναι τιμιωτάτην οὐκ ἠρκέσθη μόναις ταῖς φαινομέναις ἐν τοῖς στοιχείοις δυνάμεσιν ἀλλὰ καὶ τὴν αἰτίαν ἐπιζητεῖ τῆς γενέσεως αὐτῶν, ἄχρηστον ἰατρῷ σκέμμα.[95]
>
> Plato, however, as one who would view theoretical philosophy as the most valuable, was not satisfied simply with the observed powers in the elements but also sought the cause of their generation, an inquiry useless to the physician.[96]

Unlike in *PHP* 9, Plato is not the exponent of a practical kind of knowledge that is supplemented by a theory of nature, but the reverse.[97] The quotation limits doctors to the observable (φαινομέναις), the actions of the

[92] See *Prop.Plac.* 14.5; LG, p. 134 l. 11.
[93] In addition to the dialogue's account of the elements (53c4–57d6), *PHP* 8 engages with the text's aetiology of bodily disease (81e6–86a8), explanation of respiration (79a5–c7), and claim that drink goes into the lungs (70d7–e2).
[94] See *PHP* 8.2.14–17: De Lacy (2005), p. 492 l. 30–p. 494 l. 10.
[95] *PHP* 8.3.2–3: De Lacy (2005), p. 494 ll. 30–3.
[96] De Lacy (2005), 495.
[97] Cf. Hippocrates as the exponent of a 'practical *technē*' at *PHP* 8.3.2: De Lacy (2005), p. 494 ll. 29–30.

elements on the body. Notwithstanding this restriction, Galen provides a detailed summary of the *Timaeus*' explanation of the elements' powers, which connects the way in which they interact with one another to their geometrical shape (53c–57b).[98]

A subsequent criticism of Plato indicates that Galen may have a polemical motive for wishing to distance medicine from physical theory in the above passage. While transitioning to a discussion of the humours, Galen highlights Plato's erroneous conceptualization of health at *Ti.* 82a3–4, where it is defined as elemental instead of humoural balance.[99] Furthermore, Galen attributes Plato's failure to consider the impact of age on humoural balance to his lack of medical experience.[100] Citing these missteps, Galen weakens Plato's – and perhaps all theoretical philosophers' – epistemic authority over the body. The epistemological gap that Galen creates between medicine and physical theory helps him to challenge the assumption that philosophers' understanding of the macrocosm encompasses the human body. The narrower boundary that he places between medicine and philosophy appears to work as a defence strategy to safeguard doctors' control of the body.

Expansion from Reduction: Medicine in *QAM*

Because Galen performs his boundary work in moments of tension, where occasionally differing rhetorical goals are at stake, his corpus seems to contain multiple possibilities for what medicine can be. *QAM*, a transgressive text in terms of its openness to exploring subjects beyond medicine's boundaries (at least according to certain passages from *PHP* and *Prop.Plac.*, for instance), offers a more expansive figuration of the discipline than the iterations examined above. The way in which modern scholars such as Donini write about the tract's two interrelated claims suggests that Galen is breaching his own epistemological norms by dealing with the problem of the corporeality of the soul:

> Galen goes so far as to affirm that the soul and its parts actually *are* the temperaments of organs in which they reside; and on the basis of this he derives a further thesis, apparently completely novel, namely that one

98 *PHP* 8.3.5–13: De Lacy (2005), p. 496 l. 4–p. 498 l. 8.

99 *PHP* 8.4.24–30: De Lacy (2005), p. 505 ll. 3–19.

100 *PHP* 8.6.33–4: De Lacy (2005), p. 518 ll. 28–30: 'But perhaps he was unable to give a precise account of these matters, as they require experience and he did not occupy himself with the works of medicine' (ἀλλ' ἴσως οὐκ ἠδύνατο περὶ τῶν τοιούτων ἀκριβῶς διελθεῖν ἐμπειρίας δεομένων, αὐτὸς οὐκ ὢν τρίβων τῶν ἔργων τῆς ἰατρικῆς).

should look to doctors rather than philosophers to see to the education or re-education of men with a view to leading them towards virtue.[101]

On this interpretation of *QAM*, Galen espouses a reductive materialism that denies the ontological independence of all parts of the soul, both rational and irrational (irascible and desiderative). In support of his position, Galen makes reference to the debilitating effects of melancholy and lethargy, diseases generated from humoural build-up, on mental activities (for example, memory and understanding) to dispute the rational soul's separateness from the body – the real point of contention in the text.[102] For Donini, this flattening of the physical and psychic legitimizes doctors' intervention in moral life, for they are able to alter temperament and thus restore the innate operations of the soul, which assist in the acquisition of virtue.[103]

Subtler readings of *QAM* allege that Galen does not ascribe demonstrative status to any of the treatise's conclusions or that he only endorses the irrational soul's corporeality and mortality.[104] The characterization of *QAM* as an epistemological outlier has been questioned as well, with links being drawn to *Hipp.Elem.*, *Sem.*, and *UP*, in which the text's titular thesis – that the capacities of the soul follow the mixtures of the body – is supposedly prefigured.[105] Irrespective of these ongoing debates about the strength of *QAM*'s argument and its relationship to other Galenic works, there seems to be consensus that its aim is to elevate the medical profession above all others, especially philosophy.[106] While *QAM* specifically targets a group of 'self-styled Platonists' (τινας τῶν Πλατωνικοὺς μὲν ἑαυτοὺς ὀνομαζόντων, 4.805K), who think that the soul is neither helped nor harmed by the body, it acknowledges that its *logos* may appear to be 'destructive to the good things [coming] out of philosophy' (ἀναιρετικὸς ὅδ' ὁ λόγος ἐστὶ τῶν ἐκ φιλοσοφίας καλῶν, 4.814K).[107] Galen makes this comment after famously declaring that people should come to him to learn what to eat and drink to modulate their character traits.[108] Even if Galen

[101] Donini (2008), 196.

[102] See *QAM* 4.776–7K; Singer (2013a), 382. At *QAM* 772–4K (Singer 2013a: 378–81), Galen very summarily dispenses with the idea that the desiderative and irascible parts of the soul are immortal.

[103] See *QAM* 4.787–9K. Cf. Ballester (1988), 131: 'Galen does not see how to extend, as a physiologist, the competence of his scientific knowledge, which is only justified at the level of the somatic elements, to the terrain of the asomatic. What he does [in *QAM*] is extend in some way the field of the *physis* to spiritual and moral realities.'

[104] See Singer (2013b), 343; Havrda (2017), 85–6.

[105] See Havrda (2017), 70–7.

[106] See, e.g., Ballester (1988), 129; Gill (2010), 166; Singer (2013b), 344.

[107] On *QAM*'s quarrel with contemporary Platonists, see Jouanna (2009), 199.

[108] *QAM* 4.807–8K: 'So, then, let those who are unhappy with the notion that nourishment has the power to make some self-controlled, some more undisciplined, some more restrained, some more unrestrained, as well as brave, timid, gentle, kind, quarrelsome and argumentative – let them now

does not say that doctors can produce virtue in their patients, *QAM* wrests territory from philosophy in giving medical practitioners the power to dispose individuals to a certain way of life by shaping their character through dietary regimen. The text puts doctors at the foundation of ethics with its suggestion that medicine can make people more receptive to virtue training; in so doing, it decentres ethical philosophers from their sphere of expertise. For what Galen strikes an apologetic tone is his 'destruction' of philosophy's self-sufficiency in regulating conduct, one of its probable 'goods'.

In this section I direct attention to Galen's selective reading of *Ti.* 86a–90d, the dialogue's account of psychic illness, in *QAM*. Plato is one of several ancient authorities – including Hippocrates, Aristotle, and Chrysippus – whom Galen cites to substantiate *QAM*'s rooting of moral and mental failings in bodily defectiveness, but the *Timaeus*, in particular, is crucial for his notion that doctors have a role in ethical training.[109] Nonetheless, as will be shown, the dialogue's supposed approval of doctors' participation in the treatment of psychic maladies emerges from an interpretation that shifts focus away from Plato's own minimization of medicine's contribution to moral life. Galen quotes from *Ti.* 86a–90d in blocks (86e5–87a8, 86c4–d6, 86d6–e4, 87b3–6, 87b3–9), which advance two main arguments: (1) all diseases of the soul are the result of bodily causes; thus, (2) people should not be blamed for their moral and intellectual shortcomings.[110] Although I do not wish to wade into the contentious issue of how the *Timaeus* envisions the body–soul relationship, I find Gill's explanation, which commits Plato to neither psychological materialism nor strict dualism, helpful for understanding why a breakdown in one affects the other: the body and soul constitute a proportionate structure, so a defect in one part disrupts the whole.[111] Proportion, or health, is restored when the movements of the body and soul are harmonized.

At *QAM* 4.813K Galen identifies in the *Timaeus* three areas – 'nurture' (τροφή), 'practices' (ἐπιτηδεύματα), and 'studies' (μαθήματα) – where an

have some self-control, and come to me to learn what they should eat and drink' (Singer 2013a: 401–2, νῦν γοῦν οἱ δυσχεραίνοντες τροφῇ <ὅτι> δύναται τοὺς μὲν σωφρονεστέρους, τοὺς δ' ἀκολαστοτέρους ἐργάζεσθαι καὶ τοὺς μὲν ἐγκρατεστέρους, τοὺς δ' ἀκρατεστέρους καὶ θαρσαλέους καὶ δειλοὺς ἡμέρους τε καὶ πρᾴους ἐριστικούς τε καὶ φιλονείκους, ἡκέτωσαν πρός με μαθησόμενοι, τίνα μὲν ἐσθίειν αὐτοὺς χρή, τίνα δὲ πίνειν).

109 Besides the *Timaeus*, Galen also refers to *Laws* (see 4.806–12K). On Galen's appeal to authority in *QAM*, see Lloyd (1988).

110 See *QAM* 4.789–91, 812–13K; Singer (2013), 391–2, 403–4. As I mentioned above (p. 35n24), I follow Gill's (2000: 59–60) 'strong' reading of *Ti.* 86a–90d that attributes all (rather than a group of) psychic diseases to bodily disruption.

111 See Gill (2010), 70–3. For a modern reading that finds materialist lines of thought in the *Timaeus*, see Carone (2005).

intervention can be made to remedy vice.[112] Although the passage does gloss the latter terms (with the first meaning gymnastics and music and the second geometry and mathematics), it concentrates on the sense of 'nurture'. Galen refers to the word, which he takes to denote 'food, gruels, and drink', as evidence that Plato recognized a need for doctors, as prescribers of regimen, in the disciplining of character.[113] He also lists wine and drugs as something additional to daily regimen that can hinder the growth of vice by bringing the body into 'good mixture' (εὐχυμία) and therefore balancing the motions of the soul.[114] The *Timaeus*, however, strongly advises against the use of drugs, or anything that is external to the body, to stabilize psychic and bodily movements, for it insists that 'no person in their right mind' (οὐδαμῶς τῷ νοῦν ἔχοντι) should tolerate 'medical purging by means of drugs' (τὸ τῆς φαρμακευτικῆς καθάρσεως γιγνόμενον ἰατρικόν), except in the 'occasional instance of dire need' (σφόδρα ποτὲ ἀναγκαζομένῳ).[115] Unlike *QAM*, which does not impose a hierarchy on its three approaches to restoring equilibrium, the dialogue gives priority to study and exercise inasmuch as they are movements induced within and by oneself (ἐν ἑαυτῷ ὑφ' αὑτοῦ, 89a1–2).[116]

Plato's inferior ranking of drugs as both a bodily and psychic therapy serves to undermine doctors' claim to be the best producers of health. The dialogue's promotion of gymnastics, mathematics, and intellectual enquiry in general (τινα ἄλλην σφόδρα μελέτην διανοίᾳ κατεργαζόμενον, *Ti.* 88c1–2) – all subjects that, in Plato's view, are propaedeutic to philosophy – seems to grant the title to philosophers.[117] In foregrounding drugs as a medical treatment, the *Timaeus* may be capitalizing on current anxieties about their harsh effects to convince the reader to entrust their health to philosophers instead of doctors.[118] Perhaps, for a similar purpose, the dialogue also brings up medicine's diagnostic imprecision, for which

112 See Singer (2013a), 404. Cf. *Ti.* 87b6–9.

113 On this reading of *trophē*, see Lloyd (1988), 20–3.

114 *QAM* 4.821–22K; Singer (2013a), 408–9, whose emendation of εὐθυμία ['cheerfulness'] to εὐχυμία I follow. As Singer (2013a: 408n167) observes, this passage maintains that the body and soul can have a mutually beneficial effect on one another – a reciprocal relation which receives more detailed attention in *San. Tu.* (6.40–2K).

115 *Ti.* 89b1–3; Zeyl (2000), 85.

116 *Ti.* 88b2–89a8 also distinguishes between types of passive movements: it ranks the motion generated by swaying vehicles (αἰωρήσεων, 89a7) higher than the purging produced by drugs.

117 For the gymnasium as a philosophical space in antiquity and gymnastics' role in Plato's educational scheme, see, e.g., Reid (2011), 56–68; Wilburn (2013), 83–7. On mathematics' importance in Plato, see White (2006).

118 Without access to anaesthetics, let alone reliable analgesics, medical treatment throughout Graeco-Roman antiquity often caused considerable pain. See Girard (1990) and Harris (2018), 65–6, who discuss the toxicity and violent effects of Hippocratic pharmaceutical remedies such as hellebore.

near-contemporary medical writings, such as the Hippocratic *Ancient Medicine*, had to apologize in their responses to attacks on the profession's credibility.[119] After introducing its conceptualization of disease as disproportion between body and soul, the *Timaeus* declares that doctors are liable to misinterpret symptoms indicative of an over-powerful soul:

> ὡς ὅταν τε ἐν αὐτῷ ψυχὴ κρείττων οὖσα σώματος περιθύμως ἴσχῃ, διασείουσα πᾶν αὐτὸ ἔνδοθεν νόσων ἐμπίμπλησι, καὶ ὅταν εἴς τινας μαθήσεις καὶ ζητήσεις συντόνως ἴῃ, κατατήκει, διδαχάς τ' αὖ καὶ μάχας ἐν λόγοις ποιουμένη δημοσίᾳ καὶ ἰδίᾳ δι' ἐρίδων καὶ φιλονικίας γιγνομένων διάπυρον αὐτὸ ποιοῦσα σαλεύει, καὶ ῥεύματα ἐπάγουσα, τῶν λεγομένων ἰατρῶν ἀπατῶσα τοὺς πλείστους, τἀναίτια αἰτιᾶσθαι ποιεῖ (87e6–88a7).

> When within it there is a soul more powerful than the body and this soul gets excited, it churns the whole being and fills it from inside with diseases, and when it concentrates on one or another course of study or inquiry, it wears the body out. And again, when the soul engages in public or private teaching sessions or verbal battles, the disputes and contentions that then occur cause the soul to fire the body up and rock it back and forth, so inducing discharges that trick most so-called doctors into making misguided diagnoses.[120]

Ignorant that the soul's strength is a factor in health, doctors lack the causal know-how to read bodily phenomena. That is, their partial knowledge of health impedes them from reaching the correct conclusions about what is happening inside (ἐν αὐτῷ) their patients from, in this case, very visible and therefore semiotically loaded symptoms – effluvia (ῥεύματα).[121] On the basis of their inability to make the logical leaps required in their practice (from visible to invisible and symptom to cause), the dialogue contests doctors' right to their own professional appellation.

The sole place in his extant corpus where Galen comes close to addressing Plato's negative appraisal of doctors' diagnostic competence is his commentary on *Ti.* 88a1–7 in book four of *Plat. Tim.*, which is fragmentary in Arabic. In an extract quoted in Maimonides' *Medical Aphorisms* (24.58), Galen reports that, of cases of body–soul mismatch, he personally has seen only a few people whose souls were more powerful than their bodies, one of whom was the celebrated orator Aelius Aristides (second century CE).[122] While the full exegesis of the passage may have responded more directly to

[119] See the Introduction (p. 6) above. [120] Zeyl (2000), 83.
[121] On the semiotic weight of effluvia and other phenomena in Hippocratic medicine, in primarily a prognostic context, see Holmes (2010), 154–9.
[122] See Bos (2017), p. 101 [English], p. 102 ll. 7–12 [Arabic]. On Maimonides' engagement with *Plat. Tim.*, see p. 174 below.

Plato's rebuke, Galen's surviving comments try to absolve him of the philosopher's criticism rather than push back against it: Galen's own recognition of the disproportion between Aristides' soul and body shows that he is not one of the 'so-called doctors' (τῶν λεγομένων ἰατρῶν), whom Plato censures. In contrast, cherry-picking text from around *Ti.* 88a1–7, *QAM* appears to omit this portion of the dialogue as it marginalizes doctors in the very realm in which the tract wishes to establish their centrality: human health, encompassing both the body and soul.

Neither the *Timaeus* nor *QAM* aim to expel their disciplinary rival from participating in the preservation of bodily and psychic health; instead, their disputes, as I have argued, are about carving out a larger as well as more primary role for their disciplines in the process.[123] Whereas the former displaces medicine from the nexus of human health because of its lesser diagnostic and therapeutic abilities, the latter situates it there by making the effectiveness of philosophical therapy – ethical training – seemingly contingent on temperament. Galen redirects the *Timaeus*' tactic to increase philosophy's reach, through its mutual implication of the body and soul in health, to extend medicine into the ethical. As with the other episodes of boundary work studied above, Galen's expansion of medicine ensues from a weakening of philosophy's autonomy, which allows the discipline to occupy spaces of knowledge otherwise closed off to it.

Thinking with and beyond the Body: Vegetative Sensation in *Plat.Tim.*

The human body has been the site so far where Galen's contest with philosophy, and resultant constitutive refiguring of medicine, has unfolded. What is at issue in this rivalry is epistemic authority over the body as an object to be understood and treated. I have shown that the *Timaeus* gives Galen the opportunity to raise the stakes even further. By drawing on the dialogue's theorization of the reciprocal relationship

[123] Cf. *Aff.Dig.* and *San.Tu.*, which seem to advocate for the traditional distribution of care that allocates the soul to philosophers and the body to doctors. While *Aff.Dig.* appears to ignore medicine's contribution to psychic health, it does acknowledge that sleep (de Boer 1937: p. 53 l. 4) and 'natural intelligence' (φύσει συνετός, de Boer 1937: p. 45 l. 11), both of which seem to have a qualitative basis in Galen (see *Caus.Symp.* 7.141–3K and *UP* 8.13; Helmreich 1907: p. 488 l. 24–p. 489 l. 2), affect a person's capacity to receive ethical training. *San.Tu.* (Koch 1923: p. 19 ll. 24–30) lists food, drink, exercise, music, and sights as having the potential to destroy the *ēthos* of the soul, but then goes on to say that doctors should only be concerned with shaping character in so far as moral deviancy has an impact on bodily health. These passages dovetail with Singer's (2017: 173–6; 2018: 392–3) conclusion that the division of care in these texts is not neat.

between body and soul, he can broaden medicine's claim to epistemic authority to include psychic matters.[124] This penultimate section looks at how Galen enters into a very different site of controversy, which takes him beyond the confines of the human body: the debate about the sensitive ability of plants. As with the identity of the hegemonic organ, the nature of vegetative sensation was a subject of ongoing dispute in the philosophical schools, so Galen's engagement with this question in *Plat. Tim.* – not to mention his assertion that medicine provides the conceptual resources to resolve it – is polemically charged. Because the *Timaeus* does not posit a significant disjunct between human and plant bodies, it provides implicit justification for Galen's application of his theory of the natural faculties, which the eponymous *Nat.Fac.* frames as a product of his medical background, to plant life. While Galen focuses on what medicine has to offer to philosophy, my analysis of his appeal to the Stoic notion of 'appropriation' (οἰκείωσις) to make his own idea of the natural faculties intelligible in the context of vegetative sensation exposes the bidirectionality of the exchange.

Before I examine Galen's response to a problem that *Prop.Plac.* characterizes as inessential to medicine, I will first call attention to the passage in the *Timaeus* that was the focal point for this controversy about vegetative sensation.[125] At 76e7–77e5, Timaeus interrupts his narrative of the lesser gods' construction of the human body to talk about plant life, which serves as a preface to his account of digestion and respiration. The reason for this interlude is that it makes sense causally to explain what humans eat before describing the parts of the body and processes that deal with food.[126] The dialogue proposes that plants, as nourishment, are teleologically subordinate to humans, but it also declares that both entities have a kindred nature (τῆς γὰρ ἀνθρωπίνης συγγενῆ φύσεως φύσιν [...] φυτεύουσιν, 77a3–5). Plants and humans are akin because they are not only composed of the same four elements but also possess the 'third kind of soul' (τοῦ τρίτου ψυχῆς εἴδους, 77b3–4), which in the latter sits between the midriff and navel (or the liver in Galen).[127] Through their share in the appetitive soul, Plato seems to establish a homology between plants and humans; accordingly, study of the former provides insight into the latter, and vice versa. In particular, Plato and subsequent philosophers viewed plants as a means to investigate the minimum condition for animation – that is, what makes

[124] The dialogue also suggests several times (e.g. at 36d8–e3, 69b8–70a2) that the body provides a place for the soul to exist.

[125] See p. 35 above. [126] Cornford (1937), 302.

[127] See De Lacy (1988), 46, for Galen's location of the third part of the soul in the liver.

humans alive – as these creatures are the simplest form of life.[128] As I will discuss, the *Timaeus*' attribution of a rudimentary type of sensation to plants elicited criticism from Aristotelians and Stoics, who denied that the basic state of animation involves cognition of any sort.[129]

A Greek fragment from book three of *Plat. Tim.* (3.2) contains Galen's most extensive remarks on vegetative sensation; there, he addresses two key claims made at *Ti.* 76e7–77e5 that I will now review before looking at his exegesis.[130] Timaeus begins his interlude on plant life with the argument that plants should be counted as ζῷα because they 'partake in life' (ζῆν, 77b1–2). The term ζῷον can designate either a 'living thing' or more specifically an 'animal'.[131] The force of Timaeus' claim seems to be that, as creatures that 'live' (ζῆν), plants are alive in a similar way to animals, and so must have souls.[132] Therefore, Timaeus is not saying that plants are animals but rather that they are comparable in certain respects. Nonetheless, Aristotle and later thinkers, including Galen, seem to have taken the passage to mean that plants are animals because it ascribes sensation to them – the text's second controversial point.

The dialogue relates that the appetitive (or third kind of) soul in plants has a perceptive capacity, but it is 'totally devoid of opinion, reasoning, and intelligence and instead has a share in sensation, pleasant and painful, with desire' (ᾧ δόξης μὲν λογισμοῦ τε καὶ νοῦ μέτεστιν τὸ μηδέν, αἰσθήσεως δὲ ἡδείας καὶ ἀλγεινῆς μετὰ ἐπιθυμιῶν, 77b5–6). Although Timaeus does not specify the context in which plants feel pleasure and pain, Galen, as will be shown, interprets the statement to refer to the perception of nutriment. Pleasure and pain are 'forward-looking psychological states' that presuppose an ability to store sensory experiences, so plants seem to have an additional cognitive resource at their disposal, memory.[133] With regard to the appetitive soul in humans, Plato writes at *Ti.* 71a3–e2 that the logical soul uses the anticipation of pleasure and the threat of pain to persuade this lower part, which is incapable of grasping rational accounts, to follow its commands. The text implies that the appetitive soul has developed a sense

[128] See Das (2017a), 207.

[129] The Stoics held that plants are intermediate beings – neither inanimate nor fully animate – because they are governed by 'natural breath' (πνεῦμα φυσικόν) or 'nature' (φύσις) rather than soul. See Long and Sedley (1987), vol. I, 284, 319–20.

[130] Schröder (1934), p. 10 l. 4–p. 13 l. 7.

[131] *LSJ*, s.v. ζῷον, I.

[132] For the difficulties in translating ζῷον in this passage, see Carpenter (2010), 283. See Repici (2000), 61–5, who surveys classical Greek thinkers' views on plants as ζῷα.

[133] Lorenz (2012), 243, 248–51. *Ti.* 64b3–6 suggests that sensation involves intelligence (τὸ φρόνιμον) as well. Carpenter (2010) argues that, while plants do not possess individual intellects, they perceive by virtue of the intelligence of the World Soul.

for what tends to happen in pleasant and painful circumstances based on past incidents. The *Philebus* (35a–d), which treats pleasure in more detail, maintains that the logical soul does not endow the appetitive soul with the capacity for sensory memory, as animals, which are bereft of reason, exercise this power too.[134]

Similar to Plato, Aristotle links appetite (ὄρεξις) with sensation – as well as imagination and movement – but he denies that plants experience it.[135] At *DA* 415b23 he puts forward that plants are governed by the 'nutritive soul' (θρεπτικὴ ψυχή), which is responsible for biological processes. Galen's commentary on *Ti.* 76e7–77e5 is mainly a critical response to Aristotle's divorcing of the nutritive and sensitive faculties in plants.[136] It is not clear with which Aristotelian texts Galen is engaging when he sets out to prove in *Plat. Tim.* that plants are ζῷα on the basis of their capacity for sensation and movement, which, according to Aristotle, makes a creature an animal instead of just a living thing. In addition to his criticisms in *DA*, Aristotle appears to have attacked Plato's conception of vegetative life in his lost *On Plants* (Περὶ Φυτῶν), which Nicolaus of Damascus (b. *c.* 64 BCE) partially summarized in his identically entitled treatise.[137] Probably following Aristotle's earlier work, Nicolaus takes issue with the suggestion, which he ascribes to Plato, Anaxagoras, and Empedocles, that plants are 'animals' (*ḥayawānāt*) because they perceive sensations such as pain and pleasure.[138] Rashed draws attention to chapters 15–18 of *Avoiding Distress* to demonstrate that Galen owned a copy of Aristotle's *On Plants*, which was a rare text by the second century CE, before a large portion of his library was destroyed by the fire at Rome's Temple of Peace in 192.[139] As *Plat. Tim.* seems to pre-date the fire of 192, it is tempting to see *On Plants* as the specific target of Galen's criticism.

In his commentary, Galen offers a three-pronged defence of 'Plato's' classification of plants as 'animals' (ζῷα) by proving that they meet Aristotle's criteria for this category: they possess (1) the capacity for movement, (2) a soul, and (3) sensation. He argues:

[134] Lorenz (2012), 251. [135] See *DA* 414b1–3, 432b8–33b32. [136] See *DA* 415a2–3.

[137] Nicolaus' text survives in an Arabic translation, which is based on an earlier Syriac version, produced by Isḥāq ibn Ḥunayn and Ṯābit ibn Qurra; it was subsequently rendered into Hebrew, Latin, and Greek. On this work and its relationship to Aristotle's lost treatise, see Drossaart Lulofs (1957); Drossaart Lulofs and Poortman (1989).

[138] Drossaart Lulofs and Poortman (1989), p. 127 ll. 12–14, p. 129 ll. 1–2. The Arabic *ḥayawān* (sing.) is synonymous with the Greek ζῷον, for it can mean both a 'living thing' and an 'animal'. See *WGAÜ, Supplement*, s.v. ζῷον.

[139] Rashed (2011), 62–8. As Nutton (2009) and Nicholls (2011: 125–30) note, Galen lost not only manuscripts of his own and other authors' works but also drugs, gold, household items, and loan documents in the fire.

> ἃ δὴ <καὶ> πρόσθεν ἐδείκνυμεν εὐλόγως ὑπ' αὐτοῦ ζῷα κεκλῆσθαι. προϋποκειμένου γὰρ τοῦ τὴν ψυχὴν ἀρχὴν εἶναι κινήσεως, ὁμολογουμένου δὲ καὶ τοῦ τὰ φυτὰ τὴν ἀρχὴν κινήσεως ἔχειν ἐν ἑαυτοῖς, ἔμψυχα προσηκόντως ὀνομασθήσεται· τὸ δὲ ἔμψυχον σῶμα πάντες ἄνθρωποι καλοῦσι ζῷον. εἰ δὲ καὶ Ἀριστοτέλης βούλοιτο μὴ μόνον τῷ ἔμψυχον εἶναι τὸ σῶμα ζῷον ὀνομάζεσθαι προσηκόντως, ἀλλὰ χρῆναι προστίθεσθαι τούτῳ <τὸ> αἰσθητικόν, οὐδὲ τούτου στερεῖται τὰ φυτά. δέδεικται γὰρ ἡμῖν ἐν τοῖς τῶν φυσικῶν δυνάμεων ὑπομνήμασι γνωριστικὴν δύναμιν ἔχειν αὐτὰ τῶν τ' οἰκείων οὐσιῶν, ὑφ' ὧν τρέφεται, τῶν τ' ἀλλοτρίων, ὑφ' ὧν βλάπτεται, καὶ διὰ τοῦτο τὰς μὲν οἰκείας ἕλκειν, τὰς δ' ἀλλοτρίας ἀποστρέφεσθαι καὶ ἀπωθεῖσθαι, καὶ διὰ τοῦτ' οὖν ὁ Πλάτων εἶπεν αἰσθήσεως γένους ἰδίου μετέχειν τὰ φυτά· τὸ γὰρ οἰκεῖόν τε καὶ ἀλλότριον γνωρίζει.[140]

> Earlier, we demonstrated that he called [plants] animals with good reason. Because it is assumed that the soul is the principle of movement, and because it is agreed that plants have in themselves a principle of movement, they are rightly called ensouled. Everyone calls an ensouled body an animal. But even if Aristotle should wish that a body rightly be called an 'animal' not only because it is ensouled, but also perception must be added to it, plants are not deprived of this either. It was shown by us in [our] writings on the natural faculties that they possess a faculty of discriminating the substances appropriate to them, by which they are nourished, and [the substances] foreign to them, by which they are harmed. They attract those things that are appropriate but turn away and reject those that are foreign. For this reason, Plato said that plants take part in their own kind of perception, for they discriminate between what is appropriate and foreign.

Galen first attempts to establish that plants are ensouled, although Aristotle does not debate this point but rather disagrees with Plato about the powers available to their form of soul. He utilizes Plato's famous premise 'the soul is the principle (ἀρχή) of movement', which appears at *Phaedrus* 245c5–246a2 and *Laws* 896e8–897a4, to demonstrate that plants, whose ability to move is indisputable, have a soul. In the subsequent section of his exegesis, owing to his misinterpretation of *Ti.* 77b7–c3, Galen has to address Plato's apparent denial of movement to plants.[141] He understands the dialogue's description of plants' inability to 'revolve within and about itself, repelling movement without and exercising its own inherent movement' (στραφέντι δ' αὐτῷ ἐν ἑαυτῷ περὶ ἑαυτό, τὴν μὲν ἔξωθεν ἀπωσαμένῳ κίνησιν, τῇ δ' οἰκείᾳ χρησαμένῳ) to refer to physical motion rather than psychic rotations

[140] Schröder (1934), p. 11 ll. 8–20.
[141] See Schröder (1934), p. 12 l. 27–p. 13 l. 2.

(περίοδοι), which give rise to reason and opinion.[142] To save the validity of his argument that plants are ensouled because they move, Galen proposes that the *Timaeus* only denies locomotion (μεταβατική) to them rather than other kinds of movement such as upward and downward growth.[143]

The latter half of the above quotation tackles the thornier question of the nature of vegetative sensation. Galen does not seem to observe Aristotle's distinction between the sensitive and nutritive faculties, for he contends that plants' 'kind of sensation' (αἰσθήσεως γένους) involves the discrimination (γνωριστικὴν δύναμιν; γνωρίζει) between 'appropriate' (οἰκεῖον) and 'foreign' (ἀλλότριον) nutriment. He appeals to his doctrine of the natural faculties to articulate how this sensitive ability is manifest in plants' attraction (ἕλκειν) of beneficial and rejection (ἀποστρέφεσθαι καὶ ἀπωθεῖσθαι) of harmful food. The discussion in *Nat.Fac.* of how attraction and expulsion contribute to nutrition and govern other processes, along with the retentive and alterative powers, is mainly developed with reference to the human (and animal) body. While *Nat.Fac.* may have the totalizing ambition to extend its theory's relevance to the macrocosmic by illustrating how its titular powers operate at a basic level both in and outside the body, it presents this explanatory model as issuing from Galen's medical knowledge.

Besides stressing the utmost utility of the tract's information to medicine (τῶν χρησιμωτάτων εἰς τὴν τέχνην), Galen has recourse to his own clinical experience to demonstrate the existence of the natural faculties and their activities in the body.[144] For example, in his description of the eliminative faculty he makes use of the case of a stillbirth to argue that this power accounts for the opening of the mouth of the uterus, which remains closed during pregnancy, and the movement of the epigastric muscles, which work to expel the dead foetus.[145] As in *PHP*, Galen integrates vignettes from his practice into theoretical expositions to impress on the reader the conceptual resources that medicine gives him: through his treatment of the body he gains insight, unavailable to the disciplinary outsider, that helps him to refine previous schemata or develop his own for

[142] Plato discusses the circular movement of reason and opinion in his account of the creation of the World Soul (*Ti.* 37a–b). On the grammatical reasons behind Galen's misreading of this passage, see Ferrari (1998), 27; Wilberding (2014), 252–6.

[143] Galen achieves this reading by emending Plato's text; on this emendation, see Skemp (1947), 57.

[144] *Nat.Fac.* 2.8. Cf. *Nat.Fac.* 1.2, where Galen characterizes the production of blood from digested bread as an 'example from the subject matter of medicine' (τῆς ἰατρικῆς ὕλης . . . τὸ παράδειγμα) that offers evidence of the alterative faculty.

[145] *Nat.Fac.* 3.3. While Galen is present at the stillbirth, a midwife is primarily assisting the patient. During the course of the delivery, she confers with Galen, who does not appear to be in the same room, about the patient's progress. For another reference to Galen's clinical practice, see *Nat.Fac.* 2.8.

understanding it and the world in which it is embedded. Notwithstanding *Nat.Fac.*'s focus on the body, Galen is not concerned with apologizing for his extension of his theory of the natural faculties to the broader cosmos, because the derivation of these powers from the primary, universal qualities moistness, dryness, coldness, and warmth seems to justify the leap.[146] Nonetheless, the homology that the *Timaeus* establishes between plant and human through their participation in the appetitive soul, which is in charge of the body's nourishment (70d7–e7), offers additional legitimization for Galen's application of his theory of human nutrition to plants in *Plat. Tim.*

Wilberding cites Galen's attribution of the power of attraction to inanimate bodies, such as wheat and magnets, as evidence that *Plat. Tim.* seeks to downplay Plato's association of plants with a degree of perceptual awareness.[147] *Nat.Fac.* suggests that an entity does not require a soul and thus sensation to be able to attract what is appropriate (οἰκεῖον) to them. Wilberding compares Galen's position on vegetative sensation to that of Porphyry (*c.* 234–305/10 CE), who hypothesizes that the bodies of plants are driven by certain physical processes towards a natural state.[148] On this view, these creatures' 'pleasure' consists in the benefit that they derive from their assimilation of the nutriment taken from the soil.[149] Galen is certainly at pains in his commentary to distinguish how humans and plants perceive, because the latter lack the sensory equipment – a nervous system – to feel pleasure and pain in the same way as the former.[150] Nonetheless, *pace* Wilberding, stripping plants of any sensory power seems to ignore Galen's emphasis in his commentary on plants' ability to discriminate, or to make choices. Moreover, critical of atomism's reduction of life to chance and necessity, *Nat.Fac.* does not espouse a deterministic understanding of nature; intentionality, in various forms, is behind natural processes.[151]

With their root γνω- having the basic meaning 'to know', the terms γνωριστικήν and γνωρίζει at *Plat. Tim.* 3.2 appear to indicate that plants have an innate knowledge of what is beneficial and harmful to them. In *Nat.Fac.* Galen only uses the verb γνωρίζει (and its derivatives) to describe deliberation in humans.[152] While the absence of a brain (or mind) in plants makes it impossible for them to make decisions as humans do, the γνω-words signal that something more complex underlies the power of attraction in them than in inanimate bodies. As Holmes argues, *Nat.Fac.*

146 See *Nat.Fac.* 1.6.
147 Wilberding (2014), 257–8. See also *Nat.Fac.* 1.14, 3.15.
148 *To Gaurus on How Embryos Are Ensouled* 4; Wilberding (2011), 35–6. See also Wilberding (2014), 265.
149 Wilberding (2014), 266.
150 Wilberding (2014), 262.
151 See Holmes (2014, 2015).
152 *Nat.Fac.* 2.2, 2.4, 2.6, and 2.8.

accounts for the purposefulness of attraction in inanimate and non-conscious bodies by appealing to the Stoic conception of sympathy, which is a kind of immanent intelligence in nature, whereas animals exercise their own judgement.[153] *Nat.Fac.* categorizes plants as non-conscious life, but *Plat.Tim.* stresses their animality – so sympathy, at least in this text, does not seem to account fully for their ability to differentiate between types of nutriment.[154] I will now show that another Stoic idea, οἰκείωσις, may have provided the conceptual framework for Galen's theory of how plants, animals without the cognitive resources of higher animals, can exhibit knowingness. As with his use of sympathy in *Nat.Fac.*, Galen does not acknowledge his engagement with the notion of οἰκείωσις in *Plat.Tim.* Even so, other works such as *PHP* offer evidence of his familiarity with the idea.

The Stoics developed the concept of οἰκείωσις, which is often translated as 'appropriation' or 'familiarization', to explain the innate impulse in irrational creatures – animals (ζῷα) and children – towards self-preservation.[155] An oft-cited passage in Diogenes Laërtius (*fl.* third century CE) outlines how οἰκείωσις informs an appreciation in animals of the difference between harmful and beneficial endeavours:

> Τὴν δὲ πρώτην ὁρμήν φασι τὸ ζῷον ἴσχειν ἐπὶ τὸ τηρεῖν ἑαυτό, οἰκειούσης αὐτῷ τῆς φύσεως ἀπ' ἀρχῆς· καθά φησιν ὁ Χρύσιππος ἐν τῷ πρώτῳ περὶ Τελῶν, πρῶτον οἰκεῖον λέγων εἶναι παντὶ ζῴῳ τὴν αὑτοῦ σύστασιν καὶ τὴν ταύτης συνείδησιν. οὔτε γὰρ ἀλλοτριῶσαι εἰκὸς ἦν αὐτῷ τὸ ζῷον, οὔτε ποιήσασαν αὐτὸ μήτε ἀλλοτριῶσαι μήτε [οὐκ] οἰκειῶσαι. ἀπολείπεται τοίνυν λέγειν, συστησαμένην αὐτὸ οἰκειῶσαι πρὸς ἑαυτό. οὕτω γὰρ τά τε βλάπτοντα διωθεῖται καὶ τὰ οἰκεῖα προσίεται.[156]

> [The Stoics] say that an animal has self-preservation as the object of its first impulse, because nature from the beginning appropriates it, as Chrysippus says in the first book of *On Ends*. The first thing appropriate to every animal is its own constitution and the consciousness of this. For nature was not likely either to alienate the animal itself, or to make it and then neither alienate it nor appropriate it. So, it remains to say that in constituting the animal, nature appropriated it [the

[153] Holmes (2014: 239) relates that the notion of sympathy did not originate with the Stoics; however, their formulation of sympathy as an expression of an organizing intelligence in the cosmos seems to mirror Galen's understanding of it. For a fuller study of the impact of Stoicism on Galen's natural philosophy, see Gill (2010).

[154] See *Nat.Fac.* 1.1.

[155] On this concept in general, see Pembroke (1971); Kerferd (1972); Inwood (1985), 182–201; Engberg-Pedersen (1990); Striker (1996); Gill (2006), 36–42; Martin (2015), 343–7.

[156] Diogenes Laërtius, *Lives of Eminent Philosophers* 7.85=*SVF* 3.178.

animal] to itself. This is why the animal rejects what is harmful and accepts what is appropriate.[157]

While the impulse towards self-preservation involves a series of interconnected motives, the core condition of οἰκείωσις is an implicit understanding in the newborn animal of its own constitution and what preserves it.[158] This awareness is behind the animal's disposition to pursue things that are conducive, or 'appropriate' (τὰ οἰκεῖα), to its health and to reject things that are 'harmful' (τά [. . .] βλάπτοντα). Diogenes, who cites here Galen's Stoic nemesis Chrysippus, calls the animal's understanding of itself συνείδησις, 'self-consciousness' or 'self-awareness'.[159] The term συνείδησις does not describe a Cartesian concept of 'I-centred' self-consciousness, in which only humans participate, but a form of bodily comprehension. In other words, as Martin observes, Stoic self-consciousness is 'not knowledge that I exist but an understanding of what kind of being I am, and specifically what kind of body I have and what benefits it'.[160]

In book five of *PHP* Galen deploys the Stoic doctrine of οἰκείωσις subversively against Chrysippus' theory of a unitary soul in support of Plato's tripartite psychology.[161] He refutes Chrysippus' claim that humans are appropriated (n. οἰκείωσιν) only to what is good (τὸ καλόν) because we possess reason alone by drawing attention to our 'natural appropriation' (οἰκειώσεων φύσει) to pleasure and alienation (ἀλλοτρίωσιν) from pain.[162] To pre-empt the argument that this appropriation to pleasure is due to reason, Galen refers to the impulse (pl. ὁρμάς) towards pleasure in non-rational creatures, namely small children and animals (for example, quails and crocodiles), to prove that it comes from another source, the appetitive soul.[163] As this pattern of behaviour does not disappear when children come of age and become rational, he concludes, contrary to Chrysippus, that reason does not remove the

157 Long and Sedley (1987), vol. I, 346. Cf. Cicero, *On Ends* 3.16.

158 Gill (2006), 38; Martin (2015), 355–60.

159 At *On Ends* 3.16, Cicero uses the phrase *sensum sui* (lit. 'a sense of oneself') to convey συνείδησις.

160 Martin (2015), 360. Cf. Long (1996), 258–60, who identifies Stoic self-consciousness with proprioception, which refers to the awareness that an organism has of the relative position of its body's parts.

161 See *PHP* 5.5.1–8: De Lacy (2005), p. 316 l. 21–p. 318 l. 19. The term οἰκείωσις, which De Lacy translates as a 'feeling of kinship', and related forms (e.g. οἰκειοῦσθαι), appear five times in the passage (on which, see Tieleman 2003: 221). On Chrysippus' and other early Stoics' understanding of οἰκείωσις, see Tieleman (1996), 177–85.

162 Tieleman (2003: 221) writes that this is a 'gross oversimplification' of Chrysippus' position, which states that οἰκείωσις covers all types of appropriate behaviour in non-rational and rational animals.

163 Galen does not address why pleasure is a basic impulse (ὁρμή) as opposed to an epiphenomenon, as Chrysippus maintains in *On Ends* (see *SVF* 3.178).

appetitive part of the soul.[164] This passage of *PHP* does not explain how the appetitive soul familiarizes non-rational animals with what is pleasant to them; for his polemical purposes it is enough to establish that neither reason nor the body (by itself) has anything to do with the impulse towards pleasure.

This connection of οἰκείωσις with the appetitive soul paves the way for Galen's examination of vegetative sensation in *Plat. Tim.* The Stoics only apply the concept of appropriation (οἰκείωσις) to humans and animals because they deny that plants possess a soul.[165] Galen, on the other hand, hews to Plato's categorization of plants as ζῷα in describing how they 'attract those things that are appropriate (τὰς μὲν οἰκείας ἕλκειν), but turn away and reject those that are foreign (τὰς δ' ἀλλοτρίας ἀποστρέφεσθαι καὶ ἀπωθεῖσθαι)'. Even though he does not invoke directly the notion of appropriation (οἰκείωσις), his language strongly resembles Diogenes' summary of Chrysippus' theory. Interpreting *Plat. Tim.* 3.2 in the light of Stoic appropriation (οἰκείωσις), the 'apprehending faculty' (γνωριστικὴν δύναμιν) associated with the appetitive soul that enables plants to pursue what is 'appropriate' seems to correspond to what the Stoics call συνείδησις ('self-awareness') with reference to ensouled animals. In this way, plants, which are without a logical soul and a brain, can have a 'kind of sensation' (αἰσθήσεως γένος).

As I have proposed, the homologous relationship that the *Timaeus* articulates between plants and humans (both are bodies 'akin' in their possession of the same basic soul) seems to sanction Galen's broadening of his expertise to include vegetative life. The impetus for Galen's leap from human to plant is the pursuit of intellectual prestige that the philosophical controversy about vegetative sensation will confer on him and medicine, from whose disciplinary perspective he presents himself as writing when commenting on the *Timaeus*' 'medical' (ἰατρικῶς) statements in *Plat. Tim.* Through this leap, Galen enacts arguably his most radical piece of boundary work, his 'universalization' of medicine. He shows that his explanatory model of the natural faculties, which *Nat.Fac.* depicts as a theoretical outcome of his medical study and experience, applies to all bodies in the cosmos: human, animal, plant, and the inanimate. Despite this claim for the macrocosmic relevance of the natural faculties, Galen's interpretation of vegetative sensation – plants' attraction of beneficial and repulsion of

164 Tieleman (2003), 221.

165 For the view that οἰκείωσις is peculiar to humans and animals, see Seneca, *Epistles* 121 and Hierocles (first half of the second c. CE), *Elements of Ethics* 1.34–5; Ramelli (2009), p. 5 ll. 1–6.

harmful nutriment – assumes another framework for comprehending how these actions constitute perception, Stoic οἰκείωσις. As with *PHP* and *QAM*, the agenda of *Plat. Tim.*, so I have suggested, is to challenge philosophy's monopoly on epistemic authority through attacks on its self-sufficiency that insist on the discipline's need for medicine's conceptual resources. Galen appears to downplay his more synthetic approach to medicine and philosophy because it does not suit the purposes of this text, or passage (3.2), to emphasize their mutual dependence.

The Galenic Plato, a Disciplinary Problem

This chapter has examined how, in Galen's hands, Plato's *Timaeus* becomes a tool for disciplinary boundary work that aims to promote medicine's standing by expanding its territory while encroaching on philosophy's. As I have maintained, Galen's identification of 'medical statements' in the *Timaeus* serves not only to justify his right to comment on the dialogue but also to undermine philosophy's exclusive authority over the text. Similarly, while the characterization of Plato as a *medicus* in the Arabo-Latin prologue to *Com. Tim.* may not originate with Galen, its emphasis on the medical import of the philosopher's thought reflects, nonetheless, his contention that medical learning is an exegetical necessity for comprehending the dialogue. My analysis has found that Galen gives prominence to two themes in the *Timaeus*, its tripartite psychology and cosmic homology, as they seem to license his extension of medicine's boundaries.

The first half of the chapter, which treated *PHP* and *QAM*, revealed that Galen utilizes the dialogue's location of the soul in the brain, heart, and lower abdomen (or liver) to bring psychology and ethics within the doctor's purview. Both works refer to the *Timaeus*' description of a mutually reciprocal relationship between the soul and body to assert that study and care of the former requires medical knowledge and praxis. *PHP* presents anatomical knowledge, acquired from clinical practice and experimentation, as providing the most credible way to resolve psychological controversies such as the dispute regarding the identity of the ruling part of the soul. In questioning the soul's ontological independence, *QAM* links the health of the soul to that of the body, and therefore positions doctors as agents capable of contributing to psychic well-being. The second half of the chapter investigated Galen's efforts in *Plat. Tim.* to push medicine's boundaries beyond the limits of the human body. I demonstrated that he draws on the dialogue's homology, which connects human, animal, and plant life, to argue for the pertinence of his medical theories to the debate about the sensitive ability of plants, in particular, and the macrocosm, more generally.

The human body in the *Timaeus* has indistinct boundaries. The dialogue's tripartite psychology and aforementioned homology obscure the parameters between body and soul and between human body and cosmos. The body's entanglement at the psychic and cosmic levels allows Galen to reformulate medicine to include topics to which philosophers traditionally laid claim. As the following chapters of this book will illustrate, Galen's interpretations of Plato's *Timaeus* posed a disciplinary opportunity or problem for Islamicate thinkers. Ḥunayn ibn Isḥāq and Abū Bakr al-Rāzī, on whom the next two chapters centre, criticize Galen (either implicitly or explicitly) for not taking sufficient account of the broader theoretical ramifications of the Timaean doctrines that he treats. Galen, they assert, did not extend the boundaries of medicine far enough. The final two chapters, on the other hand, focus on Avicenna's and Maimonides' attempts to reinforce the epistemic authority of philosophy by disentangling and restoring the 'proper' boundaries between the soul, body, and cosmos. As part of their recuperative projects, both authors attack Galen's theories that take their departure from the *Timaeus*.

It is worth keeping in mind that demarcating medicine from philosophy was all the more challenging in the medieval Islamicate world because many Arabic writers read their Plato through Galen. I observed in the Introduction that the first four books of Galen's Platonic synopses offered Arabic readers a more comprehensive overview of the *Timaeus*, *Republic*, and *Laws* than other available sources such as the *Theology of Aristotle*.[166] While I have been arguing that Galen's medical reading of the *Timaeus* has the self-serving end of bestowing epistemic authority on himself and his lifework as a doctor, his interpretation had a formative role in shaping medieval Islamicate perceptions of Plato. The 'Plato medicus' of the Arabo-Latin prologue of *Com. Tim.* is one legacy of Galen's reworking of Platonic authority; later conflations of Plato's views with Galen's is another – a point to which I will return in subsequent chapters.

As a coda to this chapter, I want to close with an example from al-Bīrūnī's *The Book Confirming What Pertains to India, Whether Rational or Despicable* that encapsulates how Galen's boundary work with the *Timaeus* provoked a refiguring of disciplinary knowledge and authority. The composition attributes the idea from *Plat. Tim.* 3.2 that plants have 'a faculty

[166] See the Introduction (pp. 22–3).

that distinguishes (*al-quwwa al-mumayyiza*) between what is beneficial to them (*mulāʾim*) and what is harmful (*muḫālif*) to them' to Plato without citing Galen.[167] In associating Plato with a Galenic theory that combines conceptions of nutrition and Stoic self-awareness, al-Bīrūnī's text makes all the more emphatic Galen's own collapsing of the philosophical and medical as seen in Timaean works such as *Plat. Tim.* Its elision of the Galenic and Platonic also shows how, even in the medieval Islamicate world, Galen continued to ventriloquize through Plato a way of approaching the cosmos that enfolds his expertise into it by denying the separateness of medicine and philosophy.

[167] See Sachau (1887), p. 21 ll. 18–19. On the possible impact of Galen on other Arabic discussions of plant life, see Das (2017a).

CHAPTER 2

From the Heavens to the Body: Ḥunayn's Ophthalmology

For many medieval and modern scholars Ḥunayn ibn Isḥāq (d. 260/873 or 264/877) represents the acme of the Graeco-Arabic translation movement.[1] An Arab Christian from al-Ḥīra in south-central Iraq, Ḥunayn was fluent in Arabic and Syriac and knew Greek, possibly first as a liturgical language.[2] His famous *Epistle* (*Risāla*) to the astrologer ʿAlī ibn Yaḥyā (b. 200–1/815–16) relates that he spent a significant portion of his career working on or supervising the translation of more than a hundred Galenic titles into either Syriac or Arabic for his Christian and Muslim patrons at the ʿAbbāsid court in Baghdad.[3] Produced with philological precision as well as readability in mind, these Galenic translations commanded substantial sums of money during Ḥunayn's lifetime.[4] Moreover, after his death they were one of the primary means through which later medieval Islamicate authors – including those discussed in this book – could read a less abridged form of Galen. Although Ḥunayn is best known for his translations of Galen, bibliographers such as Ibn al-Nadīm write that he

[1] Gutas (1998: 142–50) observes that modern scholars tend to divide the Graeco-Arabic translation movement into three phases: an early, literal phase of translation; the more refined intermediate phase of Ḥunayn and his circle; and the later phase of the Baghdad Peripatetic school's revisions of earlier translations. As he argues, this classification goes back to Ḫalīl ibn Aybak al-Ṣafadī's (d. 764/1363) account – now considered baseless – of a development of translation styles from the *ad verbum* approach of, e.g., Ibn al-Biṭrīq (*fl. c.* 200/815) to the *ad sensum* method of Ḥunayn.

[2] Gutas (1998), 136. Cf. Ibn Abī Uṣaybiʿa (590–669/1194–1270), who writes that Ḥunayn studied Greek in Constantinople after a failed attempt to learn medicine from Yūḥannā ibn Māsawayh (d. 243/857) in Baghdad. See *The Best Accounts of the Classes of Physicians* (*ʿUyūn al-anbāʾ fī ṭabaqāt al-aṭibbāʾ*): Riḍā (1965), p. 257 l. 19–p. 258 l. 25. On Ḥunayn's medical career, see below (pp. 70–1).

[3] For the Arabic text of Ḥunayn's *Epistle*, see Bergsträsser (1925) with corrections from Bergsträsser (1932). Lamoreaux (2016) has produced a new edition of the *Epistle* after re-examining the two Istanbul MSS (Ayasofya 3631 and 3590) that preserve Ḥunayn's letter. His edition improves on Bergsträsser's, and it provides the first English translation of the Arabic text. On Ḥunayn's patrons, see Micheau (1997).

[4] See Overwien (2012) and Cooper (2016), who discuss how Ḥunayn and his associates adapted their source texts to produce more reader-friendly translations. On the wages that Ḥunayn and his circle received, see Gutas (1998), 139.

rendered into Arabic works from Plato, Aristotle, and other medical writers such as Paul of Aegina.[5]

As I explained in the Introduction, none of Plato's dialogues appear to have been translated into Arabic during the Middle Ages.[6] Arnzen has argued that the Platonic 'translations' which Ibn al-Nadīm and other bibliographers ascribe to Ḥunayn probably refer to Arabic versions of Middle Platonic and Neoplatonic exegeses of the dialogues.[7] Even if Ḥunayn cannot be credited with translating the *Timaeus* and other dialogues into Arabic, his circle's translations of Galen made a certain kind of Platonism accessible to readers of Arabic. While there is no evidence from Ḥunayn's extant writings that he read the original *Timaeus*, he seems to have had sufficient knowledge of the dialogue, whether gleaned from sources such as Galen, Aristotle, or even Proclus, to be able to supplement a lacuna at the beginning of Galen's *Plat. Tim.*[8] This chapter investigates how Ḥunayn utilized his circle's Arabic translations of Galen's interpretations of the *Timaeus* to create an elite ophthalmology that rivals 'generalist' medicine and philosophy in their claim to epistemic authority over the body and cosmos.

Ḥunayn wrote on a diverse range of subjects, but his main area of interest was medicine.[9] In addition to his job as a translator, Ḥunayn practised medicine, which he studied formally in Baghdad under the physician Yūḥannā ibn Māsawayh and may have learned first from his apothecary father.[10] In a text purporting to be his autobiography, Ḥunayn, who is presented as the first-person narrator, complains about his efforts to win recognition from his medical colleagues at the ʿAbbāsid court.[11] These

[5] Flügel (1871), vol. I, 245–52, 293. Ḥunayn's son, Isḥāq ibn Ḥunayn, appears to have been responsible for most of the Arabic translations of Aristotle produced in the circle: see Peters (1968). Summaries of Aristotle's *On the Heavens* and *Meteorology* are attributed to Ḥunayn; see respectively Gutman (2003), xv–xvii and Lettinck (1999). For Ḥunayn's translation of Paul of Aegina's *Pragmateia*, see Pormann (2004).

[6] See the Introduction, pp. 22–3. [7] Arnzen (2012).

[8] Ḥunayn's introduction to Galen's *Timaeus* commentary does not survive. From his *Epistle* we learn that Ḥunayn acquired a defective Greek manuscript of Galen's exegesis and that he 'supplied what was lacking at the beginning [of book one]' (*tammamtu nuqṣānan fī awwalihi*) (Bergsträsser 1925: p. 50 ll. 3–7=Lamoreaux 2016: p. 125 l. 6). See Arnzen (2013), who discusses how Ḥunayn translated for a patron a section of Proclus' commentary on the *Timaeus* (89e3–90c7) to elucidate the Platonic material in Galen's treatise *On Habits* (Περὶ ἐθῶν).

[9] For a list of Ḥunayn's works, see Ibn Abī Uṣaybiʿa: Riḍā (1965), p. 270, l. 29–p. 274, l. 10.

[10] On Ḥunayn's medical education, see Ibn al-Qifṭī, *History of Learned Men* (*Tāʾrīḫ al-ḥukamāʾ*): Lippert (1903), p. 174 l. 6–p. 175 l. 16.

[11] This text is preserved in Ibn Abī Uṣaybiʿa: see Riḍā (1965), p. 264 l. 16–p. 270 l. 28=Cooperson (2001), 109–14. Strohmaier (1965) claims that one of Ḥunayn's pupils wrote this 'autobiography' to defend Ḥunayn against charges of iconoclasm, for which he was tortured and jailed. On Ḥunayn's iconoclasm, see Cooperson (1997).

doctors cite Ḥunayn's career as a translator, which they disparage as the occupation of a 'tradesperson' (*ṣāniʿ*), to justify their refusal to admit him into their ranks; just as a smith supplies a knight with his sword, so Ḥunayn's task is to supply them with the tools – his translations – to better their craft.[12] Regardless of the veracity of the narrative, its report of Ḥunayn's struggle to establish his credibility as a medical authority sets him apart from Galen and the other authors in this book, who take for granted their professional identities as doctors. Ḥunayn became renowned, in particular, for his contributions to ophthalmology, which Galen blamed for legitimizing what he viewed as a troubling tendency among contemporary doctors in Rome and other metropolises. As I will discuss, Galen attacked the specialization of medicine into independent sub-fields, of which ophthalmology was the most well established, for fracturing the unity of the discipline and consequently endangering the health of patients.

This chapter calls attention to Ḥunayn's *Ten Treatises on the Eye* (*Kitāb al-ʿAšr maqālāt fī l-ʿayn*), which brought him posthumous fame for his expertise in the 'art of ophthalmology' (*ṣināʿat al-kuḥl*).[13] Composed over a period of more than thirty years, the ten tracts cover ocular anatomy and physiology (treatises 1–3), diseases (treatises 4–6), and drugs (treatises 7–10).[14] My analysis concentrates on Ḥunayn's boundary work in treatises one and three of *Ten Treatises on the Eye*, where he constructs an alternative to Galen's limiting conception of ophthalmology that has the theoretical capacity to vie with philosophy and 'generalist' medicine for the right to study the subject of vision. I argue that Ḥunayn's appeal to book seven of *PHP*, which Galen frames as a defence of Plato's description of the visual process at *Ti.* 45b2–46a2, allows him to make a connection crucial for justifying his inclusion of vision within the specialism's purview. Ḥunayn reads Galen's interpretation of the dialogue's link between the eyes and brain as providing implicit support for his expansion of ophthalmology's jurisdiction to encompass enquiries into sensation.

12 Riḍā (1965), p. 265 ll. 14–17.

13 See Ibn al-Qifṭī: Lippert (1903), p. 171 l. 4. In the introduction to his edition of *Ten Treatises on the Eye*, Meyerhof (1928: xlix–lii) expresses uncertainty as to whether the final redaction of the text comes from Ḥunayn or Ḥubayš. I follow subsequent scholars (e.g., Eastwood 1982; Pormann 2004: 115; Savage-Smith 2007: 151) in referring to Ḥunayn as the author of the work. Ḥunayn also composed another ophthalmological treatise (in *quaestiones* format) called *Questions Concerning the Eye* (*Kitāb al-Masāʾil fī l-ʿayn*), which consists of extracts from the first six books of *Ten Treatises on the Eye*. For a French translation of this work, see Sbath and Meyerhof (1938) (reprinted in Sezgin 1986: 745–897).

14 At the beginning of the tenth tract, Ḥunayn relates that he collected all the treatises into one volume for his nephew and fellow translator Ḥubayš. See Meyerhof (1928), p. 192 ll. 4–10 [Arabic], p. 125 [English].

I want to emphasize that *Ten Treatises on the Eye* does not openly respond to Galen's critique of medical specialization. The second part of this chapter, however, foregrounds Ḥunayn's attempts through his revisions of his Galenic source material to confer prestige on ophthalmology by privileging the eye as a cosmic organ. Building on Eastwood's reading of *Ten Treatises on the Eye*, I propose that Ḥunayn deploys Galen's teleological conception of the body's design in *UP*, which takes inspiration from the *Timaeus*, to develop an ocular anatomy that reflects the order of the macrocosm.[15] He also appears to mobilize Galen's description in *PHP* 7 of the *Timaeus*' association of the senses with the four elements for the same purpose of underscoring the eye's special affinity with the cosmos. In a similar way to Plato's *Timaeus*, where macrocosmic principles are used to elucidate the workings of the body, Ḥunayn applies a 'top-down' explanatory approach to the study of the eye. In so doing, he suggests that the specialism is unintelligible to practitioners lacking preliminary training in philosophy. I maintain that this protraction of an eye doctor's education may serve two possible aims: (1) to elevate not only the intellectual but also the socio-cultural standing of ophthalmology by putting its study beyond the means of non-elite practitioners; and (2) to establish a new epistemological hierarchy, in which philosophy is ancillary to the acquisition of specialist knowledge. This section contends that Ḥunayn, through his engagement with the Timaean aspects of *UP* and *PHP*, is able to reconfigure ophthalmology as an elite field of knowledge that is best able to provide investigators of natural reality an access point to both the body and cosmos.

Teleology, Anatomy, and Vision in Plato's *Timaeus*

To preface my explanation of Galen and Ḥunayn's descriptions of the eye and its function, I review in this section Plato's visual theory in the *Timaeus*. I do not offer a comprehensive summary of the dialogue's complex notion of vision, but rather I mention the features that are central to my argument in the second half of this chapter. Timaeus refers to the visual process at 45b2–46a2, which forms part of the dialogue's portrayal of the works of reason (29d7–47e2), to illustrate that the Demiurge and the lesser gods constructed everything with a purpose in mind.[16] The eyes,

[15] Eastwood (1982).

[16] See *Ti.* 44c3–d2. As Johansen (2004: 108) observes, the purpose of each part of the body is the principal good that it produces for humans.

which were the first organs to be created, exist so that humans can observe the planets, or 'orbits of intelligence in the heavens' (ἐν οὐρανῷ τοῦ νοῦ [. . .] περιόδους), and harmonize the rotations of their own souls with them.[17] Timaeus emphasizes the importance of the eyes by presenting them as the first organs of the body and as tools for philosophical enquiry. As I will show later, while Ḥunayn passes over the philosophical benefits of vision, he stresses the primacy of the eyes but not in terms of temporal priority.

Timaeus' theory of vision appears to operate on two physiological principles, which underlie Galen and Ḥunayn's explanations too. It assumes that (1) vision involves fire and that (2) the visual stream coalesces with daylight because 'like attracts like'. The dialogue relates that vision results from the coalescence of two streams of fire, flowing from the eyes and from the colours of external objects:

> τῶν δὲ ὀργάνων πρῶτον μὲν φωσφόρα συνετεκτήναντο ὄμματα, τοιᾷδε ἐνδήσαντες αἰτίᾳ. τοῦ πυρὸς ὅσον τὸ μὲν κάειν οὐκ ἔσχε, τὸ δὲ παρέχειν φῶς ἥμερον, οἰκεῖον ἑκάστης ἡμέρας, σῶμα ἐμηχανήσαντο γίγνεσθαι. τὸ γὰρ ἐντὸς ἡμῶν ἀδελφὸν ὂν τούτου πῦρ εἰλικρινὲς ἐποίησαν διὰ τῶν ὀμμάτων ῥεῖν λεῖον καὶ πυκνὸν ὅλον μέν, μάλιστα δὲ τὸ μέσον συμπιλήσαντες τῶν ὀμμάτων, ὥστε τὸ μὲν ἄλλο ὅσον παχύτερον στέγειν πᾶν, τὸ τοιοῦτον δὲ μόνον αὐτὸ καθαρὸν διηθεῖν. ὅταν οὖν μεθημερινὸν ᾖ φῶς περὶ τὸ τῆς ὄψεως ῥεῦμα, τότε ἐκπῖπτον ὅμοιον πρὸς ὅμοιον, συμπαγὲς γενόμενον, ἓν σῶμα οἰκειωθὲν συνέστη κατὰ τὴν τῶν ὀμμάτων εὐθυωρίαν, ὅπηπερ ἂν ἀντερείδῃ τὸ προσπῖπτον ἔνδοθεν πρὸς ὃ τῶν ἔξω συνέπεσεν. ὁμοιοπαθὲς δὴ δι' ὁμοιότητα πᾶν γενόμενον, ὅτου τε ἂν αὐτό ποτε ἐφάπτηται καὶ ὃ ἂν ἄλλο ἐκείνου, τούτων τὰς κινήσεις διαδιδὸν εἰς ἅπαν τὸ σῶμα μέχρι τῆς ψυχῆς αἴσθησιν παρέσχετο ταύτην ᾗ δὴ ὁρᾶν φαμεν.[18]
>
> First of the organs [the gods] fashioned the eyes to conduct light. They fastened them [within the head] for the following reason. They contrived that such fire as was not for burning but for providing a gentle light should become the proper body of each day. For the pure fire within us, akin to that fire, they made to flow through the eyes: so they made the eyes – [the eye] as whole but its middle [i.e. pupil] in particular – close-textured, smooth, and dense, to enable [them] to keep out all the other, coarser stuff, and let the other kind of fire pass through pure by itself. Now whenever daylight

[17] *Ti.* 47b6–c4. This regular movement mirrors the revolutions of the World Soul's 'circle of the same', which gives rise to rational thought (37c1–3). Thus, by bringing their soul in line with the motions of the planets, a person can achieve certain knowledge. Baltussen (2000: 105) describes Timaeus' account of vision at 45b2–46a2 as teleological rather than physiological.

[18] *Ti.* 45b2–d3.

> surrounds the visual stream, like makes contact with like and coalesces with it to make up a single homogeneous body aligned with the direction of the eyes. This happens whenever the internal fire strikes and presses against an external object [with which] it has connected. And because this body of fire has become uniform throughout and thus uniformly affected, it transmits the motions of whatever it comes in contact with as well as whatever comes in contact with it, to and through the whole body until it reaches the soul. This brings about the sensation [which] we call 'seeing'.[19]

Three kinds of fires contribute to the process of vision: daylight, fire in the eyes, and flames from visible objects.[20] Timaeus breaks down vision into three stages, during the first of which a non-burning fire issues from the eyes. Next, this ocular fire coalesces with daylight to become a body that extends along the line of vision and meets with visible objects, or more precisely, the flames that they emit. When the visual stream comes into contact with an object, this meeting produces a motion that is transmitted back through the current to the eyes – and ultimately to the rational soul located in the head.

According to the above passage, the lesser gods made the eyes finely porous to create a point of exit for the internal fire but also to prevent air, water, and earth, whose particles are larger than fire's, from entering them.[21] This statement about the structure of the eye constitutes Timaeus' anatomy of the organ. Its brevity notwithstanding, subsequent ancient and medieval authors (even critics of Plato's theory) adopted the teleological slant of this 'anatomy', which links design with function. Both Galen and Ḥunayn also find in this passage from the *Timaeus* support for their encephalocentric positions, because it seems to describe a special relationship between the eyes and the head, the 'vessel' (κύτος, 45a7) of the rational soul. In particular, they draw on its suggestion that the gods placed the eyes in the same location as the rational soul to facilitate communication between them as proof of the brain's sensory role.[22]

Famously, Aristotle attacked Plato's doctrine of vision when advancing his own intromissive theory at *De Anima* 2.7 (418a27–419a25) and *De Sensu et Sensibilibus* 2–3 (437a19–440b26), which state that the eyes receive effluences from visual objects.[23] As Galen formulates his own theory of

[19] I have followed the translation of Zeyl (2000: 33) with minor modification in light of Cornford's (1937: 152–3) translation.

[20] In the passage quoted above, Timaeus does not make explicit mention of the flames that stream off external objects. It is at *Ti.* 67c4–68d7 that he explains how the size of these flames' particles contract and dilate the visual current and thus produce different colour sensations.

[21] On the sizes of the four elements, see *Ti.* 56a3–5. [22] See also *Ti.* 45a7–b2.

[23] For a detailed treatment of Aristotle's theory of vision, see Johansen (1997), 23–147.

vision in *PHP* 7 as a defence of Plato's, it is worth outlining the Aristotelian criticisms that he has to address. To refute the theory of the *Timaeus*, Aristotle attempts to disprove the claims that vision involves fire and an attraction of like to like. In *Sens.*, Aristotle cites the fact that our eyes do not act like lanterns at night as proof against fire's participation in vision.[24] Moreover, he appeals to his own observation, derived from animal dissections, that the eyes exude water, not fire, when they decay as further evidence against Plato's position.[25] As for the dialogue's hypothesis that we perceive like by like, or fire by fire, Aristotle dismisses this idea at *DA* 417a3–9 by raising the following question: if we perceive by like acting on like, what prevents a sense organ such as the eye from perceiving itself, for its internal fire could act on itself?[26] He rejects the fundamental principle of attraction that, according to the *Timaeus*, is not only responsible for vision but also brought together the 'traces' (ἴχνη) of the elements before the birth of the cosmos, when Necessity was the governing force.[27]

The significance of the eyes seems to be connected with Timaeus' depiction of them as paradigmatic products of the joint work of Intellect (the Demiurge) and Necessity. The anatomy of the eye is emblematic of the purposiveness of the Demiurge's and lesser gods' creation, and the mechanics of vision function on the same primordial principle that shaped the pre-cosmic world. Vision's capacity to regulate psychic motions, on the other hand, cannot account for its – and by extension, the eyes' – superior status because hearing achieves the same effect by communicating speech and musical harmony to the soul.[28] Timaeus seems to characterize the eyes as microcosms in that studying their structure and function offers insight into the different forces at work in the macrocosm. The dialogue emphasizes this cosmic analogy by relating that the gods designed the head, the seat of the eyes, in imitation of the shape of the revolving World Soul.[29] While I will examine below how both Galen and Ḥunayn exploit the *Timaeus*' linkage of the eye and the macrocosm to extend the epistemic

[24] *Sens.* 437b12–25. In this passage, Aristotle argues more broadly that light cannot be fire because rain and cold do not extinguish it, whereas these conditions put out flames and other fiery bodies.

[25] *Sens.* 438a18–19.

[26] See also *GC* 323b21–3. Johansen (1997: 71–3) and Kalderon (2015: 152–3) identify the target of Aristotle's criticism of the like-by-like principle as Empedocles. Nonetheless, Aristotle appears to think that Empedocles and the *Timaeus* advance the same doctrine of vision (Johansen 1997: 54, 61, 86), so Plato may also be a second target. See below (pp. 96–7) for Galen's association of Empedocles' like-by-like principle with the *Timaeus*' theory of vision.

[27] *Ti.* 52d4–53c3. See Johansen (2004), 111–12.

[28] On hearing's contribution to the governance of the soul, see *Ti.* 47c4–e2.

[29] *Ti.* 44d3–6.

reach of their respective fields, I now turn to the former's efforts to restore medicine's dominion over the organ.

Ophthalmology as Fragmented Knowledge

As will become clear below, Galen follows Plato's *Timaeus* in assigning unique importance to the eye, but he speaks strongly against it being the object of specialized practice. The purpose of the present discussion is to uncover how Galen's disapproval of ophthalmology as a separate sub-field is rooted in his conviction that medical specialization threatens the unity of medicine. Galen is preceded in his polemic against medical specialization by the early imperial medical writers Cornelius Celsus (first century CE) and Scribonius Largus (first century CE), who criticized the professionalization of surgery that took place in the late Hellenistic period and the consequential development of distinct sub-groups of practitioners.[30] Of the medical specialisms that concretized during this period, eye surgery, and ocular therapy more generally, established itself relatively early, around the first century BCE.[31] Its practitioners (Gr. ὀφθαλμικοί; Lat. *medici ocularii*), perhaps in a similar way to other specialist doctors, came to ophthalmology first rather than after training in generalist medicine – although occasionally the reverse was true.[32] Unlike Galen, who singles out eye doctors (among others) in his critique, Celsus and Scribonius assert the unity of medicine and concomitantly prioritize the 'generalist' doctor's expertise, which encompasses all branches of the discipline, over those who focus on surgery or dietetics alone.[33] In a move that further marginalizes specialists from the sphere of legitimate medical practice, Scribonius withholds the title of 'doctor' (*medicus*) from anyone lacking a holistic grasp of medicine.[34] Anxiety about the generalist's position in the medical marketplace might be behind the two men's hostile responses to the specialization of medicine, for doctors now had to compete for patients with rivals not only from different sects (for example, Empiricism, Methodism, and Pneumatism) but also with proficiency in performing specific procedures on individual parts of the body.

The Parts of the Medical Art (*PAM*), which survives in a third/ninth-century Arabic version and a fourteenth-century Latin translation of a lost

30 See Mudry (1985); von Staden (2002), 41–2.

31 Jackson (1996: 2232) credits the early development of ophthalmology as a specialty to the importance of vision, the vulnerability of the eyes to disease and injury, and their relative accessibility. See also von Staden (2002), 42–3.

32 Nutton (1972), 23–4. 33 See Jackson (1996), 2232. 34 Mudry (1985), 331.

Greek exemplar, contains Galen's most extensive comments about the undesirability of medical specialization, which he presents as a socio-economic fact of urban life.[35] While Galen recognizes that certain 'single branch specialists' (Arab. *yuʿāliğu min al-ṭibb fannan wāḥidan*; Lat. *qui quamcumque artem operatur*), including oculists (lit. 'those who cut eyes': Arab. *qaddāḥī al-aʿyun*; Lat. *oculos … incidens*), spend their careers as itinerant practitioners in the countryside, the majority of them work in Rome, Alexandria, and other urban centres.[36] The large populations of these cities, Galen remarks, supply even those unable to learn medicine in its entirety with a sufficient client base to earn a living. Another treatise, *Opt.Med.Cogn.*, attributes the proliferation of medical malpractice to the anonymity produced by Rome's immense population, as well as to the greed of its inhabitants.[37] By reading *PAM* in the light of *Opt.Med.Cogn.*, Galen's localization of medical specialization in cities takes on an added significance beyond the descriptive: the phenomenon becomes emblematic of a failure in professional standards.

In a two-pronged attack targeting medical specialization on theoretical and practical grounds, *PAM* characterizes specialist knowledge as cut off from the unified wholes of medicine and the body. The pedagogical aim of *PAM* is to teach the reader how to organize medicine into its correct constituent parts through the logical method of division (διαίρεσις). It is in the context of his description of excessive divisions of the discipline that Galen introduces his arguments against medical specialization. He gives particular attention to 'the art of the oculist' (Arab. *ṣināʿat aṣḥāb ʿilāğ al-ʿayn*; Lat. *optalmicorum*), because, being the most long-standing specialized practice, it has the greatest claim to respectability. To weaken the legitimacy of this and all other specialisms, Galen alleges that, in separating their expertise from medicine, 'single-branch specialists' undermine medicine's logical coherency. He writes:

> إن عد عاد هذه النتف الصغار الكثيرة أجزاء من صناعة الطب، على ما قد يتسم الآن برومية خاصة حتى يسموا بعض الأطباء معالجي الأسنان ويسموا بعضهم معالجي الآذان ويسموا بعضهم معالجي المقعدة. أفضى القول إلى حيرة أعظم من هذه على أنّ أصحاب هذا الشأن أيضا قد وجدوا فرصة من اسم قد وضع لا منذ قريب لكن منذ مدة من الزمان بعيدة جدا، وهي صناعة أصحاب علاج العين. فإنّه إن كانت العينان مفردة بطبيب على حدته لما خرج من الواجب أن يكون للأسنان أيضا طبيب آخر مفرد على حدته وآخر للأذنين وآخرون لكل واحد من أعضاء البدن. فيجب من

[35] The authenticity of *PAM* has been disputed. Having access to only the Latin version of *PAM*, Kühn (1828) argued that the text was a forgery by the Greek doctor Niccolò da Reggio (*c.* 1280–1350). For a persuasive defence of Galen's authorship, see von Staden (2002), 23–8. For the Arabic text, see Lyons (1969), and for the Latin, see Schöne (1911).

[36] Lyons (1969), p. 26 l. 21–p. 28 l. 18. Cf. da Reggio's Latin version: Schöne (1911), 25.

[37] See *Opt.Med.Cogn.* 1.12–13: Iskandar (1988), 47.

ذلك أن يكون عدد الأطباء بعدد أعضاء البدن. وإذ كان أيضا بعض الأطباء قد يسمون قداحي الأعين وبعضهم بطاطي القيل وبعضهم مخرجي الحصى وبعضهم على مثال آخر شبيه بهذا. فقد يجب أن تصير عدة الأطباء أكثر كثيرا من عدد أعضاء البدن. وذلك أنّه ليس إنّما يوجد لكل واحد من الأعضاء طبيب مفرد على حدته فقط لكن قد يوجد لكل واحدة من علل كل واحد من الأعضاء طبيب مفرد على حدته.[38]

> Thus, it may happen that these many small bits are counted as parts of the art of medicine, and so one finds, especially in Rome nowadays, some doctors who call themselves dentists, others otologists, and others proctologists. This argument, however, leads to even greater perplexity, although its proponents find an opportune defence provided them by a title that is not recent but of very long standing, namely the art of the oculist. For if the eyes have a specialist to deal with them, it follows that there should be a specialist for the teeth, another for the ears, and others for each part of the body. So, it follows that there should be as many doctors as there are parts of the body. But one also finds some doctors who call themselves couchers of cataracts, others cutters of hernias, or lithotomists, and there are others who have different [titles] on the same pattern. Thus, it follows that the number of doctors should very much exceed the number of the parts of the body. For not only will there be a specialist to deal with each part of the body individually, but each of the ailments of each of these parts will have its own specialist.[39]

According to Galen, the division of medicine into sub-fields concerned with individual parts of the body as well as the disorders afflicting them creates a logical impasse – 'perplexity' (Arab. *ḥayra*; Lat. *aporia*) – for two reasons. First, as specialisms are not parts of medicine but something more fragmentary (they are 'bits': Arab. *nutaf*; Lat. *particulas*), these sub-divisions give a distorted impression of the discipline's components and the relations between them, which the method of division is supposed to uncover.[40] Furthermore, the line of reasoning put forward by specialists to justify their practice unnaturally multiplies medicine with its suggestion that there could be more doctors than parts of the body. The charge underlying these observations is that the divisions imposed on medicine by specialists destroy the discipline's unity by making it impossible to comprehend its innumerable fragmented parts all together, through, for instance, the logical procedure of 'collection' (σύνθεσις).[41]

38 Lyons (1969), p. 26 l. 21–p. 28 l. 9=Schöne (1911), 25.

39 Lyons (1969), 27, 29.

40 See Schöne (1911), 25. At *PHP* 9.5.11–38 (De Lacy 2005: p. 566 l. 10–p. 572 l. 15) and *HVA* 15.446–49K, Galen, following Plato, considers division to be a logical method common to all *technai* by which an accurate conception of a *technē* can be reached.

41 See *PHP* 9.5.13–14 (De Lacy 2005: p. 566 ll. 18–26), which describes division and collection as a twofold 'journey' (ὁδοιπορία). Galen summarizes how, in division, one descends from the most general genus of a thing down to its indivisible units by way of the intervening *differentiae*, whereas, in collection, one returns from the lowest species to the first genus.

Developing further his critique of medical specialization, Galen warns at *PAM* 4.3–4 that specialized practice may result in negative therapeutic outcomes because it is based on a piecemeal understanding of the body. To demonstrate that the parts of the body cannot be treated in isolation, he turns once again to the 'art of the oculist' and explains how cataract couching requires knowledge about the general care of the body.[42] Presented with a cataract patient suffering from repletion (Arab. *imtilāʾ*; Lat. *plethoricum*), the oculist, Galen maintains, will inflame the tunics that they are piercing and 'communicate' (n. Arab. *mušāraka*; Lat. *compassionem*) the pain in the eyes to the head if they lack expertise in the 'preparatory art' (Arab. *al-ṣināʿa allatī tataqaddamu*; Lat. *preparative artis*) – one of the 'elements' (Arab. *arkān*; Lat. *elementa*) of medicine whose objective is to purge the body of superfluities. This hypothetical example underscores the complex interplay of factors that contribute to disease and the interconnectedness of the body to deny the autonomy of specialisms such as ophthalmology. Through his questioning of specialists' competence to cure the parts of the body over which they claim mastery, Galen reaffirms the generalist doctor's control of the entire body. His boundary work subsumes ophthalmology into the broader field of medical knowledge.

In what seems like a concession to the primacy that Galen affords to the generalist's holistic comprehension, Ḥunayn, as the second half of this chapter will argue, invokes the eyes' connectedness to the body and macrocosm to compel ophthalmologists to train in medicine and philosophy. Ḥunayn's aim in forging these epistemic links is not to absorb ophthalmic expertise into medicine – thus denying the specialism the capacity to stand alone, as Galen seeks to do – but to expand its theoretical potential. With a grounding in medicine and philosophy, the eye doctor of *Ten Treatises on the Eye* has the conceptual framework to interpret fully the data to which he is privy as a specialist of an organ that represents a juncture between the body and cosmos. In contrast to the standard course of study mentioned above, where specialists occasionally retrained to become general practitioners in Graeco-Roman antiquity (but not vice versa), Ḥunayn makes specialized rather than general knowledge the *telos* of his medical education. His scheme seems to prefigure modern medical hierarchies in subordinating general medicine (as well as philosophy) to specialisms by reducing the former to a propaedeutic to the latter.[43]

[42] Lyons (1969), p. 32 l. 18–p. 34 l.5=Schöne (1911), 28.

[43] The preference shown by young doctors in North America, western Europe, and Australia for careers in medical specialities has been the subject of many opinion pieces in medical journals and

There may be an elitist subtext to Galen's criticism of medical specialization and Ḥunayn's reconfiguration of ophthalmology. Both men express concern about the social respectability of their occupations. I have already touched on Galen's anxiety about enhancing medicine's – and by extension, his own – standing, and Ḥunayn's 'autobiography' complains about his equation with a 'tradesperson' (*ṣāniʿ*) for his translational work at court, at least.[44] Galen and Ḥunayn's respective promotion of a general medicine and ophthalmology that requires lengthy training and the means to fund it may serve to distance their practices from their non-elite peers', who perhaps viewed medical specialization as a more feasible path. Funerary inscriptions, chiefly from imperial Rome, reveal that oculists were mostly slaves or freedpersons, although they could amass substantial wealth.[45] The backgrounds of the majority of self-styled 'doctors' (Gr. ἰατροί; Lat. *medici*) do not appear to have been very different, but the social gamut of these practitioners did include knights (*equites*), whereas no oculist seems to have reached such an elevated status.[46] Little research has been done on the social position of doctors, let alone oculists (sing. *kaḥḥāl/a*), in ʿAbbāsid Baghdad; nonetheless, evidence from subsequent periods indicates that, as with the first group, the latter were regarded as skilled labourers, even if they were sometimes poor.[47] To defend their claim to elite status, Galen and Ḥunayn construct their medical occupations as elite practices beyond the reach of the greater number of doctors and specialists, in particular, who had neither the time nor money (and possibly freedom) for protracted study.

'The Most Divine Organ' at the Service of Medicine

Notwithstanding his theoretical and therapeutic objections to ophthalmology as an independent sub-field, Galen composed a now-lost treatise

popular publications over the past twenty years. For a recent example, see Dalen, Ryan, and Alpert (2017), who list prestige as a possible motivation to specialize.

44 See the Introduction (pp. 6–10), Chapter 1, and pp. 70–1 above.

45 See Fischer (1980); Jackson (1996), 2233. While these studies concentrate on the social status of eye doctors, their conclusions probably hold true for other specialists.

46 On the social status of physicians in the imperial period, see Hirt Raj (1987), who focuses on the western provinces of the Roman Empire. Executed for being the lover of the emperor Claudius' wife Messalina, Vettius Valens (d. 48 CE) is an example of a physician who held the rank of *eques* (see De Rohden and Dessau 1897: vol. III, p. 414 no. 343).

47 Rosenthal (1978) remains the most extensive study of the social status of the physician during ʿAbbāsid rule. He concludes that doctors, on the whole, were comparable economically to shopkeepers (484). For the social classification of eye doctors in the medieval Islamicate world from the third/ninth to tenth/fifteenth centuries, see Shatzmiller (1994), 140. See also Goitein (1963: 190), who draws attention to a Geniza document that lists a woman oculist as a receiver of alms.

on ocular disorders for a beginner eye specialist.[48] The work probably did not deal with the subject of vision, because, in keeping with Galen's reductive notion of ophthalmological expertise, oculists' partial knowledge of the body precludes them from examining an activity that interfaces the eyes with the brain. As I will discuss in what follows, Galen utilizes this organic link to position the generalist doctor as the expert most capable of determining how vision operates. Furthermore, the *Timaeus*' connection of the eyes with the macrocosm allows him to make the methodological assertion that medicine offers a truthful way to investigate the natural world – a line of reasoning that Ḥunayn would appropriate. Galen's explanations of vision show that this declaration is designed to deprivilege philosophy as the exclusive authority on both the process itself and the realms that it bridges (body and cosmos). Employing an argumentative tactic familiar from his disputes over the hegemonic organ, Galen, in the passages analysed below, highlights what anatomy, as informed by medical practice, can uncover about activities that trouble the body's boundaries.[49]

Galen does not devote any of his works to vision, but treats the subject throughout his corpus.[50] Cross-references give the impression that these individual discussions make up a coherent explanation of the visual process.[51] Boudon-Millot notes that *UP* 10 and *PHP* 7, which contain Galen's most extensive surviving comments on vision, take different approaches to explicating this sense – even if Ḥunayn would later compose out of them a unified Galenic account of sight.[52] *UP* (10.12) has recourse to geometrical proofs to advance an extramissive conception of vision, where rectilinear lines stretching from the eyes to the perceived object form a visual cone. *PHP* (7.4–8), on the other hand, proposes that vision results from the interaction of pneuma and the outside air. While the former theory draws heavily on Euclid and the latter on Stoic and

[48] On the lost *On the Diseases of the Eyes* (Περὶ τῶν ἐν ὀφθαλμοῖς παθῶν), see *Lib.Prop.* 2.2 (Boudon-Millot 2007: p. 140 ll. 17–19); Savage-Smith (2002), 132–8; Zipser (2009). Cf. the Hippocratic *On Sight* (Περὶ ὄψιος), which discusses the treatment of various ocular afflictions; see Craik (2006: 3–116; 2015: 259–61) for details about the date, authorship, and contents of the work.

[49] For Galen's appeal to anatomy to defend his position on the hegemonic organ debate, see pp. 42–8 above.

[50] See, e.g., *UP* 10.3–13, *PHP* 7, *Caus.Symp.* 1.6.1–4, and *Com.Tim.* §§ 7, 16. Galen also treated vision in book thirteen of *DD*. Fragments from book two of *Plat.Tim.* (Larrain 1992: 174–5), which discuss pain and the senses, refer to vision and certain anatomical features of the eye, and thus indicate that Galen probably covered the topic in his commentary.

[51] At *UP* 8.6 Galen refers to his analysis of vision in *PHP* 7; at *Com.Tim.* § 7 he refers to *PHP* 7 and *DD* 13; at *PHP* 7.4.4 he refers to *DD*; and at *Caus.Symp.* 7.91K he refers to *PHP* 7 and *UP* 10.

[52] Boudon-Millot (2004).

Aristotelian thought, they both derive certain aspects from Plato's *Timaeus* as well.[53]

Galen prefaces his geometrical description of vision in *UP* by recounting a dream of his that rebuked him for planning to neglect the subject of vision in the text. The dream characterizes the eye along Timaean lines in that it portrays the organ and its sensory function as paradigms of the Demiurge's providence:

> ἐνύπνιον δέ τι μεταξὺ μεμψάμενον, ὡς εἰς μὲν τὸ θειότατον ὄργανον ἀδικοῖμι, περὶ δὲ τὸν δημιουργὸν ἀσεβοῖμι παραλιπὼν ἀνεξήγητον ἔργον μέγα τῆς εἰς τὰ ζῷα προνοίας αὐτοῦ.[54]
>
> Some intervening dream censured [me] because I was unjust to the most divine organ and was behaving impiously towards the Demiurge in leaving unexplained the great work of his providence for animals.[55]

As in the *Timaeus*, Galen's dream elevates the eye over all other organs owing to the benefits that vision bestows on animals; it leaves unspecified whether these benefits relate to the pursuit of philosophy, though. Galen also omits the dialogue's suggestion that the eyes were the first organs to be created by the gods, probably because this distinction goes against his own views about foetal development.[56] The passage seems to define the organ's 'godliness' in terms of its function rather than temporal priority.[57] Designed to further the welfare of animals, the eyes are proof of the teleological nature of the human body and the cosmos in which it is embedded.

Galen discloses in *UP* 17, his 'Hymn to Nature (or the Demiurge)', that he wrote this book to demonstrate to doctors and philosophers the forethought and skill underlying all of creation.[58] He reasons that anatomical study can provide proof of the providential nature of the cosmos, for, if one were to find evidence of divine wisdom in the body, it would follow that a similar intelligence is at work in the heavens.[59] Thus, anatomy produces powerful counter-evidence against the conception of a cosmos governed by random interactions of corpuscles – as advanced by atomists, one of the philosophical groups against which *UP* silently polemicizes.[60] Contemporary Aristotelians,

[53] On the various influences on Galen's visual theories, see Boudon-Millot (2012), 556–9.
[54] *UP* 10.12: Helmreich (1909), p. 93 ll. 5–9. [55] May (1968), vol. II, 490–1 [modified].
[56] Galen speculates that the liver forms first in embryos: see *Prop.Plac.* 11.2 (LG, p. 104 l. 2–p. 106 l. 5) and *Foet.Form.* 3.9 (Nickel 2001: p. 66 ll. 19–32).
[57] Cf. Boudon-Millot (2002b), 65.
[58] See Helmreich (1909), 437–51=May (1968), vol. II, 724–33.
[59] Helmreich (1909), p. 447 ll. 16–21= May (1968), vol. II, 731.
[60] Galen's critique includes the mechanistic explanations of Erasistrateans and Asclepiadeans: see Hankinson (1998b), 388–91.

at least those lacking the rigorous anatomical training advocated by Aristotle, may be another group at which Galen directs his protreptic to anatomy.[61] While Galen reports at *Lib.Prop.* 3.12 that *UP* had an enthusiastic reception among many Peripatetics in Rome, several individuals, whose names and philosophical affiliations are not identified, slandered the book.[62] Galen's infamous exchange with the Peripatetic philosopher Alexander of Damascus, which occurred after the publication of *UP*, indicates that leading intellectuals with Aristotelian leanings did dispute his anatomical findings.[63] On Galen's retelling of their confrontation, however, Alexander makes no substantive criticism of his demonstration of the production of voice – the topic on which Galen was invited to lecture in public – but tries to invalidate the anatomical display by raising an epistemological question about the reliability of the senses. The narrative attributes Alexander's hostility not only to his irritable temper but also to his insecurity about his imperfect command of anatomy, which seems to have inhibited him from challenging Galen at his own game of dissection.

Galen's use of language with overt Aristotelian resonances in *UP* offers further evidence that its didactic message is aimed at Peripatetics especially. Galen repeats the phrase 'nature does nothing in vain' (ἡ φύσις οὐδὲν ποιεῖ μάτην), as well as variants of it, which appear throughout Aristotle's biological writings, to describe the purposiveness of the parts of the body and remind the reader of the anatomical heritage of Aristotelianism.[64] Here, it serves Galen to exploit Aristotle's authority to enhance the credibility of anatomy as a method of discovery and demonstration, whereas in *PHP* he minimizes the philosopher's anatomical skill to delegitimize his cardiocentric thesis.[65] Despite this Aristotelian framing, the teleology of *UP* departs from Aristotle's in its assumption of the direction of a provident god; his unmoved mover (*Met.* Λ) is too remote to be

[61] Galen wrote *UP* for the senator and ex-consul Flavius Boethus, who had Peripatetic leanings (*Inst. Log.* 7.2; *Praen.* 5.10). As mentioned in Chapter 1 (p. 42), Galen dedicated the first six books of *PHP* to Boethus, in addition to eight other works dealing with anatomy. On Boethus' patronage of Galen and his interests in anatomy, see Johnson (2010), 78–80; Mattern (2013), 139–86.

[62] See Boudon-Millot (2007), p. 143 l. 24–p. 144 l. 7. On Galen's quarrels with contemporary Peripatetics, see van der Eijk (2009), 276–8.

[63] See *Praen.* 5.9–15: Nutton (1979), p. 96 l. 5–p. 98 l. 8. On Galen's altercation with Alexander, which seems to have taken place in the late 170s (Nutton 1979: 189), see Gleason (2009), 97–8.

[64] See Jouanna (2012), 287–312, who examines how Aristotle and other earlier thinkers shaped Galen's understanding of nature. Galen also draws on Aristotle when outlining the meaning of 'use' (χρεία) in *UP*: see Furley and Wilkie (1984), 58–70; Schiefsky (2007). See also *UP* 8.3 (Helmreich 1907: p. 449 ll. 14–21=May 1968: vol. I, 389), where Galen criticizes Aristotle for ignoring anatomical evidence in his arguments for the heart's primary sensory role.

[65] See Chapter 1 (pp. 42–4) above.

interested in the welfare of certain species.[66] Galen's teleology, however, appears to be Timaean because of its stress on god's role in fashioning a body that functions for the benefit of humans and possesses beauty. As Hankinson remarks, Galen's recognition in *UP* of anomalous conditions such as polydactyly (when individuals are born with more than five fingers on a hand) signals that he does not understand the creator god to be omnipotent or even omnicompetent.[67] Nonetheless, the rare occurrence of these 'non-normative' body parts means that they are exceptions to the general rule of divine agential design.[68]

Galen's discussion of ocular anatomy in *UP* aims to show how divine forethought is discernible in not just the functioning but also the structure of the eyes – a point on which Ḥunayn would expand.[69] Additionally, the work deploys the notion of the body's teleological design to advance a Platonic thesis with which an Aristotelian (and Stoic) reader would disagree: that the brain is responsible for sensation. In particular, Galen draws on the *Timaeus*' idea that the organs exist in a system of dependence to argue for a hierarchical relationship between the eyes and brain.[70] Adapting the dialogue's declaration that the head and the organs in it were created to serve the soul (*Ti.* 46e7–47c4), Galen proposes that the brain was situated in the head to serve the eyes.[71] He interprets the spatial proximity between the eyes and brain as evidence that the former organ depends on the latter for its sensory power.

At *PA* 656a27–657a12 Aristotle attacks the proponents of this 'proximity argument' as inept for maintaining that the brain is the seat of sensation

[66] On the differences between Galen and Aristotle's teleologies, see Hankinson (1988, 1989); Chiaradonna (2009a), 246. As Hankinson (1989: 214) comments, Aristotle does not seem to take the statement 'nature does nothing in vain' literally, for he assigns no functional purpose to the gall bladder (*PA* 677a12–19).

[67] Hankinson (1998b), 391. See *UP* 17.1: Helmreich (1909), p. 444 l. 3–p. 445 l. 2=May (1968), vol. II, 728–9.

[68] Cf. *QAM* 4.815–16K (Singer 2013a: 405–6), where Galen states that certain people as well as animals (scorpions, poisonous spiders, and vipers) are wicked by virtue of their mixture. The text, however, does not blame god for these creatures' wickedness. While medieval critics such as al-Rāzī (see p. 125 below) attack Galen for lacking a theodicy, *QAM*'s attribution of innate wickedness to mixture can be interpreted as a move to safeguard god's benevolence. Havrda (2017: 80–1) explains that the demiurgic power only gives form to the homoiomerous parts, whose capacities are determined by mixture. Similar to Plato's Demiurge (*Ti.* 30a2–c1), Galen's god is constrained by the properties of their creative material, so another cause is responsible for the mixtures that make some living things irredeemably bad.

[69] *UP* 10.2–6: Helmreich (1909), 56–78=May (1968), vol. II, 465–80.

[70] See Broadie (2012), 252, who gives other examples of relations of dependence in Timaeus' anatomy.

[71] *UP* 8.5: Helmreich (1907), p. 460 ll. 15–20. On this passage, see Boudon-Millot (2002b), 66. Cf. *UP* 1.2 (Helmreich 1907: p. 1 ll. 13–16=May 1968: vol. I, 67), where Galen emphasizes that all the parts of the body function for the sake of the soul.

when they cannot discover the real reason why four of the five sense organs (eyes, ears, nose, and tongue) are in the head. According to him, the sense organs that process complex sensory data require pure blood to perceive precisely, so they have been placed in the brain because it generates this type of blood owing to its lack of heat.[72] Galen refers to his conception of a provident as well as economical Demiurge to refute Aristotle's assignment of a refrigeratory rather than sensory role to the brain. He retorts that if the brain's purpose is to prevent blood from overheating and losing its sensitive power, why was the organ not placed closer to the heart, which is responsible for the body's heat and blood?[73] Anatomical study reveals that most of the sense organs are located in the head because the nerves – and thus sensation – originate in the brain.[74] Galen subversively uses anatomy and teleology, which *UP* identifies as key aspects of Aristotle's thought, to persuade his Aristotelian readership that their forerunner's cardiocentrism contravenes methodologies and tenets from their own philosophical tradition. As in *PHP*, Galen incorporates cases from his clinical practice into the narrative of *UP* to convey that it was through his work as a doctor that he honed the anatomical expertise that he now leverages to answer questions about divine providence and sensation.[75] Thus, *UP* constitutes more of a protreptic to medicine than to anatomy per se, for it is a means to acquiring a superior grasp of the latter.

Book seven of *PHP* brings up vision for the similar purpose of defending Plato's attribution of sensation to the brain. Galen refers to the visual process to explain how psychic pneuma alters the nerves in the brain to produce sensation.[76] Galen's hypothesis of a visual medium – the external air – in this book led Meyerhof to equate his theory of vision (as well as Ḥunayn's, which derives almost verbatim from *PHP* 7) with that of Aristotle, who argues that the sensation takes place through a transparent medium stretching from the eyes to the visible object.[77] Aristotle may have posited that the external air acts as a medium in vision, but Galen is distinct

[72] *PA* 656b3–7. According to Aristotle, as heat 'ousts' (ἐκκόπτει) the sensory activity innate in blood, cold promotes sensation.

[73] *UP* 8.2: Helmreich (1907), p. 445 l. 14–p. 449 l. 13=May (1968), vol. I, 387–9.

[74] See *UP* 8.6: Helmreich (1907), pp. 461–72=May (1968), vol. I, 398–407.

[75] On the cases at *UP* 4.9, 5.4, and 14.11 (Helmreich 1907: p. 209 l. 26–p. 210 l. 16, p. 258 ll. 20–8; Helmreich 1909: p. 322 l. 9–p. 323 l. 4=May 1968: vol. I, 214–15, 251, vol. II, 645–6), which includes the treatment of a nearly disembowelled gladiator in Pergamum, see Mattern (2008), 174.

[76] See *PHP* 7.4.2–3 and 7.5.31–3. For a more detailed discussion of the role of pneuma in Galen's physiology, see Chapter 1 (p. 46) and Chapter 4 (pp. 153–4).

[77] See Meyerhof (1928), xli–xlii. There, he also notes that Aristotle, Galen, and Ḥunayn integrate Plato's idea of a 'meeting' (συναύγεια) of the visual streams into their theories.

in conceiving of it as an instrument that is rendered sensitive when pneuma encounters it after exiting the eyes following its passage through the brain.[78] Galen attributes the pneuma's capacity to change the visual medium to like acting on like, which recalls the 'like attracts like' principle of the *Timaeus*.

In *PHP* 7 Galen is at pains to situate his theory of vision in relation to Plato's account in the *Timaeus*.[79] He quotes from *Ti.* 45b2–c2 and 58c5–d1, both of which emphasize the contribution of fire to sight.[80] As his interpretation of these passages makes clear, Galen does not understand Plato to mean literally that the eye contains fire, but rather that the organ's nature is luminous, similar to pure fire.[81] The dialogue calls the type of fire in the eye φῶς ('light'), and Galen chooses a derivative of the word (φωτοειδής, 'light-like') to refer to the pneuma responsible for vision, which is the 'organ' of sensation par excellence.[82] In so doing, Galen suggests an equivalence between his own pneumatic conception of vision and Plato's elementary theory. Galen also has recourse to *Ti.* 45c2–d3, which outlines the meeting of the internal ocular fire and daylight, to articulate how pneuma interacts with the medium of vision.[83] Sunlight illuminates air, making it luminous and thus akin in nature to pneuma. The luminosity of both the pneuma and the air allows them to merge into one sympathetic instrument (ὁμοιοπαθὲς ὄργανον) that transmits the colour of visible objects back to the brain.[84]

Galen's theory of vision in *PHP* 7 has two apparent objectives: to refute the Stoic, Epicurean, and Aristotelian explanations of the sense, and to substantiate further his encephalocentric model of sensation, which the text sets in opposition to the cardiocentric positions of Aristotle and Chrysippus.[85] By bringing pneuma into his account of vision, Galen has the conceptual framework to elaborate precisely how the brain is involved

[78] See *PHP* 7.7.22–6: De Lacy (2005), p. 474 ll. 15–29.

[79] The late antique Greek writers Nemesius and Meletius interpret the Aristotelian aspects of Galen's theory, specifically the notion that air acts as a visual medium, as Platonic. See respectively Nemesius, *On the Nature of Man* (van der Eijk and Sharples 2008: 105) and Meletius Monachus, *Nature of Man* (Migne 1860: col. 1177a). On Meletius' dependence on Nemesius, see Telfer (1955), 217.

[80] *PHP* 7.6.3–7: De Lacy (2005), p. 462 l. 27–p. 464 l. 7.

[81] *PHP* 7.6.7: De Lacy (2005), p. 464 ll. 7–8. On Galen's dismissal of the Platonic description of colours as fiery particles, see Ierodiakonou (2014), 241.

[82] See *PHP* 7.7.25: De Lacy (2005), p. 474 ll. 20–2. Galen famously calls pneuma 'the first instrument of the soul' (ὄργανον [. . .] τὸ πρῶτον αὐτὸ τῆς ψυχῆς) at 7.3.24. On the role of pneuma in vision in Galen, see Ierodiakonou (2014), 241–7.

[83] He quotes the passage at *PHP* 7.6.8–9: De Lacy (2005), p. 464 ll. 9–15.

[84] *PHP* 7.7.19–26: De Lacy (2005), p. 474 ll. 3–29.

[85] See Chapter 1, pp. 42–6.

with this and other forms of sensation, which the *Timaeus* leaves unexplained. Therefore, the eyes represent for Galen a battleground where what is at stake is the nature of sensation – if not the structure of the soul itself.[86] He gives doctors sway over this domain because their command of anatomy makes them more credible contributors to issues dealing with the organs and their functions as opposed to philosophers, who, lacking both extensive and practical contact with the human body, cannot match their expertise. The following section considers how Ḥunayn invests ophthalmology with the same authority as Galen's 'generalist' medicine to investigate the visual process by reconceptualizing the specialism in such a way that it can withstand his criticisms.

Ḥunayn's Ophthalmology

Eastwood remarks that, in contrast to Galen's discussions of vision in *UP* and *PHP*, Ḥunayn's *Ten Treatises on the Eye* is more concerned with developing a visual theory that is useful for medical practice than with engaging in polemics.[87] His characterization of Galen as 'the philosophical controversialist' and Ḥunayn as 'the medical teacher' underscores this distinction between the two authors' rhetorical aims.[88] Ḥunayn's silence regarding the identity of his sources, at least in the anatomical and physiological chapters of *Ten Treatises on the Eye*, certainly implies that he is uninterested in drawing attention to his allegiance to or departure from earlier authorities.[89] For the same reason, he may also have omitted the explicit references in his Galenic source texts to Plato's *Timaeus*, and paraphrased them instead. Nonetheless, the absence of any overt criticism of prior ocular theories in *Ten Treatises on the Eye* does not necessarily mean that Ḥunayn fully endorses those presented within his book. In the *Doubts about Galen* (*al-Šukūk ʿalā Ǧālīnūs*), which will be examined in the next chapter, Abū Bakr al-Rāzī records that Ḥunayn wrote a tract (now lost) which attacked Galen's conception of the visual medium in *PHP* 7 – specifically, the claim that ocular pneuma renders the outside air

[86] As the initial sections of *PHP* 7 stress, the attribution of sensation to the brain invalidates the Aristotelian and Stoic theory of a unitary soul, which regards the heart as the source of all psychic powers, including perception. See *PHP* 7.1–3: De Lacy (2005) p. 428 l. 1–p. 448 l. 3.

[87] Eastwood (1982), 57–8. [88] Eastwood (1982), 37.

[89] In treatise ten, Ḥunayn identifies some of the authors (e.g., Paccius, Galen, and Paul of Aegina) of the compound recipes from which he is quoting. See, e.g., Meyerhof (1928), 140 [English], 208 [Arabic]; 143 [English], 211 [Arabic]; 144 [English], 213 [Arabic]. Moreover, the incipit of the text (Meyerhof 1928: 1 [English], 69 [Arabic]), which may not be original to Ḥunayn, announces that the material follows the opinions of Hippocrates and Galen.

sensitive.[90] Ḥunayn does not set out in *Ten Treatises on the Eye* to expound his own position on the enduring controversy about the mechanics of vision.

This collection of treatises participates, however, in a subtler polemic with Galen's objections to ophthalmology and medical specialization in general. I discussed above how Galen censures eye doctors and other specialists for their fragmentary knowledge of the body, which threatens the unity of medicine and even the health of patients. My analysis will show that Ḥunayn, perhaps responding to Galen's criticisms, develops an ophthalmology that takes into consideration the interconnectedness of the body. His decision to treat vision in treatise three also suggests that his boundary work may have the more ambitious aim of promoting ophthalmology as a claimant to epistemic authority over the natural world vis-à-vis medicine and philosophy. To this end, Galen's interpretations of the *Timaeus*' teleological description of the body and elemental theory of vision give Ḥunayn the means with which to argue for a connection between the eye and the cosmos. Therefore, just as Galen exploits the links that the dialogue draws between the human body and macrocosm to expand what constitutes medical knowledge, so Ḥunayn joins the eye to these two larger systems to increase the epistemic scope of ophthalmology.

Before reviewing the Timaean aspects of *Ten Treatises on the Eye* that Ḥunayn takes from Galen, I want to look briefly at how the work reflects his broadened conception of ophthalmology at a structural level. The book can be divided into two halves, the first of which (treatises 1–4) deals with the theoretical aspects of ophthalmology and the latter (treatises 5–10) with more practical advice regarding the diagnosis and treatment of particular eye disorders. Covering ocular anatomy and the nature of the brain, treatises one and two indicate that eye specialists cannot restrict their study to the eyes alone. As Ḥunayn explains, the eyes are outgrowths of the brain and accordingly those responsible for their care must learn about this organ as well:

[90] See Koetschet (2019), p. 82 ll. 1–2. In this passage al-Rāzī notes that, despite this disagreement, Ḥunayn did not totally reject Galen's visual theory. The tract probably refers to Ḥunayn's *Treatise on his Apology for What Galen Said in the Seventh Book of the 'Book of the Opinions of Hippocrates and Plato'* (*Maqāla fī iʿtiḏārihi li-Ǧālīnūs fīmā qālahu fī l-maqāla al-sābiʿa min Kitāb Ārāʾ Abuqrāṭ wa-Aflāṭūn*), which Ibn Abī Uṣaybiʿa lists in his bibliographical entry on Ḥunayn (Riḍā 1965: p. 272 l. 17). Another small treatise entitled *On Light and its Nature* (*Fī l-ḍawʾ wa ḥaqīqatihi*), which is attributed to Ḥunayn in the manuscript tradition, suggests that Ḥunayn held an Aristotelian notion of vision. For the Arabic text of this work, see Cheikho (1899); for a German translation of it, see Prüfer and Meyerhof (1911). Arnzen (1998: 64, 716–17) disputes this text's attribution to Ḥunayn on linguistic and conceptual grounds.

قد يجب على من أراد معرفة طبيعة العين أن يكون بطبيعة الدماغ عالما، إذ كان مبدؤها منه ومنتهى فعلها يرجع إليه.[91]

> Whoever wishes to know the nature of the eye must be informed about the nature of the brain, because it [i.e. the eye] has its origin in it and the end of its activity returns to it [i.e. the brain].[92]

In *PAM*, Galen invokes the bond between the brain and eyes to discredit specialized approaches to the body: the links between the parts of the body speak against attempts to isolate them as discrete objects of care.[93] Ḥunayn, on the other hand, does not cite the relationship between the two organs as part of a rhetoric of exclusion but uses it to justify his extension of ophthalmic knowledge.[94]

Furthermore, by connecting the brain and the eye, Ḥunayn proposes that sensation is an appropriate subject of enquiry for those learning about the eyes. Following Galen and, more indirectly, Plato's *Timaeus*, he puts forward this close association between the two organs as evidence for the encephalocentric view of sensation that treatise three expounds.[95] At the beginning of the third treatise Ḥunayn goes so far as to say that complete knowledge of the condition of the eyes only comes from understanding how pneuma from the brain contributes to their activity (*fiʿl*), vision.[96] Treatise six illustrates the pertinence of this theoretical information to the diagnosis and treatment of ocular disorders: Ḥunayn attributes a range of 'latent eye affections' (*ālām al-ʿayn al-ḫafiyya*) – such as paralysis, myopia, and night blindness – to a change in the quality or quantity of the pneuma passing from the brain into the eyes.[97] This aetiology may be based on Galen's discussion of the same conditions in his lost *On the Diseases of the Eyes*, but, as I proposed above, this work probably did not encourage eye specialists to study how vision occurs, because Galen's primary purpose in broaching the subject is to polemicize against philosophers.[98]

91 Meyerhof (1928), p. 83 ll. 3–4. 92 Meyerhof (1928), 15 [modified]. 93 See p. 000 above.

94 As I remarked earlier (p. 80), Ḥunayn directs his advice to learned specialists of the eye, so his account is exclusionary in that it is elitist.

95 In his *Medical Questions* (*Masāʾil fī l-ṭibb*: Abū Rayyān, ʿArab, and Mūsa 1978: p. 9 ll. 4–6), Ḥunayn also asserts that the brain is the source of sensation.

96 Meyerhof (1928), 20 [English], 89 [Arabic].

97 Meyerhof (1928), 71–3 [English], 143–4 [Arabic].

98 Meyerhof (1928: 54n1) suggests that Galen's *On the Diagnosis of Eye Diseases* is Ḥunayn's source for treatise six. However, in his *Epistle* (Bergsträsser 1925: p. 30 ll. 10–14=Lamoreaux 2016: p. 69 ll. 10–13), Ḥunayn does not state that he translated this tract into Arabic; instead, he writes that Sergius of Rešʿaynā rendered the work into Syriac and that he himself found a Greek manuscript of the text, but did not have the time to translate it.

Ḥunayn's ophthalmological text forms a unified whole because each treatise provides the conceptual basis for its successor. The first treatise on ocular anatomy represents the core of his ophthalmology; Ḥunayn, however, has reason to treat the nature of the brain in treatise two as treatise one emphasizes the eyes' dependence on this organ.[99] Similarly, Ḥunayn can point to the brain's production of psychic pneuma as justification for his explanation of vision and other types of sensation in treatise three. Treatise four, which summarizes the information indispensable for successful medical treatment, proposes that eye-care professionals, similar to generalist doctors, must learn about not only the entire body but also 'knowledge of the thing[s] of nature' (*maʿrifat al-šay' al-ṭabīʿī*) – probably a periphrasis for physics.[100] In this respect, Ḥunayn's eye specialist appears to be almost indistinguishable from Galen's ideal doctor. By basing the study of the eye on the same principles as the broader discipline of medicine, Ḥunayn constructs an ophthalmology that is not vulnerable to the criticisms which Galen levels at the specialism in *PAM*. Moreover, this shared framework seems to enable ophthalmology to pursue the same lines of enquiry, pertaining to the body and beyond, that Galen allocates to medicine.

Cosmic Order and the Crystalline Humour

With its conception of the body as mirroring a wider natural order, Plato's *Timaeus* provides Galen with a teleology that he utilizes in *UP* to contest philosophy's monopoly on cosmic knowledge. In selecting most of his material in the first treatise of *Ten Treatises on the Eye* from *UP*, Ḥunayn produces an anatomy of the eye with a similarly pronounced teleological slant.[101] Whereas Galen makes inferences about the provident, teleological nature of creation from the structure of the human body, Ḥunayn seems to appeal to certain assumptions about the cosmos to describe ocular anatomical features such as the crystalline humour (Gr. τὸ κρυσταλλοειδὲς ὑγρόν; Arab. *al-ruṭūba al-ǧalīdiyya*), or lens. Ḥunayn diverges from

[99] See especially the subsection entitled 'the discourse on the brain' (*al-qawl ʿalā al-dimāġ*) in treatise one (Meyerhof 1928: 7 [English], 77 [Arabic]).

[100] See Meyerhof (1928), 40 [English], 112 [Arabic]. See also the note on Meyerhof (1928), 40; there, Meyerhof relates that he cannot track the Galenic source (if there is one) for the opening remarks about the knowledge involved in medical treatment. The rest of the chapter integrates passages from *CAM*, *Ars Med.*, and *MM*.

[101] In his *Epistle* (Bergsträsser 1925: p. 27 l. 13–p. 28 l. 8=Lamoreaux 2016: p. 63 ll. 4–13) Ḥunayn reports that Ḥubayš translated books one through sixteen – and he, book seventeen – of *UP* from Syriac into Arabic.

Galen not only in shifting the direction of his explanatory approach – that is, from using the body to explain the cosmos to using the cosmos to explain the body – but also by revising the text of *UP* to present a more coherent ocular anatomy. He begins with the innermost structure of the eye – the crystalline humour – and moves outwards. *Ten Treatises on the Eye* reports the following about this part of the organ:

> الرطوبة الجليدية ـ وأما الآن فنبتدئ بالقول في الرطوبة الجليدية. فنقول إنّها بيضاء صافية نيرة مستديرة ليست بمستحكمة الاستدارة بل فيها عرض، وهي في وسط العين كنقطة توهمناها في وسط كرة. أما بياضها ونورها وصفاؤها فلتقبل الاستحالة من الألوان سريعا، وذلك لأنّ الشيء الأبيض الصافي النير يسرع إلى قبول الألوان كالزجاجة الصافية وما أشبه ذلك. وأما استدارتها فلئلا يسرع إليها قبول الآلام، وذلك لأنّ كل شكل خلا المستدير تسرع إليه الآفة لما له من الزوايا. وأما عرضها فلتقبل من المحسوس أجزاء كثيرة، وذلك لأنّها لو كانت مستحكمة الاستدارة لما لقى منها المحسوس الا أجزاء يسيرة، وأما الشيء المسطح فأنّه يلقى مما يماسه أكثر مما يلقى الشيء الكري المستدير. وأما ما ذكر من أنّ موضعها في وسط العين فذلك دليل على أنّ جميع ما سواها مما في العين إنّما خلق لها، إما ليدفع عنها آفة، وإما ليؤدي إليها منفعة. ولذلك أحاطت بها الأجزاء من كل جانب وصارت هي في الوسط.[102]

> We will now begin with the discussion of the ice-like humour [i.e. crystalline humour], and we say: it is white, transparent, luminous, and round; its roundness, however, is not perfect [i.e. globe-shaped], but there is a flattening in it. It is situated in the middle of the eye, like a point which we imagine to be in the centre of the ball. Concerning its white colour, luminosity and transparency, [the purpose of these qualities is] to receive the changing of colours rapidly, since a white, transparent, luminous thing is quick to receive colours, as in the case of clear glass and similar substances. Its roundness serves [to prevent] it from being damaged, since any shape except the round one is very liable to receive injuries on account of its corners. Its flattened form enables it to receive impressions of more perceptible objects than would be the case if it were perfectly round; for a flattened body meets more of the objects which are in its path than does a perfectly spherical body. If we mentioned, moreover, that its place is in the centre of the eye, then it is a proof that all that surrounds it in the eye was created for it, either to protect it from injury or to be useful to it. Therefore, those parts surround it from all sides while it is in the middle itself.[103]

Ḥunayn has excerpted, loosely paraphrased, and combined several passages from *UP* 10.1–6, which cover the properties and function of the crystalline humour.[104] Here, as in Galen, the lens plays the most significant role in the visual process: images form on its surface when the surrounding air and pneuma

[102] Meyerhof (1928), p. 73 l. 13–p. 74 l. 9. [103] Meyerhof (1928), 3–4 [modified].

[104] For these passages, see Helmreich (1909), 55–6, 62, 75–6. Cf. MS Bibliothèque nationale de France, arabe 2853, fols. 170a, 172b, for the corresponding Arabic translation of the Greek text. I am grateful to Pauline Koetschet for sharing a copy of this manuscript with me.

from the brain collide. Akin to Aristotle's visual medium (the 'diaphanous'), the transparency of the crystalline humour, which Ḥunayn compares to 'clear glass' (*al-zuǧāǧa al-ṣāfiyya*), allows it to receive a variety of colours.[105]

Eastwood recognized that the lens has a more central position both structurally and functionally in Ḥunayn's ocular anatomy than in Galen's.[106] At *UP* 10.4 Galen appears to locate the crystalline humour at the anterior of the eye, close to the cornea.[107] *Ten Treatises on the Eye*, however, places it in the middle (*wasaṭ*) of the organ. An anatomical diagram in the oldest manuscript of the text, MS Ṭibb Taymūr 100, Dār al-Kutub (fol. 314, see Figure 1 below), depicts the part as a perfect circle surrounded by the other tunics (or layers) of the eye, which are drawn as concentric rings.[108] Ḥunayn may have followed a lost post-Galenic source in relocating the lens, but the increased centrality of the part seems to coincide with the more pronounced stress that he puts on its contribution to vision. The penultimate sentence of the above passage suggests that the tunics of the eye participate in a teleological hierarchy, where the outer layers serve the lens in either a protective or functional capacity.[109] Their activities are subordinate to the lens's task of receiving impressions of perceptible objects. This account of the eye's anatomy echoes the hierarchical conceptions of the body that Galen and the *Timaeus* put forward, according to which various relations of dependence link both larger and smaller structures. Stimulated by Galen's (and, more indirectly, Plato's) notion of teleological design, Ḥunayn modifies the description of the lens in *UP*: instead of attributing the flattened shape of the part to the economy of Nature, the above quotation maintains that this form enables the eye to accept a greater amount of what is perceived of the outside world.[110]

105 This comparison is not found in *UP*. 106 Eastwood (1982), 5–7.

107 The oldest extant Greek copy of *UP*, the tenth- or eleventh-century manuscript Vat. Urb. gr. 69, contains (fol. 118) a drawing of the eye that situates the lens towards the front of the organ. The illustration may be based on an ancient original, or the copyist may have drafted it in light of Galen's description of the eye. For a reproduction of the image, see the frontispiece in May (1968), vol. II.

108 The vitreous and albuminoid humours are illustrated as semicircles that make up a full circle, in which the lens is nested. Meyerhof (1928: 74) and Eastwood (1982: 8) rotate the folio in the Taymūr MS with the anatomical drawing so that the diagram represents a vertical cross-section of the eye. The four diagrams of the eye in the manuscript are the oldest surviving depictions of ocular anatomy. On anatomical illustrations in medieval Arabic manuscripts in general, see Savage-Smith (2007).

109 For example, Ḥunayn reports that the lens cannot take its nourishment directly from blood because the humour would stain the part's transparency. Thus, the vitreous humour exists to act as a medium through which the lens can take its nourishment without having to come into immediate contact with the blood (Meyerhof 1928: 6 [English], 75–6 [Arabic]).

110 As Eastwood (1982: 4–5) explains, Galen argues in *UP* that, if the lens were a perfect sphere, the lines coming from visible objects would not intersect certain sections of the eye. To avoid this waste of space, Nature flattened the lens.

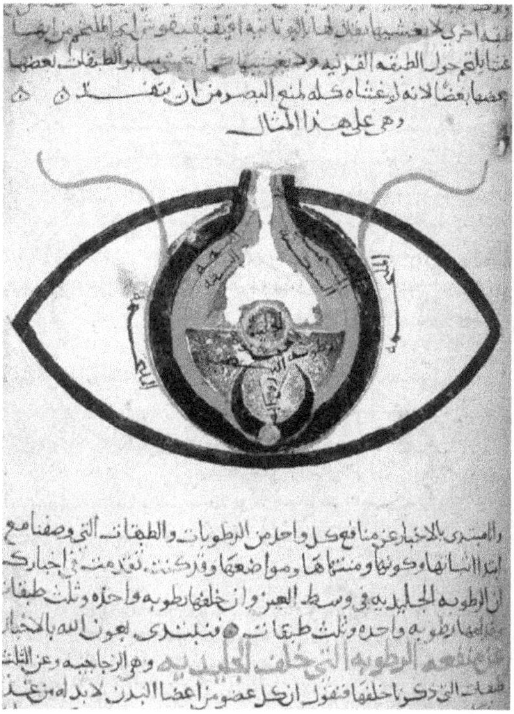

Figure 1 Anatomy of the tunics of the eye according to Ḥunayn's *Ten Treatises on the Eye* (Ṭibb Taymūr MS 100) (Source: wikicommons).

Ḥunayn cites the centrality of the crystalline humour as a 'proof' (*dalīl*) of its prime importance to the eye. He does not offer any grounds for this statement, which specifically alleges that the medial position of the lens entails that the tunics around the structure were 'created' (*ḫuliqa*) for it. He introduces it as if it were an axiom. Ḥunayn's use of a derivative of the root *ḫ-l-q*, which he employs to render δημιουργεῖν and other Timaean terms relating to divine craftsmanship in Galen, indicates that the proof may be based on his notion of cosmic order.[111] That is to say, the eye reflects a broader pattern of divine creation, which is characterized by a dominant centre and subordinate periphery. This power dynamic was at work in early ʿAbbāsid Baghdad; the city and the caliphs who lived there

[111] See, e.g., the Arabic translation of *Com. Tim.*, where δημιουργός is translated as *al-ḫāliq* (Kraus and Walzer 1951: p. 5 l. 13) and δημιουργεῖν as *ḫalaqa* (p. 9 l. 6). The root *ḫ-l-q* is also used in the Qurʾān to describe God's creative activity (see Arnaldez 1978; Peterson 2001).

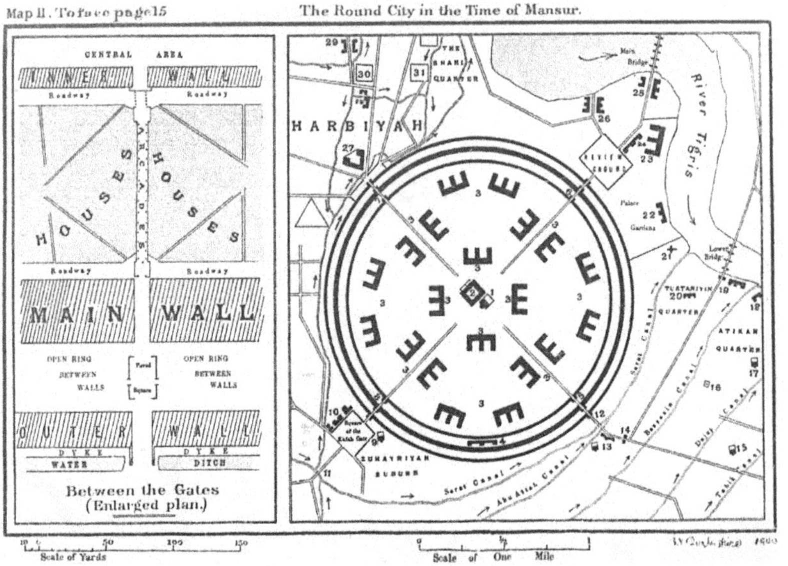

Figure 2 A map of eighth-century Baghdad's round city (G. Le Strange (1900), *Baghdad during the Abbasid caliphate from contemporary Arabic and Persian sources* London: Oxford University Press, p. 12).

represented the centre of the Muslim world and the cosmos itself.[112] It is worth noting that al-Manṣūr (r. 136–58/754–75), the second ʿAbbāsid caliph, constructed Baghdad on a circular plan, with two concentric defensive walls encircling the royal palace and mosque at the heart of the city (see Figure 2).[113] The original layout of Baghdad was a potent symbol of al-Manṣūr's centralized rule, and its resemblance to other earlier circular cities in the region, whose design supposedly mirrored a cosmic hierarchy, signifies that caliphal power encompasses both the earth and the heavens.

In mentioning Baghdad's circular plan, I am not proposing that Ḥunayn took direct inspiration from the place when outlining his anatomy of the eye, especially because caliphs after al-Manṣūr moved their palaces either away

[112] According to Gutas (1998: 28–52), the early ʿAbbāsid caliphs adopted Sasanian imperial ideology and political astrology, which emphasize the cosmic significance of the ruler, to legitimize their reign. This idea of cosmic kingship is not unique to the Sasanians but goes back at least to the Achaemenids. L'Orange (1953: 90–3) observes how certain reliefs and seals from Persepolis depict Ahuramazda and the Great King as standing in a ring, a symbol of the cosmos.

[113] See Lassner (1970), 121–46, 207, who reconstructs the city on the basis of medieval sources.

from the city centre or from the city altogether.[114] Instead, the reference helps to explain why Ḥunayn may not have found it necessary to establish the aforementioned 'proof' – 'Abbāsid society was structured around an individual who once resided at the very centre of the imperial capital. Furthermore, it reveals the extent to which earthly and cosmic hierarchies were intertwined for those under 'Abbāsid rule.[115] In a similar way to Plato's *Timaeus*, which depicts the eye as the paradigmatic product of the cosmic forces of Intellect and Necessity, *Ten Treatises on the Eye* portrays the organ as a model of cosmic order. Regardless of whether Ḥunayn intended his anatomy of the eye to recall al-Manṣūr's circular city, the connection certainly serves his text's body politics: the comparison appears to identify the eye as the centre of power in the body, and as a result privileges the specialist doctors concerned with its care.

Elementary Pairs

Ḥunayn expands on the notion of vision as a cosmic process, which is governed by macrocosmic principles, in his explanation of the five senses in treatises two and three. Based on *PHP* 7, the latter treatise reproduces Galen's Platonic assertion that vision and other kinds of sensation involve an attraction of like to like.[116] In the *Timaeus*, as I observed, this affinity relates to the tendency of the elements to move to their own kind: vision results from the meeting and union of three types of fire. Galen interprets this doctrine more loosely in alleging that a qualitative similarity – luminosity – accounts for the commingling of ocular pneuma and daylight in the visual process. Ḥunayn's text constructs a closer link between perception and the elements than in Galen through its suggestion that the elements determined both the creation and number of the senses. Ḥunayn states:

> وإذ كان الأمر على هذا فالصواب أن يقال: إنّ حاسة البصر نارية نورية وحاسة السمع هوائية وحاسة المذاق مائية وحاسة اللمس أرضية وحاسة الشم بخارية. وذلك أنّه لما كانت الأركان أربعة جعل لكل واحد منها حاسة بها يتعرف. وهو ما يحدث فيه من الحوادث المدركة حسا وأقرب إدراك ما عسر من بخارات حسا مفردة إذ كان البخار شيئا وسطا في طبيعته بين الهواء والماء فصارت خمسا من غير أن تكون الأركان خمسة.[117]

[114] Al-Mu'taṣim (r. 218–27/833–42), who ruled during Ḥunayn's lifetime, broke away from Baghdad completely by transferring the capital to Sāmarrā', which lies sixty miles north of the city (Lassner 1970: 154).

[115] Cf. al-Ma'mūn (r. 196–227/812–33), who situated himself as the central political and religious authority of 'Abbāsid society (Gutas 1998: 75–104).

[116] Ḥunayn prepared the Syriac translation of *PHP* from which Ḥubayš composed his Arabic version (Bergsträsser 1925: p. 26 l. 16–p. 27 l. 4=Lamoreaux 2016: p. 61 ll. 1–8).

[117] Meyerhof (1928), p. 110 ll. 5–12.

> Because the situation is like this, it is correct (*ṣawāb*) to say that the sense of vision is fiery (*nāriyya*) and luminous (*nūriyya*), the sense of hearing airy (*hawā'iyya*), the sense of taste watery (*mā'iyya*), the sense of touch earthy (*arḍiyya*), and the sense of smell vapoury (*buḫāriyya*). As there are four elements, a sense was made for each one of them by which each is recognized – namely the phenomena arising in them that are perceptible to the senses. Something approximate to perception is what arises from vapour and is perceived in an unusual [way], because the nature of vapour is halfway between air and water. Thus, there are five [senses] without the existence of five elements.[118]

The passage subordinates the creation of the senses to the creation of the elements. With the exception of smell, Ḥunayn pairs each sense with an element and cites these elementary bonds as the reason for their separation. Accordingly, vision and taste are distinct senses because they are matched respectively with fire and water. Ḥunayn denies the existence of a fifth element, the quintessence, and hews to Platonic tradition in viewing smell as a quasi-sense (*aqrab idrāk*), whose sensible object is between air and water.[119]

Ḥunayn bases his comments on *PHP* 7.5.42–6.1.[120] There, Galen quotes Empedocles, fr. DK 109B, 'By earth we perceive earth; by water, water; / air by shining air; and consuming fire by fire' (γαίῃ μὲν γὰρ γαῖαν ὀπώπαμεν, ὕδατι δ' ὕδωρ, | αἰθέρι δ' αἰθέρα δῖα, ἀτὰρ πυρὶ πῦρ ἀΐδηλον), to convey that perception arises from the alteration of similars (τῶν ὁμοίων ἀλλοιώσεως). Be that as it may, Galen does not explicitly pair off the elements with the senses, but prefaces his citation to Empedocles with the vague remark that 'it was needful' (δεόντως) that the organ of vision be luminous (αὐγοειδές), the organ of hearing airy (ἀεροειδές), and so on.[121] He comes very close to making this equation when introducing smell, which is the fifth sense 'although there are not five elements' (οὐκ ὄντων πέντε στοιχείων).[122] Ḥunayn, however, reads into the Empedocles fragment an aetiological link between the senses and the elements, which Galen does not develop. He seems to construe Galen's statement about the luminosity and airiness of the organs of sight and hearing as a 'correct' (*ṣawāb*) assumption that follows from this connection.

The adjectives that Galen employs at *PHP* 7.5.42 to describe the sense organs emphasize their qualitative kinship with, rather than direct

118 Meyerhof (1928), 37 [modified]. 119 See *Ti.* 66d4–e4 and below.
120 See De Lacy (2005), p. 462 ll. 1–24. 121 De Lacy (2005), p. 462 ll. 1–3.
122 De Lacy (2005), p. 462 ll. 20–1.

derivation from, the elements. To repeat what was discussed earlier, Galen – unlike the *Timaeus* – characterizes the visual stream as luminous rather than fiery. His choice of αὐγοειδές, instead of an adjective such as πυροειδές (lit. 'fire-like'), underscores the diminished role that fire plays in his theory of vision. Moreover, the suffix –ειδές (from εἶδος, 'kind') in these compound adjectives suggests that the sense organs are not literally made of air, water, earth, and vapour but belong to a category of things with a similar nature to these elements. This subtle distinction is lost in Ḥunayn's Arabic text: *nāriyya*, *nūriyya*, *hawāʾiyya*, *māʾiyya*, *arḍiyya*, and *buḫāriyya*, which derive from the roots for fire, air, water, earth, and vapour, may represent Arabic equivalents of Galen's Greek adjectives, but they do not capture the –ειδές suffix.[123] Although Ḥunayn may not have chosen these adjectives for the specific purpose of creating a more pronounced connection between the elements and sense organs, they contribute, nonetheless, to the passage's alignment of the body with the fundamental materials of the cosmos.

Treatise two seems to modify more conspicuously Galen's characterization of the sense organs as 'luminous' (αὐγοειδές), 'air-like' (ἀεροειδές), and so on. The relevant section describes the five sense objects: colour, sound, odour, flavour, and tactile qualities (for example, coldness and hardness). Ḥunayn adopts a significant part of the treatise from *UP* 8; his account of the sense objects follows roughly the sixth chapter of this book, which maintains, as in *PHP*, that sensation is an alteration of like by like. Galen writes in the chapter that the 'bright, luminous [sense organ]' (τὸ μὲν αὐγοειδές τε καὶ φωτοειδές) is altered by colours, the 'air-like [organ]' (τὸ δ' ἀερῶδες) by sound, and the 'vapour-like [organ]' (τὸ δ' ἀτμῶδες) by odours.[124] Implicit in Galen's statement is the idea that the eye, for instance, can be altered by colours because both are luminous and bright. Ḥunayn reworks this explanation in two respects: he clarifies how the sense objects are related to the four elements and proposes that the sense organs have a special affinity with certain elements on account of their respective coarseness or subtleness. His text reads:

والحواس خمس ألطفها البصر ومحسوسه النار وما كان من جنس النار أعني اللون. وأجناس النار ثلاثة، اللهب والحمرة والنور. الدليل على أنّ النور نار أنّه إذا جمع بزجاجة أو بجرم صاف أو مصقول أحرق. وبعد البصر في اللطافة السمع، ومحسوسه الهواء وما يعرض فيه أعني

[123] According to the *Glossarium Graeco-Arabicum* (http://telota.bbaw.de/glossga/), *ḥuwāʾiyya* renders ἀεροειδής in Qusṭā ibn Lūqā's translation of pseudo-Plutarch's *De Placitis Philosophorum*. Ullmann (2006: 194) also lists *nayyir*, which comes from the same root as *nāriyya* and *nūriyya*, for αὐγοειδής.

[124] Helmreich (1907), p. 464 ll. 13–17.

الصوت. لأنّ الصوت إنّما هو قرع في الهواء أو هواء متقرع، وبعد السمع الشم ومحسوسه البخار. والبخار هو شيء فيما بين الأرض والماء يلي الهواء في اللطافة. وبعد الشم المذاقة ومحسوسها الماء وما يقبل الماء. وذلك أنّ الطعوم إنّما تكون إذا خالط الماء شيئا من اليبس وعملت فيه الحرارة، سمى اليونانيون الشيء المطعوم <خولوس> وتفسيره السيال والمنصب. وأغلظ الحواس اللمس ومحسوسه الأرض وآلامها أي حالاتها، أعني الصلابة واللين والحرارة والبرودة والرطوبة واليبوسة وما يتولد عن ذلك.[125]

There are five senses and the finest (*alṭafuhā*) of them is vision. Its sensible object is fire (*al-nār*), namely what belongs to the class of fire (*min ğins al-nār*), that is, colour. There are three kinds (*ağnās*) of fire: flame (*al-lahab*), red heat (*al-ḥumra*), and light (*al-nūr*). The proof (*al-dalīl*) of the fact that light is fire is that, when it is concentrated in a glass or in a transparent or shining body, it causes burning. Next to vision the finest sense is that of hearing; its sensible object is the air (*al-huwā'*), namely what occurs in it, that is, sound, because sound is only a blow in the air or beaten air. After hearing comes the sense of smell; its sensible object is vapour (*al-buḫār*). Vapour is something between earth (*al-arḍ*) and water (*al-mā'*) and is not far behind the air in rarity (*al-laṭāfa*). After the sense of smell follows that of taste; its sensible object is water, namely what it absorbs [into itself]; for flavour is only possible when the water dissolves something solid and creates warmth in it. Therefore, the Greeks called the thing tasted *chylos*; its meaning is 'the distilled' and 'the poured out'. The coarsest (*ağlaẓ*) of the senses is that of touch; its sensible object is the earth, namely the feelings of it (*ālāmuhā*) or its states (*ḥālāt*), that is, hardness, softness, warmth, cold, humidity and dryness and what arises from these.[126]

Ḥunayn lists the four elements and vapour as the objects of the senses, but qualifies this identification by specifying that colour, for example, is a form of fire. *Min ğins al-nār* may represent a periphrasis for αὐγοειδές at *UP* 8.6; if so, Ḥunayn appears to stress, in line with Galen, that the sense objects are related generically to rather than made out of the four elements. Nonetheless, 'the proof' (*dalīl*) in the passage indicates that Ḥunayn regards fire as having a direct role in vision. He appears to refer to burning mirrors, which are parabolic lenses that concentrate sunlight into a small area and in so doing ignite the exposed surface, to argue that light is fire.[127]

125 Meyerhof (1928), p. 84 l. 11–p. 85 l. 4. 126 Meyerhof (1928), 16 [modified].

127 See Smith (2015), 159n80. Although Hellenistic authors such as Diocles (*fl.* 190–180 BCE) wrote about burning mirrors (πυρεῖα), Galen never mentions them in his writings. In *On Mixtures* (3.2, 1.657–8K) Galen transmits the famous account of how Archimedes burned the Roman fleet that attacked Syracuse during the second Punic War with πυρεῖα. Simms (1991) demonstrates that πυρεῖα means here 'incendiary material' rather than 'burning mirrors'. Ḥunayn, however, translated πυρεῖα as burning mirrors (*al-marāyā al-muḥriqa*) in his Arabic version of *On Mixtures* (Dold-Samplonius 2007). The works on burning mirrors by Diocles and Anthemius of Tralles (sixth century), one of the architects of the Hagia Sophia, were translated into Arabic and used by al-Kindī and other medieval optical writers (Smith 2015: 172).

Therefore, his conception of light corresponds more closely to the theory of light in Plato's *Timaeus*, which Aristotle and later Peripatetics rejected, than that of Galen, who classifies light as a luminous substance in *PHP*.[128]

Ḥunayn orders the senses in the above quotation in accordance with their 'rarity' or 'fineness' (*al-laṭāfa*). As Eastwood remarks, this scale can designate either a quantitative or qualitative distinction: it may rank the senses by their weight and density or by the composition of their substance.[129] Regardless of the ambiguity of this gradation, it forms the basis on which the senses are paired with the elements. Ḥunayn's text implies that, as vision is the finest sense, its object is fire, which is the rarest element, and hearing goes with air because both are second in fineness or rarity, and so on. Because this ranking of the elements became standard after Plato and Aristotle, Ḥunayn takes it for granted that his reader requires no rationale for it.[130] The treatise's comments about the 'rarity' of the senses seem to serve as a gloss on Galen's assertion at *UP* 8.6 that the sense organs are altered only by objects similar in nature to them. Galen, at least in *UP*, does not expand on how, for example, colour is like the 'bright, luminous [sense organ]'. To supplement this exegetical lacuna, Ḥunayn proposes that the homogeneity between vision and colour, as well as the other senses and sense objects, is based on the degree of their rareness or coarseness. By linking the sense objects with the elements, Ḥunayn does not have to work to establish that, for example, colour is 'rarer' than sound, as he can appeal to a canonical doctrine from ancient physics to support this hierarchy.

In making this equation of the sense objects with the elements, Ḥunayn draws on Galen's *Com.Tim.*, which he and his junior colleague ʿĪsā ibn Yaḥyā ibn Ibrāhīm translated into Arabic.[131] The definition of odour in the above passage demonstrates that Ḥunayn made use of Galen's summary of the dialogue, for it classifies the sense object as a mixture of earth and water rather than of air and water, as *PHP* does following *Ti.* 66d8–e2.[132]

[128] I mentioned above (p. 88n90) that a treatise entitled *On Light and its Nature* circulated under Ḥunayn's name. In contradiction to *Ten Treatises on the Eye*, the work, following Philoponus, dismisses the idea that light is a fiery body (Cheikho 1899: p. 1109 ll. 12–17).

[129] Eastwood (1982), 18–19.

[130] Cf. Plato and Aristotle, who order the elements according to their relative weights and therefore tendency to move upwards or downwards in the cosmos. See *Ti.* 63a–e and *DC* 4.3–4 (310a–312a).

[131] Bergsträsser (1925), p. 50 l. 14–p. 51 l. 2, with corrections from Bergsträsser (1932), p. 23 l. 10–11=Lamoreaux (2016), p. 125 l. 9–p. 127 l. 2. In particular, Ḥunayn has drawn on Galen's description of the sense objects at *Com.Tim.* §§ 15–16: Kraus and Walzer (1951), p. 19 l. 15–p. 22 l. 13.

[132] Eastwood (1982), 17n53. Cf. *PHP* 7.6.1 (De Lacy 2005: p. 462 ll. 20–4) and *Com.Tim.* § 15 (Kraus and Walzer 1951: p. 20 ll. 11–13). See also Eastwood (1981), who examines Galen's varying accounts of the elements involved in smell.

Furthermore, Ḥunayn's list of species of fire parallels Galen's in *Com. Tim.*, which is based on *Ti.* 58c5–d1. Ḥunayn and the Arabic version of *Com. Tim.* differ, on the other hand, in that the former reads *al-nūr* instead of *al-ḍaw'* for φλόξ ('light').[133] To emphasize vision's association with fire, Ḥunayn may have selected *al-nūr* rather than *al-ḍaw'* because it derives from the root for fire (*n-w-r*). This method of employing Galen to explain Galen reflects the translation practices of Ḥunayn's circle.[134] In this particular case, Ḥunayn has appealed to a Galenic exegesis of Plato's *Timaeus* to flesh out Galen's theory of sensation in *UP*, which also has roots in the *Timaeus*. Thus, Ḥunayn's incorporation of material from *Com. Tim.* into the *Ten Treatises on the Eye* results in the development of a doctrine of sensation which appears to be more Timaean than Galen's. The dialogue's conception of the eye as possessing the same teleological structure, operating on the same principles, and composed of the same fundamental materials as the macrocosm, helps Ḥunayn to establish ophthalmologists as stakeholders in cosmic knowledge.

Conclusion: The Eye, a Cosmic and Disciplinary Threshold

As I have shown, *Ten Treatises on the Eye* does not treat the eye as an independent unit but situates it in relation to the larger systems of the body and cosmos. In the passages examined so far, Ḥunayn's composition constructs a relationship between the eye and macrocosm by discussing how purposeful design and the elementary principle of like to like are at work even at this corporeal level. The *Timaeus* elevates the eye as a paradigm of cosmic creation because it operates due to these principles, which are governed by Intellect and Necessity. Galen, on the other hand, refers to the organ's exemplary teleological structure as the sole reason for its superior status. When concluding his account of vision at the end of treatise three, Ḥunayn goes further than both of these sources in assigning a special cosmic significance to the eye. For him, vision, unlike other forms of sensory perception, is a process that involves the supra-lunary realm, the planets and fixed stars. He maintains that the 'heavenly bodies' are responsible for the colours that we see:

133 *Ten Treatises on the Eye* also reads *al-ḥumra* instead of *al-ǧamra* ('embers') for διάπυρος (lit. 'red-hot'), but this change may be due to a scribal error because these terms only differ orthographically by one diacritical dot.

134 See Overwien (2012), 157–61.

حتى يكاد أن يكون به تغير الهواء من قبل هذه الثلاثة تغيرا لازما له. أعني من نور الشمس ومن الألوان الناضرة المشرقة التي للأجسام العلوية ومن الروح الباصر الصادم له عند خروجه من الحدقتين.[135]

> Thus, the air is considerably and necessarily altered by the influence of these three things: sunlight, the colours radiating and shining from the heavenly bodies (*al-ağsām al-ʿulwiyya*), and the optic pneuma which strikes it on leaving the pupils.[136]

Three levels of creation – the body, the world, and the heavens – converge at the eye. At the organ's surface, the optic pneuma exiting the body comingles with the air, which has been transformed by sunlight and the 'heavenly bodies', to form a continuous path of transmission from the brain to the perceived object.[137] The eye functions as a threshold through which the body can reach out into the macrocosm, and vice versa.

Galen, on whom Ḥunayn draws in treatise three to articulate his text's theory of vision, does not acknowledge that the planets and fixed stars have a role in the visual process. Prior to the above quotation, Ḥunayn summarizes Galen's 'clear proof' (*dalāla bayyina*) at *PHP* 7.7.1–4 of the importance of bright air for colour perception: namely, how, if a person were to recline under a tree in this type of air, the tree's colour would envelop them.[138] According to Galen, daylight, bright air, and pneuma are the three requirements for vision.[139] Ḥunayn's elder contemporary al-Kindī (*c.* 185–252/801–66) alleges that the 'light of the stars' (*ḍiyāʾ kawkabī*) contributes to the colour of the sky, so the idea that the 'heavenly bodies' determine, to some extent, human perception of colour was current at the very least.[140] Ḥunayn departs from Galen and even Plato in considering the bond between the eyes and macrocosm to be more than analogical. That is to say, these organs not only serve as corporeal examples of the teleological order and mechanical principles

[135] Meyerhof (1928), p. 111 ll. 6–9. [136] Meyerhof (1928), 38 [modified].
[137] See Meyerhof (1928), 37 [English], p. 109 l. 18–p. 110 l. 4 [Arabic].
[138] Cf. De Lacy (2005), p. 470 ll. 3–17; Meyerhof (1928), p. 110 ll. 11–20 [English translation at 38].
[139] Cf. Nemesius, who writes at *On the Nature of Man* 8 (van der Eijk and Sharples 2008: 109) that vision requires 'an unimpaired sense-organ, suitable movement and suitable distance, and clear and bright air' (ἀβλαβοῦς αἰσθητηρίου, συμμέτρου κινήσεως καὶ διαστήματος, ἀέρος καθαροῦ καὶ λαμπροῦ).
[140] See al-Kindī's *Cause of the Blue Colour of the Sky* (*Fī ʿillat al-lawn al-lāzuwardī allāḏī yurā fī l-ğaww fī ğihat al-samāʾ wa yaẓunnu annahu lawn al-samāʾ*): Spies (1937), p. 14 ll. 1–5 [English translation at 17]. Another point of contact between Ḥunayn and al-Kindī's explanations of colour, which is suggestive of a shared lost source, is that both of them refer to glass (*zuğāğa*) to demonstrate how transparency is involved in colour perception. Cf. p. 91 above and Spies (1937), p. 14 ll. 10–11 [English translation at 18].

of the macrocosm but also function because their inner substance, pneuma, is transformed by the macrocosm, or heavens. While the *Timaeus* associates the eyes with the heavens by alleging that the former was created to observe the latter, it does not attribute to the stars or planets any direct influence on the visual process.[141]

Situated in the body but also facing out towards the cosmos, the eye in *Ten Treatises of the Eye* is a space that offers opportunities for disciplinary boundary work. Against Galen's characterization of ophthalmology as knowledge cut off from the complex of medicine, Ḥunayn construes the specialism as a unified system that extends from the body to the heavens – domains over which doctors and philosophers asserted their authority. As this chapter has shown, Ḥunayn co-opts Galen's tactic of using Plato's *Timaeus* to expand medicine's parameters to perform his own boundary work. Through Galen's writings he appeals to the dialogue's identification of the brain as the seat of sensation to argue that, as the eyes are outgrowths of this organ, bodily perception falls within the specialism's remit. In so doing, Ḥunayn subverts and turns to his own advantage Galen's exclusionary rhetoric in *PAM*, which invokes the eye's participation in the larger network of the body to attack the division of medicine into sub-fields dedicated to the care of individual organs. Furthermore, the *Timaeus*' notion of teleological design and principle of like to like (as filtered through Galen) allows Ḥunayn to make two reciprocal arguments that serve to entangle the specialized study of the eye and philosophy. Ḥunayn implies that the anatomical structure and function of the eyes are inexplicable without understanding the order and elements of the cosmos, but he also leaves the impression that the organ's involvement with both the sub- and supra-lunary worlds gives its specialists privileged access to knowledge of these realities.

I have proposed that this representation of philosophy as a preliminary to ophthalmology works to weaken its claim to higher epistemic standing. Ḥunayn's idealized education in *Ten Treatises on the Eye* promotes specialized knowledge over philosophy and general medicine by reducing the two fields to steps in its acquisition. This shift in the past educational pattern – where specialization, as the more accessible course of study, tended to precede general training for many practitioners – generates an elite ophthalmology that requires a considerable expenditure of time and money to learn. Ḥunayn seems to erase the specialism's non-elite associations, and thus enhance its prestige and authority, by endowing it with the

[141] See *Ti.* 47a1–c6.

same intellectual underpinnings as Galenic medicine. The wide circulation of *Ten Treatises on the Eye* among a diverse range of pre-modern Islamicate and European readers (eye doctors, philosophers, and mathematicians) testifies to the success of Ḥunayn's rehabilitation and expansion of ophthalmology as a respectable pursuit that cuts across traditional disciplinary lines.[142]

[142] For later Arabic, Persian, and Latin ophthalmological writers' use of the text, see Hirschberg (1908), 34–7. On its contribution to optics, see Lindberg (1976) *passim*.

CHAPTER 3

Al-Rāzī: The 'Arab Galen' and his Plato, New Disciplinary Ideals

The critical reception of Abū Bakr Muḥammad ibn Zakariyyā᾽ al-Rāzī (251–*c.* 313/865–*c.* 925) in the medieval period reflects a contemporary anxiety about maintaining a distinct boundary between medicine and philosophy.[1] Al-Rāzī's detractors censured him for writing on the 'divine science' (*ilāhiyyāt*, 'metaphysics' or 'theology'), the superior part of philosophy according to the medieval hierarchy of the sciences, when his expertise lay in medicine.[2] Avicenna, whose own views about the relationship between medicine and philosophy will be discussed in the next chapter, retorts in an epistolary exchange with al-Bīrūnī, who was more sympathetic to al-Rāzī's philosophical endeavours, that

محمد بن زكرياء الرازي المتكلف الفضولي في شروحه في الإلاهيات وتجاوز قدره في بط الجراح والنظر في الأبوال والبرازات.[3]

> Muḥammad ibn Zakariyyā᾽ al-Rāzī [was] misleading and meddlesome when he explained metaphysics (*al-ilāhiyyāt*).[4] He exceeded (*taǧāwaza*) his capacity for sewing wounds and examining urines and faeces.

In his letter to Samuel ibn Tibbon, the Hebrew translator of the *Guide for the Perplexed* (*Dalālat al-ḥā᾽irīn*), Maimonides offers a similar, though less caustic, evaluation of al-Rāzī's work on metaphysics:

[1] Al-Rāzī's bibliographer, Abū l-Rayḥān al-Bīrūnī (Kraus 1936b: p. 6 ll. 1–3) gives 5 Šaʿbān 313/26 October 925 for al-Rāzī's death date. For other (more improbable) dates for his death, see Kahl (2015), 2n2.

[2] On this hierarchy and its late antique provenance, see the Introduction (pp. 19–22).

[3] *Questions and Answers* (*al-As᾽ila wa l-aǧwiba*): Naṣr and Muḥaqqiq (1995), p. 13 ll. 10–13. Similar to al-Rāzī, al-Bīrūnī opposed key Aristotelian tenets such as the eternity of the world, which he challenged Avicenna to defend in their correspondence. Furthermore, while contemporary and later Islamicate authors condemned al-Rāzī's theological writings as heretical, al-Bīrūnī writes, 'I do not believe that he set out to delude but rather was deluded himself' (*lastu aʿtaqidu fīhī muḫādaʿatan inḫidāʿan*: Kraus 1936b: p. 4 ll. 11–12) after reading the works of Mani (*c.* 216–74 CE). On these charges of heresy, see below.

[4] Avicenna appears to be referring here to al-Rāzī's discussion of metaphysics in his lost *Book of the Divine Science* (*Kitāb al-ʿIlm al-ilāhī*). For the medieval witnesses to this text, see Kraus (1939), 165–90.

והחכמה האלהית לאלראזי הוא ספר אין בו תועלת כי ראזי רופא היה לבד.[5]

The *Metaphysics* of al-Rāzī is a useless book because al-Rāzī was only a doctor.

Finally, the philosopher al-ʿĀmirī (d. 381/992), a near-contemporary of al-Rāzī, dismisses those who hold that medical expertise implies an ability to handle philosophical subjects:

والعجب من أهل زماننا أنّهم متى رأوا إنسانا قرأ كتاب أقليدس وضبط أصول المنطق، وصفوه بالحكمة، وإن كان خلوا من العلوم الإلهية؛ حتى أنّهم ينسبون محمد بن زكريا الرازي لمهارته في الطب إليها – هذا، أعزك الله، مع صنوف هذيانه في القدماء الخمسة وفي الأرواح الفاسدة.[6]

The extraordinary thing about the people of our own time is that when they see that a person has read Euclid's book [i.e. the *Elements*] and mastered the principles of logic, they attribute wisdom to him even if he completely lacks knowledge of the divine sciences [i.e. metaphysics]. Thus, they ascribe wisdom to Muḥammad ibn Zakariyyāʾ al-Rāzī because of his proficiency in medicine – (God bless you!) in spite of his various ravings about the five eternals and corrupt spirits.[7]

These three authors pigeonhole al-Rāzī as a doctor, and they characterize his foray into metaphysics as a disciplinary transgression: coming from the inferior science of medicine, al-Rāzī was incapable of answering philosophical questions. They cite his medical career as part of a polemical strategy to discredit his metaphysical theories, with which they disagree.

Echoing this medieval assessment, Kraus and Pines give more weight to al-Rāzī's medical accomplishments and write, in their entry on him in the *Encyclopaedia of Islam*, that 'Rāzī is above all a physician and he is rightly regarded as the greatest physician of Islām'.[8] The fragmentary state of al-Rāzī's philosophical treatises, in contrast to the wide circulation of his medical texts in Arabic, Hebrew, Latin, and European vernaculars, seems to indicate that they had a limited readership in the Middle Ages.[9] Al-Rāzī's alleged rejection of prophecy – a heretical position for a Muslim or

[5] Originally composed in Arabic, this letter survives in several Hebrew versions, two of which have been edited by Marx (1935: 375–81). I reproduce Marx's (1935: 378) transcription of the passage in Codex Adler 2013.

[6] *On the Afterlife* (*Kitāb al-Amad ʿalā al-abad*): Rowson (1988), p. 74 ll. 15–18.

[7] The translation is from Stroumsa (1999), 92 [with minor modifications].

[8] Kraus and Pines (2012).

[9] On the formative role of al-Rāzī's medical works in medicine in the medieval East and West, see Jacquart (1996), 970–5, 978; Pormann and Savage-Smith (2007), 163–4.

any adherent of a revealed religion – is often cited as the reason for the unpopularity of and outright hostility to his philosophical ideas.[10]

Considering his eminence in medicine, it may come as a surprise that al-Rāzī was a relative latecomer to the field. As his name reveals, al-Rāzī was born in the ancient Iranian city of Rayy, where he dedicated his youthful studies to philosophy, alchemy, literature, and music.[11] Ibn Abī Uṣaybiʿa reports that al-Rāzī was inspired to take up medicine in his thirties after seeing a boy with two faces in a hospital in Rayy.[12] Regardless of the veracity of this account, al-Rāzī quickly gained a reputation for his medical learning and was put in charge of the large hospital in Rayy. He travelled to Baghdad some time in the 280s/late 890s, and directed at least one hospital there.[13] Towards the end of his life, and suffering from blindness due to cataracts, al-Rāzī returned to his native city, where he died in his early sixties after purportedly refusing medical treatment for his infirmity.[14]

Al-Rāzī appears to have earned the sobriquet 'the Arab Galen' (*Ǧālīnūs al-ʿarab*) because of his intense preoccupation with medicine.[15] While the designation is complimentary in this context, in the eyes of some of his successors al-Rāzī was too similar to Galen: he made the same disciplinary mistakes. As the following two chapters will show, Avicenna and Maimonides admonish Galen not only for entering into philosophical debates that were beyond his medical expertise but also for claiming that these debates were relevant to medicine.[16] These criticisms mirror those

10 See Kraus (1939), who has collected the fragments and testimonia of the surviving philosophical texts by al-Rāzī. In this chapter I will not address whether al-Rāzī actually held heretical views about prophecy. Modern scholars disagree about his position on prophecy and his religiosity in general. For instance, Mahdi (1996: 150) proposes that, if al-Rāzī rejected the validity of prophecy, 'one cannot call him a Muslim philosopher in the proper sense of the term'. Stroumsa (1999: 13–14) cautions that al-Rāzī's dismissal of prophecy does not necessarily imply radical apostasy; instead, she presents him as a 'freethinker', or sceptic of revealed religions. Cf. Rashed (2008: 179), who argues that al-Rāzī is not anti-prophetic but rather critical of the possibility of miracles.

11 On al-Rāzī's life and for a list of his works, see al-Bīrūnī's *List of al-Rāzī's Books* (*Fihrist kutub al-Rāzī*): Kraus (1936b); Ullmann (1970), 129–37; Sezgin (1970), 274–94; Goodman (1995); Kahl (2015), 1–2.

12 Riḍā (1965), p. 414 l. 24–p. 415 l. 10. Ibn Abī Uṣaybiʿa identifies the source of this story as the *Book on Hospitals* (*Kitāb fī l-Bīmāristānāt*) by Abū Saʿīd Manṣūr b. ʿĪsā, who was nicknamed 'the ascetic of the scholars' (*zāhid al-ʿulamāʾ*).

13 Kahl (2015: 2n27) proposes that al-Rāzī may have headed either the Barāmika or Muʿtaḍidī hospitals, or possibly both. At the time of al-Rāzī's arrival in Baghdad only the Barāmika hospital, which was built during the reign of Hārūn al-Rašīd (r. 170–93/786–809), was in service. Al-Rāzī, however, appears to have been involved in the selection of the site of the Muʿtaḍidī hospital, which was founded around 287/900.

14 Al-Bīrūnī (Kraus 1936b, p. 5 ll. 8–14) relates that an oculist from Ṭabaristān (a province in northern Iran) travelled to Rayy to treat al-Rāzī's cataract. Al-Rāzī allegedly declined the treatment out of fear of the pain that the procedure would cause.

15 Riḍā (1965), p. 415 l. 10.

16 See Chapters 4 and 5.

targeted at al-Rāzī in the above passages – although it is important to note that, despite his pagan beliefs, Galen was not maligned for his religious views as was the Muslim al-Rāzī.[17] This chapter will examine al-Rāzī's attempts to present himself, a doctor with a command of the 'divine science', as the most reliable investigator of the cosmos in contrast to Galen's limited philosopher-doctor. In so doing, it will highlight how al-Rāzī undermines his predecessor's credibility by claiming to have a better understanding of Plato's *Timaeus*.

My analysis will demonstrate that Galen was a model that al-Rāzī set out not just to imitate but to surpass. Al-Rāzī held that science was progressive, and therefore he did not view Galen as the final point, or 'seal' (*ḫātam*), in the development of the medical tradition.[18] He invokes the idea of scientific progress to justify his own critical approach to Galen's theories in the *Doubts about Galen* (*al-Šukūk ʿalā Ǧālīnūs*), with which this chapter will primarily deal.[19] Shihadeh classifies al-Rāzī's book as an 'aporetic commentary', a type of exegesis that identifies weak points in a system of thought with the aim of either making it more robust or replacing it with an alternative.[20] As I will explain, the *Doubts* represents al-Rāzī's effort to reshape Galenic medicine by extending its philosophical scope. In particular, I will show how al-Rāzī argues for the relevance of medicine to certain metaphysical issues, and vice versa, when disputing Galen's readings of several doctrines from the *Timaeus*. Chapter 1 suggested that Galen appeals to the dialogue in his 'Timaean' works to redefine medicine's epistemic purview; I will illustrate here that al-Rāzī similarly views the text as an instrument which he can utilize to accomplish his own disciplinary boundary work.

Chiefly, this chapter will argue that, because the *Timaeus* is central to both Galen and al-Rāzī's disciplinary projects, al-Rāzī tries to weaken the

[17] As Strohmaier (1968, 2012) has demonstrated, Ḥunayn and his associates often altered or even omitted from their Galenic translations material that would be offensive to monotheistic readers, so these efforts shaped Galen's Islamicate reception.

[18] In the *Chronology of Doctors* (*Taʾrīḫ al-aṭibbāʾ*), Isḥāq ibn Ḥunayn refers to Galen as the 'seal' of the ancient medical tradition, which recalls Muḥammad's title as the 'seal of the prophets' (*ḫātam al-nabiyyīn*). For the passage, see Rosenthal (1954), 65. On the significance of this description of Galen, see Das (2017b), 175–6.

[19] See Koetschet (2019), p. 4 l. 16–p. 6 l. 13. For an English translation of this passage, see McGinnis and Reisman (2007), 50. In what follows I refer to Koetschet's (2019) Arabic text of the *Doubts about Galen* (hereafter *Doubts*), which improves on the previous editions of Muḥaqqiq (2005) and ʿAbd al-Ġanī (2009). I wish to thank Pauline Koetschet for sharing over the years her research on and thoughts about the *Doubts*, which have greatly informed my own interpretation of the work.

[20] See Shihadeh (2015), 45–6. The aporetic commentary is a genre of exegesis that goes back at least to late antiquity; see, e.g., Damascius' (sixth century) *Doubts and Solutions Concerning First Principles*, which is part of the commentary tradition on Plato's *Parmenides*. See Rappe (2010) for an English translation of Damascius' text and an analysis of his dialectical strategy.

epistemic authority of his precursor – and therefore his vision of medicine – by pointing out the flaws in his interpretations of Plato. My examination of the *Doubts*' attack on Galen's position on cosmic creation will suggest that al-Rāzī depicts him as an Aristotelian to separate him further from Plato. Moreover, in considering al-Rāzī's response to Galen and later Galenists' opinions about pleasure and the immortality of the soul, I will contend that he champions a more metaphysical reading of Plato, which links questions about the body and the cosmos to the nature of God. To understand how al-Rāzī defines his Platonism, the first part of this chapter will review the ideas that he attributes to Plato and the possible sources for them. I should stress, however, that this survey is not intended to be exhaustive, if this is even achievable given the fragmentary state of al-Rāzī's philosophical oeuvre. It will become clear that, as with the other Islamicate authors examined in this book, Galen is an important source of al-Rāzī's knowledge of Plato and the *Timaeus*. Therefore, the Platonism that the *Doubts* formulates in opposition to Galen's Platonism – what I call al-Rāzī's 'anti-Platonism' – also relies on Galenic interpretations of Plato.

Apart from his prefatory remarks apologizing for his critique of Galen, al-Rāzī does not state how the *Doubts* advances a more expansive medicine. In general, the book seems unsystematic in that there is no explanation of the selection and order of the Galenic texts treated in it.[21] Before moving on to al-Rāzī's disputes with Galen and later followers' readings of Plato's *Timaeus*, I will discuss his conception of medicine in the tracts *The Philosopher's Way of Life* (*al-Sīra al-falsafiyya*), *The Guide* (*Kitāb al-Muršid*, also referred to as *The Book of Aphorisms*, *Kitāb al-Fuṣūl*), and the *Secret of the Art of Medicine* (*Sirr ṣināʿat al-ṭibb*) to contextualize his boundary work in the *Doubts*. My aim is to demonstrate that, by criticizing Galen's interpretation of Plato, al-Rāzī sets out in the *Doubts* to produce a medicine where doctors are epistemic authorities over not only the physical but also the metaphysical.

The Platonism of al-Rāzī

Although al-Rāzī's theory of scientific progress asserts that later thinkers are better equipped to perfect their disciplines, he prefers Plato and the 'ancient philosophers' (*qudamāʾ al-falāsifa*) over Aristotle and his

[21] An exception to this silence is al-Rāzī's comments about the first work that he critiques – *On Demonstration*. He writes that he has started with *DD* because 'it is the most important and most useful book ever, after the books of divine revelation' (Koetschet 2019: p. 6 ll. 16–17; McGinnis and Reisman 2007: 51).

commentators.[22] According to the historian Ṣāʿid al-Andalusī (420–62/1029–70), al-Rāzī supposedly attacked Aristotle for perverting the teachings of Plato and earlier philosophers. In his *Book of the Categories of Nations* (*Kitāb Ṭabaqāt al-umam*), Ṣāʿid connects al-Rāzī's strong opposition to Aristotle with his support of the 'old natural philosophy' (*al-falsafa al-ṭabīʿiyya al-qadīma*), which stems from Pythagoras:

وممن صنف في ذلك أبو بكر محمد بن زكرياء الرازي وكان شديد الانحراف عن أرسطاطاليس وعائبا له في مفارقة معلمه أفلاطون وغيره من متقدمي الفلاسفة في كثير من آرائهم، وكان يزعم أنّه أفسد الفلسفة وغير كثيرا من أصولها. وما أظن الرازي أحنقه على أرسطاطاليس وحداه إلى تنقصه إلا ما أباه أرسطاطاليس.[23]

> Belonging to this group [i.e. the adherents of the old natural philosophy] is Abū Bakr Muḥammad ibn Zakariyyāʾ al-Rāzī. He vehemently turned against Aristotle and faulted him for disagreeing with most of the opinions of his teacher Plato and the other philosophers who preceded him [i.e. Plato]. He claimed that [Aristotle] corrupted philosophy and altered most of its principles. I believe that al-Rāzī bore malice towards and criticized Aristotle only because the [early philosophers'] views were in conflict with Aristotle's.

As the passage relates, al-Rāzī seems to have accused Aristotle of fundamentally changing the philosophy of Plato and the Presocratics for the worse. Ṣāʿid himself was partial to Aristotle, so this report may represent a polemical exaggeration of al-Rāzī's attitude.[24] Al-Rāzī's criticism of standard Aristotelian positions, such as the eternity of the cosmos, does not necessarily imply a sweeping rejection of Aristotle's thought, as Ṣāʿid appears to assume.[25] For instance, unlike Ḥunayn's stance in the *Ten Treatises on the Eye*, al-Rāzī holds an intromissive theory of vision, which shows influence from late antique readings of Aristotle's *De Anima*.[26] Thus, notwithstanding the claims of Ṣāʿid and even al-Rāzī himself, al-Rāzī's philosophy is not 'untainted' by the Aristotelian tradition.[27]

[22] In the *Doubts* (Koetschet 2019: p. 6 ll. 7–13), al-Rāzī acknowledges that his theory could be interpreted as claiming that all later scientists are superior to the ancients. However, he asserts that later scholars have mainly refined the discoveries of their forerunners. See also Mahdi (1996), 151.

[23] Kraus (1939), § 7, p. 180 l. 2–p. 181 l. 6.

[24] After recounting al-Rāzī's philosophical views, Ṣāʿid eulogizes Aristotle for purifying philosophy by removing from it the wickedness (*ḫubṯ*) of earlier scholars' views; see ʿAlwān (1985), p. 96 ll. 5–6.

[25] For al-Rāzī's views on the creation of the cosmos, see pp. 110–12, 122–8 below.

[26] See Koetschet (2017), 183–7, who identifies Themistius' paraphrase of *DA* as a possible source for al-Rāzī's explanation of colour perception.

[27] Cf. Galen's desire to separate himself from the Aristotelian tradition (see van der Eijk 2009).

While Ṣāʿid's text describes al-Rāzī as a modern exponent of the *maḏhab* ('doctrinal system' or 'school') of Pythagoras, in his surviving works al-Rāzī most closely aligns himself with Socrates and Plato.[28] He refers to Socrates as his *imām* ('leader') and presents him as his ethical model in the *Book on Spiritual Medicine* (*Kitāb fī l-Ṭibb al-rūḥānī*) and *The Philosopher's Way of Life*.[29] Nonetheless, he appears to give precedence to Plato in calling him the 'master and the great one of the philosophers' (*šayḫ al-falāsifa wa ʿaẓīmuhā*).[30] Modern scholars often characterize al-Rāzī as a Platonist, but they point out that his knowledge of Platonic ethics, physics, and metaphysics is limited to the *Timaeus*.[31] In contrast to his near contemporary al-Fārābī (d. 339/950), al-Rāzī does not demonstrate any familiarity with the *Republic* and *Laws*; the *Timaeus* is the only dialogue that he cites by name.[32] This one dialogue, however, pervades al-Rāzī's thought: its cosmogony may have inspired his theory of the five eternals (*al-qudamāʾ al-ḫamsa*), which is the basis of his metaphysics.

The reports of al-Rāzī's metaphysical views relay that he attributed the creation of the cosmos to the interaction of five eternal things: the Creator (*al-bāriʾ*), soul (*nafs*), matter (*hayūlā*), absolute time (*zamān*), and absolute space (*makān*; or in some sources, void, *ḫalāʾ*).[33] Desiring union with matter, soul initiated cosmic creation by descending into the material world, which is composed of atoms. Owing to the chaos caused by the fall of soul, the Creator intervened to rectify the damage and to check the processes set into motion. Out of compassion for soul, the Creator gave her intellect (*ʿaql*) so that she might come to realize the folly of her descent and therefore seek a way to return back to the tranquillity of the upper world.[34]

28 See Kraus (1939), § 7, p. 180 ll. 1–2.

29 For Socrates as al-Rāzī's *imām*, see *Philosopher's Way of Life*: Kraus (1939), p. 99 l. 5; Walker (1992), 65n11. On the role of Socrates in al-Rāzī's ethics, see Bar-Asher (1989a, 1989b).

30 See *Spiritual Medicine*: Kraus (1939), p. 27 l. 14.

31 See, e.g., Kraus and Pines (2012); Fakhry (1968), 17; Walker (1992), 71; Mahdi (1996), 152; Pines (1997), 86–9.

32 Al-Fārābī's *On the Principles of the Views of the Inhabitants of the Excellent State* (*Fī Mabādiʾ ārāʾ ahl al-madīna al-fāḍila*) is based on the *Republic*; see Walzer (1985) for the Arabic text and an English translation. Al-Fārābī also wrote a summary (*talḫīṣ*) of the *Laws*; for the Arabic text and a Latin translation, see Gabrieli (1952). Walzer (1985: 426) and Gutas (1997: 117–19) propose that al-Fārābī utilized Galen's synopses of the *Republic* and *Laws* in the composition of these works.

33 The terms for these principles vary slightly in the testimonia. Cf. al-Bīrūnī's list at Kraus (1939), §1, p. 195 ll. 1–2, with al-Marzūqī's (d. 421/1030) at Kraus (1939), § 3, p. 197 ll. 6–9.

34 Kraus (1939), p. 285 ll. 7–11. The Persian writer Nāṣir-i Ḫusraw (394–472/1004–80) provides a detailed summary of the role of soul in al-Rāzī's account: see Kraus (1939), p. 284 l. 6–p. 286 l. 6. In identifying the disordered element in his cosmogony as feminine, al-Rāzī is following a tradition that is also seen in the epistles of the Brethren of Purity (Iḫwān al-Ṣafāʾ, fourth/tenth century), who regard their higher psychic principle, the Universal Soul, as feminine (Netton 2002: 44).

Goodman remarks that the aim of this 'myth', and al-Rāzī's metaphysics in general, is 'to breathe new life into the program of the *Timaeus*'.[35] It should be pointed out, though, that the above account shares only superficial features with the cosmogony of the original *Timaeus*. They correspond in that both depict the world as having come into existence from pre-existing matter at some time – that is, if one adopts a literal reading of γέγονεν at *Ti.* 28b7 – and establish God (or the Demiurge), matter, and space as separate principles.[36] Furthermore, al-Rāzī also invokes the dialogue's geometrical theory of the elements (53c–55c) to support his own atomistic conception of matter.[37] The *Timaeus*, however, is far from clear on whether the Receptacle, which is identified as 'everlasting space' (τὸ τῆς χώρας ἀεί, 52a8), should be understood as void, as al-Rāzī takes 'absolute space' to mean.[38] Similarly, since antiquity exegetes have disputed whether the dialogue contains a notion of uncreated time: although time is said to have come into being with the stars and planets (38b6–39e2), this event may only indicate the creation of measured time, and so what came before was unmeasured temporal flow, or indefinite extension (which is akin to al-Rāzī's absolute time).[39] The most significant divergence between the two cosmogonies concerns the createdness of the cosmic soul. The *Timaeus* asserts that the Demiurge put together (συνεστήσατο, 35a1) and set the World Soul into the body of the cosmos (34b1–4), whereas al-Rāzī regards it as uncreated.[40]

While certain medieval sources connect al-Rāzī's five eternals with Plato, this theory must derive from some intermediary.[41] Nāṣir-i Ḫusraw accuses al-Rāzī of plagiarizing from the little-known al-Īrānšahrī (*fl.* second half of the third/ninth century), who may have developed the theory of the five eternals in the light of Plato's *Timaeus* (however it was available to

[35] Goodman (1975), 40n55. On the parallels between al-Rāzī's theory of the five eternals and the cosmogony of the *Timaeus*, see also Fakhry (1968), 19–21.

[36] See *Ti.* 27d5–29d3, 47e3–53c3.

[37] See Koetschet (2019), p. 108 ll. 2–8. Cf. Pines (1997), 86, who notes that the elementary theory of the *Timaeus* is incompatible with al-Rāzī's atomism.

[38] O'Brien (1984: 359–65) shows that the *Timaeus* is inconsistent on the existence of void: Timaeus denies its existence at 58a7, 60c1–2, and 79b1–c1 but affirms it at 58b4–7, where he describes the presence of gaps between the structures of the elements. See also Sedley (1982), 188, who compares the Receptacle with the Epicurean notion of void.

[39] The Epicurean Velleius makes this distinction at Cicero, *DND* 1.9. In modern times, Vlastos (1939) famously defended this interpretation.

[40] Cf. *Phaedo*, *Phaedrus* 245c, and *Laws* 10, which state that the soul is uncreated.

[41] Abū Ḥātim al-Rāzī (d. 322/933–4) and Faḫr al-Dīn al-Rāzī (*c.* 543–606/1149–1209) record that al-Rāzī attributed his conception of absolute time and space to Plato. For the reports of these two Rāzīs, see respectively Kraus (1936a), p. 48 ll. 9–11, p. 50 ll. 13–14; and Kraus (1939), p. 278 ll. 15–19.

him).[42] Citing the idea of the soul's longing for and descent into matter, modern commentators have argued for Gnostic, Neoplatonic (primarily Plotinian), and Plutarchan influences.[43] In the remainder of this section I will consider some of the possible sources that may have transmitted the dialogue's cosmogony and other doctrines to al-Rāzī. I will examine al-Bīrūnī's *List of al-Rāzī's Books* and other medieval bibliographies to ascertain what the titles of al-Rāzī's treatises can reveal about the nature of his Platonic resources. I will touch on the quotations that al-Rāzī explicitly attributes to the *Timaeus* to work out in what form he may have read the dialogue. Since Pines' brief but ground-breaking study of al-Rāzī's Platonic sources, no one has reconsidered his findings, especially in the light of Arnzen's research on the Arabic transmission of the *Timaeus*.[44] An exhaustive description of al-Rāzī's Platonism would be beyond the scope of this chapter, but the following partial survey is necessary to provide background for understanding his criticism of Galen and later Galenic readings of Plato in the *Doubts*.

Of the ninety-three philosophical titles given in al-Bīrūnī's *List of al-Rāzī's Books* (most of which are lost), only five have Platonic associations: *The Small Metaphysics* [lit. *The Divine Science*] *according to the Opinion of Socrates* (*al-ʿIlm al-ilāhī al-ṣaġīr ʿalā raʾy Suqrāṭ*), *Doubts about Proclus* (*al-Šukūk ʿalā Abruqlus*), *Refutation of Porphyry's Book to the Egyptian Anebo* (*Naqḍ kitāb Furfūriyūs ilā Anābū al-miṣrī*), *Commentary on the Book Timaeus* (*Tafsīr kitāb Ṭīmāwūs*), and *Summary of Plutarch's Book* (*Talḫīṣuhu li-kitāb Flūṭarḫus*).[45] The first title does not appear in the bibliographies of Ibn al-Nadīm, Ibn Abī Uṣaybiʿa, and Ibn al-Qifṭī, who refer instead to a *Small Metaphysics* (*al-ʿIlm al-ilāhī al-ṣaġīr*) or an *On Metaphysics according to the Opinion of Plato* (*Fī l-ʿIlm al-ilāhī ʿalā raʾy Aflāṭūn*).[46] Notwithstanding the variation in the titles, all the bibliographies distinguish this work from al-Rāzī's infamous larger exposition of metaphysics, entitled either the *Large Metaphysics* (*al-ʿIlm al-ilāhī al-kabīr*) or simply *Metaphysics* (*al-ʿIlm al-ilāhī*), which

[42] See Kraus (1939), p. 220 ll. 1–2. Pines (1997: 87) proposes that al-Rāzī may have followed al-Īrānšahrī's atomistic reading of the *Timaeus*. For the scant details on al-Īrānšahrī's life and works, see Kargar (2012).

[43] See, e.g., Goodman (1975), 26; Pines (1997), 86n117, 87.

[44] Pines (1997), 83–90. Pines' book was originally published in German in 1938.

[45] See respectively Kraus (1936b), p. 16 no. 114, p. 17 no. 126, p. 17 no. 128, p. 15 no. 107, and p. 16 no. 113. In addition to the last two titles listed above (which are grouped with al-Rāzī's commentaries, summaries, and epitomes), I include as 'philosophical' the works under the subheadings 'physics' (*ṭabīʿiyyāt*), 'logic' (*manṭiqiyyāt*), 'philosophical and conjectural' (*falsafiyya wa taḫmīniyya*), 'what is above nature' (*mā fawqa l-ṭabīʿa*), and 'metaphysics' (*ilāhiyyāt*).

[46] See Kraus (1939), 166–7; Pines (1997), 101–2.

discussed the theory of the five eternals.[47] As mentioned above, al-Rāzī regards Socrates almost exclusively as an ethical authority in his extant corpus, so *On Metaphysics according to the Opinion of Plato* is perhaps the more accurate title of this treatise. Medieval Arabic readers gleaned their information about the life and teachings of Socrates from earlier doxographies, some of which attribute to him metaphysical views with a strong Neoplatonic slant.[48] Therefore, al-Rāzī could have composed a treatise on 'Socratic' metaphysics based on the reports preserved in Arabic doxographies, which often incorporate late antique sources.[49]

The next two titles, *Doubts about Proclus* and *Refutation of Porphyry's Book to the Egyptian Anebo*, indicate a more definite engagement with Neoplatonism. Because Proclus was foremost known to medieval thinkers as a supporter of eternalism, the *Doubts about Proclus* probably attacked his eighteen arguments advanced in *On the Eternity of the World* in defence of this position.[50] In antiquity, the question about the world's createdness was inextricably bound to the interpretation of the cosmogony of the *Timaeus*. Thus, in the *Doubts about Proclus* al-Rāzī may have tried to undermine Proclus' eternalist reading of the dialogue to defend his own creationist account. Although Proclus' text was available in two Arabic versions, al-Rāzī may have made use of John Philoponus' *Against Proclus on the Eternity of the World*, which also circulated in Arabic and quotes in full Proclus' eighteen proofs.[51] As in the case of later Islamicate authors, Philoponus' arguments in support of creation *ex nihilo* may have inspired al-Rāzī's critique of Proclus, even if he does not subscribe to Philoponus' idea of creation.[52] Regardless of how al-Rāzī read Proclus, either *On the Eternity of the World* or *Against Proclus on the Eternity of the World* would have given him an overview of the cosmological sections of the *Timaeus* as well as the prior controversies relating to their interpretation.[53]

[47] See Kraus (1939), 165–6.

[48] See Alon (1991), 103. Most Socratic doxographical material pertains to ethics; see, e.g., al-Kindī's *Sayings of Socrates*: Adamson and Pormann (2012), 268–72.

[49] See Gutas (1975), 9–34, 436–63.

[50] Pines (1997), 106n173.

[51] On the two Arabic versions of Proclus' work, one of which is by Isḥāq ibn Ḥunayn, see Badawī (1955); Anawātī (1956). As the original Greek text of *On the Eternity of the World* is lost, modern editors rely on Philoponus' treatise to reconstruct it.

[52] On Philoponus' influence on medieval Islamicate philosophy, see, e.g., Davidson (1987), 86–116; Harvey (2004). See also Verrycken (1997), 270–81, who maintains that Philoponus supported an eternalist interpretation of Plato's cosmology in his writings before 529 – when *Against Proclus on the Eternity of the World* was published.

[53] For Philoponus' familiarity with earlier exegeses of the dialogue's cosmogony (including Galen's in *DD* 4), see Verrycken (1997), 281–7. As I will discuss below, al-Rāzī presents Galen as arguing in support of an eternalist position in *DD* 4, whereas Philoponus cites this text as espousing

Al-Rāzī appears to have targeted another Neoplatonic commentator, Porphyry (*c.* 234–305/310), in his *Refutation of Porphyry's Book to the Egyptian Anebo*. Porphyry's *Letter to the Egyptian Anebo* does not survive, but later sources, most notably Iamblichus' (*c.* 240–325) response *On the Mysteries of the Egyptians*, depict it as an attack on divination and theurgy, which includes a range of rituals to effect an encounter with a god.[54] The bibliographies of Ibn al-Nadīm and Ibn Abī Uṣaybiʿa imply that al-Rāzī actually wrote on Iamblichus' reply to Porphyry, for they record an *On the Refutation of the Book of Anebo to Porphyry, on the Explanation of the Doctrines of Aristotle on Metaphysics* (*Fī Naqḍ kitāb Anābū ilā Furfūriyūs fī šarḥ maḏāhib Arisṭālīs fī l-ʿilm al-ilāhī*).[55] Given al-Rāzī's alleged rejection of prophecy and miracles, it seems more probable that he composed a refutation of Iamblichus' defence of theurgy and divine revelation in *On the Mysteries*. Nonetheless, the description of the subject of the *Book of Anebo to Porphyry* as Aristotelian metaphysics puts into doubt al-Rāzī's access to the original text of Iamblichus, who aligns himself with the Hermetic and Platonic traditions.[56] Furthermore, the listings in Ibn al-Nadīm and Ibn Abī Uṣaybiʿa give the impression that Iamblichus replied to Porphyry as 'Anebo', when in fact he adopted the guise of Anebo's teacher 'Abamon' (*Myst.* 1.1).

The historian al-Masʿūdī (d. 354/956) and the philosopher al-Šahrastānī (d. 548/1153) offer evidence that *On the Mysteries* and the *Letter to Anebo* may have circulated in Arabic as a single work that was conflated with Porphyry's now fragmentary commentary on Plato's *Timaeus*. In his *Book of Notification and Review* (*Kitāb al-Tanbīh wa l-išrāf*), al-Masʿūdī relates that al-Rāzī wrote on 'the questions and answers' (*al-masāʾil wa l-ǧawābāt*) between Porphyry and Anebo on the 'divine sciences' (*al-ʿulūm al-ilāhiyya*, or metaphysics), and thus he signals that al-Rāzī's tract was based on both Porphyry's letter and Iamblichus' rejoinder.[57] Immediately following this information about al-Rāzī, al-Masʿūdī brings up the Arabic transmission of Plato's *Timaeus*.[58] Van Bladel observes that this apparent tangent is explicable in light of al-Šahrastānī's quotation of the *Letter to Anebo* in the

a creationist view similar to his own (*De aet. mund.* 600.3–601.16). Thus, if al-Rāzī had access to Philoponus' work, his misrepresentation of Galen's arguments in *DD* 4 is all the more striking.

[54] For the surviving material, see Sodano (1958) with qualifications from Johnson (2013), 42–4.

[55] See Flügel (1871), vol. I, p. 300 ll. 17–18; Riḍā (1965), p. 423 ll. 16–17. Cf. Ibn al-Qifṭī's entry *Book of the Exposition of the Book of Anebo to Porphyry, on the Explanation of the Doctrines of Aristotle on Metaphysics* (*Kitāb tafsīr kitāb Anābū ilā Furfūriyūs fī šarḥ maḏāhib Arisṭālīs fī l-ʿilm al-ilāhī*) at Lippert (1903), p. 274 ll. 11–12. The following analysis is indebted to van Bladel (2009), 97–100.

[56] See *Myst* 1.2. [57] de Goeje (1965), p. 162 ll. 5–15.

[58] de Goeje (1965), p. 162 l. 15–p. 163 l. 5; for an English translation of the passage, see Zimmermann (1986), 150.

Book of Religions and Sects (*Kitāb al-Milal wa l-niḥal*).[59] There, al-Šahrastānī relates that Porphyry dismissed those who ascribed to Plato a belief in the world's createdness, and cites the *Letter to Anebo* (*Risālatuhu ilā Anābū*) for Porphyry's arguments against creationism.[60] Al-Šahrastānī's text of the *Letter to Anebo* has strong parallels with a fragment of Porphyry's exegesis of *Ti.* 30a2–6, where it is explained in what sense God brought the world into existence.[61] As al-Mas'ūdī's knowledge of Porphyry's exchange with 'Anebo' (Iamblichus) appears to come from al-Rāzī, his implicit connection of the *Letter to Anebo/On the Mysteries* with Plato's *Timaeus* suggests that al-Rāzī's text of the two Neoplatonic works was also conflated with Porphyry's *Timaeus* commentary.[62]

It is not clear how much of Porphyry's commentary circulated with the *Letter to Anebo* and *On the Mysteries*, or vice versa. In detailing the content of 'Anebo's' reply to Porphyry, al-Mas'ūdī reports that it defends the doctrines of Pythagoras and Thales, the first of whom is mentioned twice by Iamblichus in *On the Mysteries* and the latter not at all.[63] These scant details suggest that al-Mas'ūdī (and perhaps al-Rāzī) may have had only a superficial acquaintance with either Iamblichus or Porphyry's compositions. The linking of 'Anebo's' response to Porphyry with Aristotelian metaphysics in the bibliographies of Ibn al-Nadīm and Ibn Abī Uṣaybi'a hint that al-Rāzī's work may have dealt at length with Porphyry's eternalist reading of the cosmogony of the *Timaeus*. Al-Šahrastānī emphasizes that Porphyry adhered to all of Aristotle's doctrines, and he seems to adduce Porphyry's eternalist position in the '*Letter to Anebo*' – or rather, his commentary on the *Timaeus* – as proof of this commitment.[64] Similar to al-Šahrastānī, al-Rāzī may have regarded Porphyry's explanation of creation in the *Timaeus* as an apology of Aristotelian metaphysics and entitled his tract accordingly.

My analysis has shown that al-Rāzī appears to have had access to at least two Neoplatonic interpretations of the initial passages of the *Timaeus*. While I have stressed al-Rāzī's departure from Proclus and Porphyry on the issue of the eternity of the world, his cosmology mirrors theirs in certain respects. For instance, as noted above, al-Rāzī's theory of the soul's descent into matter is sometimes characterized as 'Plotinian' or 'Gnostic', but Porphyry and Proclus hold this notion too. Moreover, similar to al-Rāzī, the problem of evil occupies the attention of both

[59] van Bladel (2009), 99.
[60] See Wakīl (1968), 215–17. Wakīl, or his manuscript, transcribes Anebo as Abānō.
[61] Cf. Sodano (1964), fr. 51, p. 34.
[62] van Bladel (2009), 99.
[63] See de Goeje (1965), p. 162 l. 9; *Myst.* 1.1.2.8, 1.2.6.1–2.
[64] Wakīl (1968), p. 214 ll. 19–21.

thinkers.[65] Although these are broad correspondences, a systematic study might bring to light more substantial connections between the ideas of al-Rāzī and these two Neoplatonists.

Pines points to the final pair of titles *Commentary on the Book Timaeus* and *Summary of Plutarch's Book*, which he combines into a single treatise, *On Plutarch's Commentary on the Book Timaeus* (*Fī Tafsīr Aflūṭarḫūs fī kitāb Ṭimāwūs*), to demonstrate that al-Rāzī did not depend solely on late antique Neoplatonic exegeses of Plato's dialogue.[66] Notwithstanding al-Bīrūnī's separation of the works, Pines finds grounds for the conflation in Ibn Abī Uṣaybiʿa, Ibn al-Nadīm, and Ibn al-Qifṭī, who list a *Commentary on Plutarch's Book on the Commentary on the Book Timaeus* (*Tafsīr kitāb Flūṭarḫus fī tafsīr kitāb Ṭīmāwus*).[67] He hypothesizes that the Plutarchan tract in question could be *On the Birth of the Soul in the Timaeus* (Περὶ τῆς ἐν τῷ Τιμαίῳ ψυχογονίας) or the lost *On the World's Having Come into Being According to Plato* (Περὶ τοῦ γεγονέναι κατὰ Πλάτωνα τὸν κόσμον), both of which express cosmogonic views similar to al-Rāzī's – creation in time, eternity of matter, and the fall of the soul.[68] Apart from these bibliographical listings, no other medieval Arabic source connects Plutarch's name to Plato's *Timaeus*.[69] In fact, al-Rāzī himself relays in the preface to his *Abridgement on Galen's Therapeutic Method* (*Talḫīṣuhu li-ḥīlat al-bur'*) that he summarized the pseudo-Plutarchan *Doctrines of the Philosophers* (*De Placitis Philosophorum*).[70] Al-Bīrūnī's entry *Summary of Plutarch's Book* probably refers to al-Rāzī's abridgement of the *Doctrines of the Philosophers*; thus, this identification calls into question al-Rāzī's access to a Plutarchan interpretation of the *Timaeus*. A scribal error, such as a missing space, in an earlier bibliographical source may account for why Ibn Abī Uṣaybiʿa and the others read '*Commentary on Plutarch's Book*' and '*On the Commentary on the Book Timaeus*' as a single title.[71]

[65] Porphyry treats this problem in *Philosophy from Oracles* and *On the Return of the Soul* and Proclus in *On the Existence of Evils*. These works do not appear to have been translated into Arabic. Proclus, however, touches on the subject of evil in an Arabic fragment of his commentary on the *Timaeus* (for which, see Arnzen 2013: 37), and his argument for eternalism based on God's goodness in *De aet. mund.* was very influential in the Islamicate world (see Davidson 1987: 61–2). The problem of evil was also central to *kalām* (speculative theology) theories, with which al-Rāzī was familiar: see Rashed (2000), 46–54.

[66] Pines (1997), 84, 103.

[67] See Riḍā (1965), p. 425 ll. 22–23; Flügel (1871), p. 301 l. 5; Lippert (1903), p. 285 ll. 5–6. Pines (1997: 103) misleadingly suggests that al-Bīrūnī gives the same title as the other bibliographers.

[68] Pines (1997), 86n117, 103n69.

[69] On the works of Plutarch available in Arabic, see Das and Koetschet (2019), 374–7.

[70] See Das and Koetschet (2019), 378–9.

[71] Ibn Abī Uṣaybiʿa (Riḍā (1965), p. 426 ll. 18–19) attributes to al-Rāzī a *Book on the Natural Opinions* (*Fī l-'Ārā' al-ṭabīʿiyya*), which mirrors the Arabic title of ps.-Plutarch's *Plac.Philos.* Thus, at some point in al-Rāzī's bibliographical tradition, Plutarch's name must have dropped out from the title.

Furthermore, it is not necessary to see Plutarchan influence on al-Rāzī to explain his cosmogony, for his theories of matter and soul share similarities with those of Porphyry, Proclus, and other Neoplatonists, and his belief in creation in time could have found support from Galen's *Com. Tim.*, which offers a literal reading of *Ti.* 28b7. I want to propose now that al-Rāzī's *Commentary on the Book Timaeus* may be based on a Galenic exegesis of the dialogue, either his synopsis or lemmatic commentary. Al-Bīrūnī's grouping of al-Rāzī's commentary with his treatments of Galenic works is suggestive in this respect. His section on al-Rāzī's exegetical texts lists the *Commentary on the Book Timaeus* first, then five Galenic compositions (*Epitome of the Book of the Big Pulse*, *Abridgement of the Therapeutic Method*, *Abridgement of Causes and Symptoms*, *Abridgement of the Affected Parts*, and *Abridgement of Hippocrates' Aphorisms*), and finally the *Summary of Plutarch's Book*.[72] The placement of the *Commentary on the Book Timaeus* next to the epitomes and abridgements of Galen instead of the *Summary of Plutarch's Book* seems to indicate that it has a closer relationship with the Galenic set. The omission of Galen's name from the titles of al-Rāzī's summaries of his works may explain why the *Commentary on the Book Timaeus* is not described as an exegesis of a Galenic source.

The fact that the citations attributed explicitly to 'Timaeus' in al-Rāzī's writings largely derive from Galen's *On the Medical Statements in Plato's Timaeus* gives additional credence to the above hypothesis. Of his surviving output, his medical works, especially the *Comprehensive Book*, mention the *Timaeus* by name the most.[73] Only one quotation in the *Comprehensive Book* links Galen with the dialogue, but citation markers in other passages, which signal that the Platonic source consisted of four 'chapters' or 'books' (*maqālāt*), demonstrate a more extensive use by al-Rāzī of Galen's four-volume exegesis.[74] The *Comprehensive Book* calls *On the Medical Statements*

[72] Kraus (1936b), pp. 15–16 nos. 107–13. As Ullmann (1970: 43) notes, the 'Big Pulse' (*al-Nabḍ al-kabīr*) refers to a collection of four Galenic tracts on the pulse, so the *Epitome of the Big Pulse* (*Iḫtiṣār Kitāb al-Nabḍ al-kabīr*) is probably a summary of this anthology. Al-Rāzī's lost commentary (or 'abridgement', *talḫīṣ*) on the Hippocratic *Aphorisms* appears to have been based on Galen's *Commentary on Hippocrates' 'Aphorisms'*; see Rosenthal (1966), 231–2; Pormann and Joosse (2012), 220.

[73] See al-Rāzī (1955–70), vol. I, p. 16 ll. 14–16; vol. I, p. 88 l. 19–p. 89 l. 9; vol. I, p. 92 ll. 12–16; vol. I, p. 153 ll. 15–19; vol. I, p. 175 ll. 4–10; vol. IV, p. 88 ll. 7–12; vol. VI, p. 45 ll. 10–15; vol. VIII, p. 120 ll. 4–5; vol. IX, p. 67 ll. 13–14; vol. IX, p. 72 ll. 5–6; vol. X, p. 62 l. 8–p. 63 l. 8; vol. X, p. 303 ll. 3–6; vol. XIII, p. 55 l. 3–p. 56 l. 7; vol. XIV, p. 98 l. 8–p. 99 l. 4; vol. XV, p. 111 ll. 10–14; vol. XVI, p. 101 l. 15–p. 102 l. 8; vol. XVII, p. 19 ll. 3–6; vol. XX, p. 297 l. 11; vol. XX, p. 450 l. 18–p. 451 l. 7; vol. XXI, p. 318 ll. 3–5; vol. XXIII, p. 88 ll. 4–6; vol. XXIII, p. 135 l. 6–p. 136 l. 2; vol. XXIII, p. 136 ll. 3–5. See also *On Smallpox and Measles*: Channing (1766), ll. 12–15.

[74] See al-Rāzī (1955–70), vol. X, p. 303 ll. 3–6, which preserves the lemmatic structure of Galen's *Plat. Tim.*

in Plato's Timaeus the 'Medical Timaeus' *(Ṭīmāwūs al-ṭibbī)* as well as just 'Timaeus' (*Ṭīmāwūs*), so the 'Timaeus' treated in al-Rāzī's lost commentary may be Galen's medical interpretation. Textual parallels between the discussions of pleasure and the immortality of the soul in *Spiritual Medicine*, the fragmentary *On Pleasure* (*Fī l-Laḏḏa*), and Galen's *Com. Tim.* demonstrate that al-Rāzī also formulated several of his philosophical ideas in the light of this second Galenic explanation.[75] Despite its more holistic overview of Plato's dialogue, none of al-Rāzī's extant works either identify Galen's *Com. Tim.* as the 'Timaeus' or refer to Galen as its author. Further to this point, the *Doubts* groups the abridgement with 'Plato's books' (*kutub Aflāṭun*), and thus seems to evince that the text's Galenic authorship is inconsequential to al-Rāzī.[76] This lack of any direct association of *Com. Tim.* with the *Timaeus* does not, however, preclude the possibility that al-Rāzī wrote a commentary on the source, as his works testify to his considerable interest in it, which may have culminated in a systematic examination.

My review has considered the diverse range of ancient sources that may have contributed to al-Rāzī's knowledge of Plato's *Timaeus*. By appealing to the medieval bibliographic tradition, I have shown his probable engagement with Neoplatonic interpretations of the dialogue, which stress its metaphysical significance. Listings such as the *Doubts about Proclus* indicate that Neoplatonic eternalist readings of the cosmogony of the *Timaeus* may have had a 'negative' influence on al-Rāzī by offering a position against which he could refine his own understanding of Plato's creation account. As will be discussed, al-Rāzī broaches the subject of creation several times in the *Doubts*; therefore, depending on the chronological relationship between this text and his Neoplatonic refutations, he may have modelled his critique of Galen's 'eternalist' cosmogony on his responses to Proclus – or the reverse. I have also speculated that the source underlying al-Rāzī's lost commentary on the *Timaeus* may be one of Galen's Platonic exegeses, which emphasize the importance of the dialogue not only to metaphysics but also to ethics, physics, and medicine. Al-Rāzī's citations of Galen's lemmatic commentary in his medical works suggest that, on account of his predecessor, he views the *Timaeus* as resisting strict disciplinary classification in its coverage of the heavenly and corporeal. I argued in the first chapter that one objective of Galen's exegetical project

[75] See Bar-Asher (1989a, 1989b), who shows the profound influence of Galen's *Com. Tim.* on al-Rāzī's earlier ethical thought. On the relationship between the doctrines of pleasure in al-Rāzī and Galen's abridgement, see also Kraus (1939), 139–40; Adamson (2008), 83–8.

[76] For more on this grouping, see p. 131 below.

on the *Timaeus* was to justify and advertise his dual expertise in philosophy and medicine. The next section will examine how this endeavour may have informed al-Rāzī's definition of his own disciplinary identity.

The Philosopher-Doctor, Further Entanglements

Facing criticisms of his career, al-Rāzī composed a defence, *The Philosopher's Way of Life*, in his final years, as Galen had done with *Prop. Plac.*[77] The two apologies are written from different perspectives in that Galen stresses his identity as a doctor – he claims certain knowledge of only subjects relevant to medicine – whereas al-Rāzī argues for his status as a philosopher. Unlike *Prop.Plac.*, the objections to al-Rāzī's disciplinary authority do not relate to his epistemic constancy; instead, his detractors contend that his rejection of an ascetic lifestyle disqualifies him from the philosophical rank. He appeals to the figure of the mature Socrates, who turned away from the austere habits of his youth in favour of a married, active civic life, to prove that asceticism is not obligatory for philosophers.[78] At the end of the text, al-Rāzī's résumé of his own philosophical activities, which he divides into theoretical and practical accomplishments, offers insight into his conception of the relationship between medicine and philosophy. He includes among his theoretical philosophical achievements the books *On Metaphysics*, *Spiritual Medicine*, and *Physics* (*Samʿ al-kiyān*) as well as medical compositions such as the *Book for al-Manṣūr* (*Kitāb al-Manṣūrī*), *Everyman his Own Doctor* (*Man lā yaḥḍuruhu ṭabīb*), and *On Current Drugs* (*Fī l-Adwiya al-mawǧūda*).[79] For his practical philosophical endeavours, al-Rāzī cites his role as a court physician.[80] Al-Rāzī's equation of his philosophical and medical pursuits suggests a more radical entanglement of the disciplines than in Galen, who asserts a distinction (however negotiable) between the two.[81]

The works in which al-Rāzī directly addresses what doctors should know similarly deny a foundational separation between medicine and philosophy. Leaving aside for now the relevant statements from the *Doubts about Galen*, I shall focus on al-Rāzī's definition of medical knowledge in *The Guide* and

[77] *The Philosopher's Way of Life* seems to be a late work because al-Rāzī mentions that his failing eyesight has forced him to dictate his books (Kraus 1939: p. 110 ll. 13–15).

[78] Kraus (1939), p. 99 l. 14–p. 100 l. 15. See Bar-Asher (1989a), who compares this image of Socrates with the Cynic model of him in *Spiritual Medicine*.

[79] Kraus (1939), p. 108 l. 10–p. 109 l. 7. [80] Kraus (1939), p. 109 ll. 19–20.

[81] Cf. *Lib.Prop.*, where Galen separates his medical writings from his philosophical works. At Boudon-Millot (2007), 164–73, he subdivides his philosophical output into tracts on logical demonstration, ethics, and Platonic, Aristotelian, Stoic, and Epicurean thought.

the *Secret of the Art of Medicine*, which provide an overview of the discipline for beginning doctors through a series of aphorisms.[82] Of the two, *The Guide* seems to set more restrictive parameters for medicine. Covering many of the same topics (for example, the elements, temperament, six non-naturals, and drugs), both assert that medicine encompasses the domain of nature (*ṭabīʿa*), but *The Guide* remarks that there is a limit to what doctors need to know about it. Al-Rāzī offers the following proviso when discussing how nature assists the sick body:

> يكفي الطبيب أن يعلم من الطبيعة ما قلناه، فأما ماهيتها فمختلف فيها، وهو ما يخص الفيلسوف الطبيعي والإلهي، دون الطبيب. وإن أحب محب النظر في ذلك، فليشرف على ما قلناه في صدر كتابنا في سمع الكيان.[83]

> It suffices the doctor to know what we have mentioned about nature [namely, that it works to expel disease from the body]. As for its quiddity, there is disagreement about it. This is the concern of the natural and divine philosopher, not the doctor. If one wants to inquire about this, let them look at what we mentioned at the beginning of our book *Physics*.

In placing enquiries into the reality of nature beyond medicine's purview, al-Rāzī seems to adhere to the late antique conception of the discipline as inferior to physics and metaphysics in terms of its epistemic capacities.[84] As the next chapter will reveal, Avicenna, one of al-Rāzī's most trenchant critics, also expresses reservations about doctors investigating the quiddity of nature. Unlike Avicenna, however, al-Rāzī does not cite some deficiency in doctors' intellectual framework as the reason for why they should curtail their study of nature; in fact, he gives no rationale. Moreover, he encourages the more ambitious reader to look at his treatment of the subject in his *Physics*, so his comments seem advisory rather than prescriptive. By directing the reader to one of his own books on nature, al-Rāzī conveys that doctors can pursue issues traditionally belonging to physics and metaphysics (the 'divine' philosophy); he silently contests philosophy's exclusive claim to knowledge about natural reality.

The discussion of the elementary composition of the body at the start of *The Guide* also undermines a strict demarcation between medicine and philosophy. In the tenth aphorism al-Rāzī reviews Galen's refutation of material monism – that the cosmos is composed of one element – and atomism – that it consists of small, insentient parts – in *On the Elements*

[82] For these texts' aims, see Iskandar (1961), 2; Kuhne Brabant (1982), p. 358, §§ 0.4–0.5.
[83] Iskandar (1961), p. 102, aph. 315. [84] See the Introduction, pp. 19–22.

according to Hippocrates.[85] In so doing, he signals that would-be-doctors should concern themselves with this debate about the number and nature of the elements, which Avicenna's *Canon of Medicine* would later bar them from examining.[86] Al-Rāzī dismisses as 'invalid' (*laysa yaṣiḥḥu*) the Galenic text's attack on atomism, and refers the reader to his defence of the theory in the *Doubts about Galen*, which explains how the soul, rather than the body's elementary atoms, is responsible for sensation and life.[87] While *The Guide* neglects the soul in its summary of medicine, this reference to the *Doubts* seems to put at least comprehension of the soul's relationship to the body within its boundaries. The advice to read the *Doubts*, which al-Bīrūnī characterizes as a work on physics, as part of a medical curriculum further highlights how al-Rāzī's enmeshment of medicine and philosophy works to open up a larger epistemic space for the former.[88]

The *Secret of the Art of Medicine* also recognizes that a doctor's task is to work with nature to heal the body, but it is more forthright in asserting that the knowledge enabling one to do so comes from philosophical training.[89] An aphorism in the sixth book, which relays 'indispensable information for the skilful physician' (*lā ġanāʾ li-l-ṭabīb al-māhir*), links medical competence with expertise in various parts of philosophy:

> من لم يعن بالأصول الطبيعية والعلوم الفلسفية والقوانين المنطقية والأركان الرياضية وعدل إلى اللذات الدنياوية فاتهمه لا سيما في صناعة الطب.[90]

> Whoever shows no interest in natural principles, the philosophical sciences, rules of logic, and the elements of mathematics but turns towards the pleasures of this world, mistrust them especially in the craft of medicine.

The text emphasizes that the respectability of medicine depends on its practitioners eschewing worldly pleasures in favour of philosophical study. In this respect, it echoes Galen's exhortation in *The Best Doctor is Also a Philosopher* (*Opt.Med.*) that doctors should receive a preliminary education in philosophy to restore medicine to its former authoritative status, which it enjoyed under Hippocrates.[91] Apart from the omission of ethics,

85 Iskandar (1961), pp. 20–1, aph. 10. Cf. De Lacy (1996), 60–93.

86 See Chapter 4, pp. 144–8.

87 Although Galen cites *Ti.* 56d1–57b7 in *Hipp.Elem.* to support his theory of four elements that undergo change (De Lacy 1996: p. 88 ll. 10–11), al-Rāzī does not associate Plato with this position in *The Guide*. As the *Doubts* presents Plato as an atomist, al-Rāzī's failure to mention the philosopher in aph. 10 may be part of a strategy to separate him from Galen so as to reclaim him as his own intellectual precursor.

88 See Kraus (1936b), p. 13, no. 88.

89 See Kuhne Brabant (1982), p. 389, aph. 6.78; there, al-Rāzī contrasts medicine with alchemy, whose practitioners aim to alter the order of nature.

90 Kuhne Brabant (1982), p. 384, aph. 6.07.

91 See Boudon-Millot (2007), 284–6, 90–1.

al-Rāzī's listing of physics (*al-uṣūl al-ṭabīʿiyya*), logic (*al-qawānīn al-manṭiqiyya*), and mathematics (*al-arkān al-riyāḍiyya*) as requisite philosophical subjects follows Galen's recommendations in *Opt.Med.* and *Ord. Lib.Prop.*[92] The aphorism adds, however, 'philosophical sciences' (*al-ʿulūm al-falsafiyya*), which appear to denote areas of philosophy different from those already mentioned. Ethics and metaphysics are the major parts of philosophy that are not named, so the vague phrase may refer to them or represent a kind of synecdoche for all of philosophy. Whatever its meaning, the addition of 'philosophical sciences' seems to imply that doctors need a more extensive education because medicine governs a broader domain of knowledge than Galen's writings suggest.

In the works discussed above, al-Rāzī does not draw on the *Timaeus* to articulate his definition of medicine. His appeal to the body's link with nature to argue for the relevance of philosophy to medicine recalls, nonetheless, Galen's use of the dialogue's notion of the body's entanglement in a larger cosmic system to justify his interest in subjects usually allocated to physics – for instance, the soul and elements. I have hinted that al-Rāzī views medicine as embracing not only the physical but also the metaphysical. By eliding his activities as a doctor and as a philosopher in *The Philosopher's Way of Life*, al-Rāzī seems to present himself as an alternative paradigm to Galen's more limited philosopher-doctor, and therefore a rival source of epistemic authority. To this same end, *The Guide* also highlights al-Rāzī's grasp of both physics and metaphysics to its medical readers. In what follows, I will demonstrate how the *Doubts about Galen*, through its criticisms of Galen, positions al-Rāzī's more expansive formulation of medicine as the necessary replacement for the philosophically and medically inadequate system of Galenism.

Galen, the Bad Platonist

Concerned with legitimizing its critical treatment of Galen, the preface to the *Doubts about Galen* does not comment on the text's structure, which is made up of a series of seemingly unconnected critiques of Galenic theories. A survey of the subjects tackled, which include the eternity of the world, sensation, plant life, the elements, temperament, and the corporeality of the soul, indicates that al-Rāzī may have conceived of the *Doubts* as

[92] See Boudon-Millot (2007), 99, 291. Galen famously specifies that doctors should train in geometry. See Pines (1953: 486) for al-Rāzī's criticism in the *Doubts* of Galen's reliance on geometry.

a response in part to Galen's *Prop.Plac.*, for the tract addresses all these topics in one place.[93] Nonetheless, besides starting with creation, the *Doubts* does not arrange its material in the same way as *Prop.Plac.* While Galen wrote *Prop.Plac.* to assert his epistemological consistency on a number of issues, many of which pertain to doctrines in Plato's *Timaeus*, al-Rāzī appears to use it to attack his forerunner for being inconsistent.[94] Employing a dialectical strategy, al-Rāzī sets the claims of agnosticism in *Prop.Plac.* regarding subjects supposedly beyond medicine's purview against passages from the Galenic corpus expressing viewpoints on them to prove that Galen's opinions are contradictory as well as erroneous. As *Prop.Plac.* defines medicine's epistemic contents in light of Galen's own knowledge, al-Rāzī seems to redraw the discipline's boundaries by revealing that his predecessor took a stance on philosophical questions allegedly unknowable and thus irrelevant to doctors.

Throughout the *Doubts*, al-Rāzī acknowledges in various ways the interplay between the medical and philosophical aspects of Galenic thought and intimates that Galen's shortcomings in philosophy damaged the credibility of his medicine – and vice versa. He primarily targets Galen for his faulty philosophical learning, which prevented him from comprehending the metaphysical (specifically, theological) ramifications of the physical phenomena that he observed.[95] The passages examined below will illustrate that the *Doubts* appears to attribute several of Galen's philosophical errors to his misunderstanding of Plato's *Timaeus*, which al-Rāzī interprets differently owing in part to his sources. They will show that al-Rāzī associates Galen's or later Galenists' rejection of the 'Platonic' position on creation, pleasure, and the soul with his or their failure to account for the benevolence of God.[96] Because al-Rāzī seems to base his own epistemic authority on his adherence to Plato and the 'old natural philosophers', he attempts to weaken Galen's epistemic authority by highlighting his deviation from Plato.

[93] Cf. on creation, Koetschet (2019), p. 6 l. 15–p. 18 l. 7, and LG, 60–2; on sensation, Koetschet (2019), p. 70 l. 11–p. 80 l. 3, and LG, 80–5; on plant life, Koetschet (2019), p. 84 ll. 2–13, and LG, 142–5; on the elements, Koetschet (2019), p. 106 l. 12–p. 132 l. 2, and LG, 84–7; on temperament, Koetschet (2019), p. 132 l. 4–152 l. 13, and LG, 76–81; and on the soul, Koetschet (2019), p. 36 l. 10–p. 38 l. 15, p. 219 l. 11–224 l. 6, and LG, 64–70.

[94] Al-Rāzī cites *Prop.Plac.* seven times in the *Doubts*: Koetschet (2019), p. 8 ll. 11–12, p. 16 ll. 1–2, p. 18 l. 7, p. 38 l. 5, p. 40 ll. 5–6, p. 84 l. 6, p. 94 l. 13.

[95] Cf. Koetschet (2019), p. 142 l. 10–p. 144 l. 10, where al-Rāzī recognizes that a theory at the basis of Galen's laws about temperament is philosophically sound but incorrect when applied to medicine.

[96] This line of argumentation draws on Pines (1953), 485, and Koetschet (2015), 195.

Al-Rāzī's initial critique of Galen's views on creation is the section of the *Doubts* that has attracted the most scholarly attention.[97] This interest largely stems from its citation of book four of the lost *On Demonstration (DD)*, which contained Galen's reflections on the debate about the createdness of the world that the *Timaeus* provoked. Al-Rāzī focuses on two premises from *DD* 4 that seem to establish the eternity of the world – namely, 'the universe does not corrupt' and 'anything that does not corrupt is not generated' – and contrasts them with Galen's insistence in *Prop.Plac.* that this cosmic question cannot be known for certain.[98] In defence of his own belief in a temporal origin of the world, which is never expounded in the *Doubts*, al-Rāzī alleges that Galen did not provide sufficient argumentation to verify his assertions about the incorruptibility of the cosmos.[99] As has been pointed out, al-Rāzī's depiction of Galen as holding an eternalist, Aristotelian position in *DD 4* is misleading: Philoponus' *Against Proclus on the Eternity of the World* (599.22–600.16) offers evidence that Galen argued in support of Plato's doctrine of creation in the *Timaeus.*[100] Adamson remarks that distorting Galen's reasoning in *DD* is 'part and parcel of al-Rāzī's hostile strategy' in the *Doubts.*[101] While the polemical payoff of revealing Galen's inconsistent opinions in *Prop.Plac.* and *DD* 4 may be clear, what al-Rāzī achieves by characterizing the latter work as championing eternalism is less obvious.

Al-Rāzī's decision to broach cosmogony first signals to the reader of the *Doubts* that Galen's views on the subject are key for understanding the rest of his thought and the flaws in it. In the medieval period, as in antiquity, eternalism was seen as a defining position of Aristotelianism, so al-Rāzī's reading of *DD* 4 appears to call into question Galen's Platonic credentials. Rejecting the eternity of the world, al-Rāzī presents himself as the more faithful follower of Plato, and thus implies that his interpretations of other

97 For an English translation of the passage, see McGinnis and Reisman (2007), 51–3. See Koetschet (2019), 6–19 for a French translation of it and Strohmaier (1998), 271 for a partial German translation. On the section more generally, see Pines (1953), 485; Chiaradonna (2009b); Adamson (2014), 208–10; Koetschet (2015).

98 See Koetschet (2019), p. 8 ll. 1–15.

99 In particular, al-Rāzī attacks Galen's use of astronomical observations to demonstrate that the cosmos is incorruptible. Moreover, he asserts that, to corroborate his premises, Galen needed to establish that there is nothing outside the cosmos that can cause it to corrupt. See Koetschet (2019), p. 12 l. 5–p. 14 l. 4.

100 On this testimonium from Philoponus, see Chiaradonna (2009b), 45–6. See also Koetschet (2015), 176–90, who examines how al-Rāzī identifies Galen's arguments in *DD* 4 with Aristotle's proofs against a temporal origin of the world in *DC* 270b12–17. In *On Marasmus* (*Marc.* 7.671K), Galen indicates that he did propose in *DD* 4 that the cosmos is incorruptible but adds that this conclusion does not preclude its createdness, for it is not inevitable that everything born will die. On al-Rāzī's reading of *Marc.*, see pp. 125–8 below.

101 Adamson (2014), 210.

Timaean doctrines, which later passages in the *Doubts* will treat, should be accorded more weight than Galen's.[102] Given that al-Rāzī may have made reference to Galen's *Com. Tim.* when formulating his own Platonic stance on creation, this grouping of Galen with Aristotle seems all the more rhetorically charged.[103] In line with the *Timaeus* (29d7–e2), al-Rāzī regards God's goodness as the principal cause of creation.[104] Specifically, al-Rāzī denies that God was negligent (*lā yaʿriḍu lahu sahw wa lā ġafla*) in allowing the soul to descend into the material world, for, out of mercy, the divinity gifted the soul with intellect, by which she can escape her fallen condition.[105] Accordingly, his attribution of an eternalist viewpoint to Galen allows him to make a serious theological charge against his predecessor: that Galen denies the goodness of God.[106] In making this inference about Galen's theology, al-Rāzī advances his rival system of philosophical medicine as the acceptable alternative for devout practitioners.

The opening critique of Galen does not address the theological implications of eternalism, but al-Rāzī links it with a curtailment of God's cosmological role when revisiting the subject in a later passage. He brings up Galen's claim in *DD* 4 that the cosmos is incorruptible in his discussion of the short tract *On Marasmus* (*Marc.*), which examines the cause of withering (μαρασμός) or decay in the body. *Marc.* formulates a response to this aetiological query during the course of its broader investigation into the power responsible for the life of the body, so al-Rāzī scrutinizes Galen's comments on the identity of this vital source too. Al-Rāzī writes:

> وقال في كتاب الذبول: إنّ الذبول «يلحق جميع الحيوان ضرورة لأنّه لم يوجد حيوان لا يشيخ.» وهذا مأخوذ من الاستقراء لا من طبيعة الحيوان. ثم قال: «والقول بأنّ كل متكون يفسد ليس هو حقا لامحالة لكن مقنع»، وهذا يناقض النتيجة التي إليها يجري في كتابه البرهان، التي هي أنّ كل ما لا يفسد فليس بمتكون لأنّه، إن كان يمكن أن يكون متكون لا يفسد، جاز أن يكون العالم وإن لم يفسد متكونا. وقال: «إنّ الحرارة الغريزية هي المصورة». وقال في آراء أبقراط وأفلاطن: «إنّ فلك البروج هو المصور». وقال في القوى الطبيعية: «إنّ هذه القوة أعلى وأشرف في الطبيعة»،

[102] Al-Rāzī does not mention Plato or the *Timaeus* in his discussion of creation. The *Doubts* makes explicit reference to the *Timaeus* only once (Koetschet 2019: p. 24 l. 5), and there al-Rāzī summarizes Aristotle's description of the dialogue's theory of vision at *Sens.* 437b10–13. The following analysis will show that this lack of citation belies the actual extent of al-Rāzī's engagement with the dialogue's ideas.

[103] Cf. *Secret of the Art of Medicine* 6.08 (Kuhne Brabant 1982: 384), where al-Rāzī appears to give Aristotle and Galen the same authoritative standing: 'Whenever Galen and Aristotle agree about a concept, then it is so; whenever they disagree, it is difficult to discern who is correct.'

[104] Galen summarizes this passage at *Com. Tim.* § 2; Kraus and Walzer (1951), p. 5 ll. 9–10.

[105] See Kraus (1939), 203–4, 283–5. See Rashed (2000), who demonstrates al-Rāzī's concern with the issue of divine justice, or God's goodness.

[106] As Koetschet (2015: 190–7) contends, al-Rāzī considers his own system to be superior to Galen's because it offers a theodicy.

وبنى أمره في منافع الأعضاء على أنّ البارئ عز وجل هو المصور، وقال: «إنّ قوما يتوهمون أنّ الحار الغريزي والطبيعة هو شيء واحد بعينه ولم يصيبوا».[107]

> He says in his *Book of Marasmus*: 'Marasmus takes hold of all living creatures necessarily because there is no living creature that does not grow old.' This [statement] is based on induction not on the nature of the living creature. Then he says: 'The statement that everything generated corrupts is not true absolutely but is plausible.' This contradicts the conclusion that he reaches in his *Book of Demonstration*, namely that everything which does not corrupt is not generated because, if it were possible that [something] generated does not corrupt, then it would be possible that the world is generated and, despite being generated, does not corrupt. He says: 'Innate heat is what gives form to [us].' He says in *On the Opinions of Hippocrates and Plato*: 'The zodiac is what gives form to [us].' He says in *On the Natural Faculties*: 'It is a higher and nobler power in nature.' He established in *On the Utility of the Parts* that the almighty and sublime Creator is what gives [us] form. He says: 'Some people imagine that innate heat, that is nature, is the only thing itself [that gives form] but they are wrong'.

The passage does not clarify how the inevitability of decay and the formative (*muṣawwir*) principle of the body are related topics. In juxtaposing citations from *Marc.* and *DD*, the first part of the text suggests that Galen's observations about the corruption of the body, or the ageing process, have a bearing on his cosmological beliefs. Al-Rāzī makes this jump from medicine to cosmology because Galen does so in *Marc.* There, Galen repeats his argument from *DD* 4 about the eternity of the world to question whether ageing is really a 'necessary and natural' (ἀναγκαῖόν τε καὶ κατὰ φύσιν) affection of the body. In contrast to al-Rāzī's interpretation at the beginning of the *Doubts*, at *Marc.* 7.671K Galen presents the conclusion that not everything born necessarily dies as the takeaway of his analysis in *DD*. In the above quotation al-Rāzī does not specify that his second excerpt from *Marc.* is an internal citation to *DD* 4.[108] Thus, he creates a false opposition between Galen's positions on the unavoidability of corruption in *Marc.* and *DD* 4.

The first part of the passage begins and ends with an assertion about the inevitability of corruption, so al-Rāzī implies that Galen inclined towards the opinion that generation always entails corruption. This belief is given as the reason why Galen finds the hypothesis of a generated cosmos being incorruptible implausible in *DD*. Al-Rāzī omits that Galen, turning to Plato's *Timaeus* (41d1–3) and the *Statesman* (270a, 273d), posited in *DD* 4

107 Koetschet (2019), p. 216 ll. 3–11.

108 The first quotation is loosely based on *Marc.* 7.699–70K. For an English translation of this Galenic work, see Theoharides (1971).

the existence of an extrinsic demiurgic cause which can preserve a generated thing from destruction.[109] Possibly wishing to distance Galen from this position that ascribes an active cosmological role to the Demiurge, the second part of the quotation from the *Doubts* illustrates that parts of the Galenic corpus appear to deny the divine's involvement in the formation of the cosmos. Specifically, it focuses on Galen's conflicting identifications of the formative principle, which is not defined but is the cause that gives form to matter or makes a thing 'what it is' in Platonic and Aristotelian philosophy.[110] As al-Rāzī holds with the *Timaeus* (52d–53b) that the world came into being from pre-existing matter, the formative principle would be what gave this material shape – God. Therefore, by alleging that certain Galenic texts equate the formative principle with innate heat or the zodiac, al-Rāzī suggests that Galen's cosmology has no causal function for God. That is to say, Galen's connection of the formative principle with natural entities seems to mean that the cosmos' structure is due to intrinsic forces. The passage depicts Galen's eternalist cosmology as lacking the presence of God.

As in the case of his review of Galen's cosmogonical stance in *DD* 4, al-Rāzī misrepresents the fundamental role of innate heat (Gr. ἔμφυτον θερμόν; Arab. *ḥarāra ġarīziyya*) in *Marc.* There, Galen never calls innate heat, which causes withering by dehydrating the body, a 'formative' principle, but states that its power to attract and to break down food helps to manage the body's material (τὴν ὕλην διοικεῖ, 7.675K). Restricting the influence of innate heat to the realm of the body, the treatise describes it as a 'corporeal' (σωματοειδής) rather than cosmic force that the 'demiurgic Nature' (ἡ φύσις ἡ δημιουργοῦσα) uses to create plants and animals.[111] Thus, despite al-Rāzī's statement to the contrary, *Marc.* shares the same cosmological framework as *UP*: both stress that innate heat is the tool of a higher creative principle, which is introduced as an amalgam of a personified Nature and the supreme god of Plato's *Timaeus*.[112] There is nothing in the Greek that corresponds to al-Rāzī's supposed extracts from *PHP*, *Nat.Fac.*, and even *UP*.[113] To obscure Galen's belief in a provident

109 Philoponus reports Galen's arguments in *DD* 4 about the preserving action of the Demiurge; see *De aet. mund.* 600.24–601.5. On this passage, see Chiaradonna (2009a), 248; Chiaradonna (2009b), 67–8.

110 For Aristotle's definition of the 'formal' cause, see *Phys.* 194b27–30.

111 *Marc.* 7.677K.

112 Galen designates innate heat as the 'first tool of nature' (πρῶτον ὄργανον τῆς φύσεως) at *UP* 14.6: Helmreich (1909), p. 299 ll. 6–7.

113 The Arabic versions utilized by al-Rāzī may have transmitted a different text. However, as has been amply documented, al-Rāzī often adapts his sources. On his different modes of citation, see Weisser (1991); Bryson (2001), 21–66; Garofalo (2002), 395–7; Pormann (2004), 61–92.

creator, al-Rāzī has probably distorted the views of at least *PHP*, which asserts that the human body is the product of a divine demiurge.[114]

Al-Rāzī's reading of *Marc.* and *PHP* emphasizes the dependence of Galen's cosmos on natural principles in order to insinuate that his predecessor neglected God's contribution to the world. In the above passage al-Rāzī appears to hold *UP* to be Galen's most exemplary work, where anatomical enquiry serves theology by furnishing empirical evidence of a wise creator. Nonetheless, in placing the citation of *UP* after a series of texts which at best downplay the preservative and formative powers of God, he portrays this work as an outlier.[115] He seems to view this disregard of God's benevolent management of the cosmos as a flaw that destabilizes the system of Galenism, for, as I will now demonstrate, the *Doubts* also presents it as the reason for later Galenists' misinterpretation of the Platonic theory of pleasure.

Hedonism and Two Galenic Readings of Plato

Al-Rāzī brings up the subject of pleasure when attacking Galen's assertion at *UP* 3.10 that pain is an unavoidable experience because the human body is composed of lowly material, menstrual blood and semen.[116] Galen makes this link between pain and the material substrate of the body as part of his defence of divine providence: our inferior make-up explains why we suffer despite the omnibenevolence of the Demiurge. While al-Rāzī may look favourably at *UP* in his review of Galen's varying stances on the formative principle of the body, he criticizes the aforementioned passage of the text for its apparent denial of God's omnipotence. In particular, he is uncomfortable with the suggestion that matter impedes God's ability to create life without suffering. Al-Rāzī cites Galen's theory of pleasure, which derives from the *Timaeus*, to show how Galen contradicts himself in accepting that humans have the capacity to achieve a state free from both pain and pleasure. As further grounds for his refutation of Galen's viewpoint in

[114] See *PHP* 9.8.22–9.9.3 (De Lacy 2005: p. 596 l. 5–p. 598 l. 8), where Galen refers to *Ti.* 41a7–d3 to discuss how the same god fashioned the cosmos and the body. Cf. *Critical Days* 9.911, 930–2K, which examines the connection between the zodiac and health.

[115] At Koetschet (2019), p. 44 ll. 4–6, al-Rāzī records Galen's doubts about whether animal anatomy proves the existence of a supremely wise creator, as *UP* claims. Al-Rāzī's text has Galen asking, if studying animals is a way to learn about God, what does the propensity of these creatures to harm one another say about the creator's sagacity? See also below.

[116] The following discussion expands on Schwarb (2017), 136–7. For the Galenic passage, see Helmreich (1907), p. 174 l. 19–175 l. 6=May (1968), vol. I, 189.

UP, he indicates that the treatise has led later Galenists to identify pleasure with the good – a position whose theological consequences he also proceeds to unpack. He argues:

> وأقول: إنّ هذا الكلام قد صرح فيه أنّ المواد ليست من خلق المصور وأنّ المصور لا يمكنه أن يحدث في كل مادة إلا ما لها أن يكون فيها. وإذ كان الأمر كذلك، ثم كان هذا المصور حكيما ناظرا ولم يمكنه أن يحدث من مادة ما حيوانا لا يألم ولا يموت. فالوجه في الحكم والنظر له ترك إحداثه البتة ليريحه من الألم البتة والموت والشدائد والحسرات.
>
> فإن ظن ظان أنّ جالينوس يرى أنّ ما يناله الإنسان في عمره من اللذة يترجع على ما يصل إليه من الألم أو يوازنه، فليعلم أنّ أفلاطن وسائر الطبيعيين قد أجمعوا على أنّ اللذة رجوع إلى الطبيعة بالراحة من مؤلم، وليس من الحكمة والنظر للمصور أن يخلق خلقة لا ينفك فيها من ألم. وهلا أراحة من ألم، إذ كان منفكا منه في حالته الأولى، مع أنّ هذا الكلام يناقض كلامه وكلام جميع الفلاسفة في إصلاح الأخلاق، وذلك أنّه يدعو إلى أن يكون الخير المطلوب لنفسه إنّما هي اللذة. وتتبين مضادة هذا القول لما في كتاب جالينوس في الأخلاق ولما في كتب أفلاطن خاصة وجميع أفاضل الفلاسفة. ولئن كانت اللذة أفضل ما في الحي لتكونن أفضل الحيوان أكثرها تهيؤا لإصابتها. وإن كان ذلك كذلك لتكونن البهائم أفضل من الناس بل من الكواكب بل من البارئ.[117]

I say: In this account [*UP* 3.10], he makes clear that matter is not part of the creation of the one who gave us form and that the one who gave us form can only bring into being in each matter the property that exists in it. If this is so, and [if] then the one who gave us form is wise and considerate, and it is impossible for [them] to bring into being from matter some creature that neither feels pain nor dies, there would be more appearance of wisdom and consideration, in this case, to refrain altogether from bringing it into existence so as to spare it always from pain, death, hardship, and distress.

If someone supposed that Galen believes that whatever [amount] of pleasure a person obtains in their life is a return of whatever [amount] of pain [they] attained or [that pleasure] balances [the pain], let them know that Plato and the rest of the natural philosophers agreed unanimously that pleasure is returning to a natural state free from pain. It is not in keeping with the wisdom and deliberation of the one who gave [us] form to create something and there not be in it a separation or respite from pain. Why did [the one who gave us form] not spare [the thing] from pain if it was free of [pain] in its primary condition? Nonetheless, this account contradicts [Plato's] account and the account of every philosopher on [the subject of] ethics. That is to say, he puts forward [above] that the good sought after for its own sake is pleasure. It is clear, however, that this proposal contradicts what Galen says in *On Character Traits* and what Plato, in particular, says in his books and all of the best philosophers. If pleasure is the best [thing] for a creature, then the best living things are more influenced by their afflictions. If this is so, then cattle are better than people, and more than that the stars and even the Creator!

[117] Koetschet (2019), p. 46 l. 4–p. 48 l. 2.

The first half of the passage targets the notion in *UP* that pain is intrinsic to the body, whereas the second half reveals that Galen's own understanding of pleasure posits the existence of a neutral original condition. In outlining the Galenic theory of pleasure, al-Rāzī opposes two conceptions of the sensation: the idea of a reader of Galen that pleasure is an endpoint or goal, and that of Plato and all other 'natural philosophers' (*ṭabīʿiyyīn*), who view pleasure as an experience that one has when returning to the natural state.[118] At the end of the text, al-Rāzī aligns Galen with the Platonic definition of pleasure, so his criticism in this part seems to be that Galen's teachings in *UP* have caused certain adherents to adopt a hedonism with blasphemous implications.

The two positions on pleasure that al-Rāzī contrasts appear to represent different interpretations of *Ti.* 64c8–d3, which states that the sensation is 'a sudden return to a natural condition' (τὸ δ' εἰς φύσιν ἀπιὸν πάλιν ἀθρόον ἡδύ).[119] The nameless (or perhaps imaginary) Galenist preserves the dialogue's identification of pleasure as a 'return' (*yataraǧǧaʿu*), which they take to mean recompense for pain previously felt, but leaves out its qualification that what is restored is the natural condition. This individual's theory comes close to al-Rāzī's in *Spiritual Medicine*, which alleges that a person is pleased only to the same degree (*miqdār*) that they are harmed.[120] Both the Galenist and al-Rāzī depart from the *Timaeus* in linking the intensity of pleasure with the amount of pain that preceded it, rather than with the speed of the restoration. Even so, *Spiritual Medicine* in addition to *On Pleasure* (*Fī l-Laḏḏa*), which are based on Galen's summary of the Platonic doctrine at *Com. Tim.* § 14, hold that pleasure is only experienced while the body is returning to its 'primary condition', which is neither painful nor pleasant.[121] As al-Rāzī suggests, owing to the connection at *UP* 3.10 between pain and the body's material constituents, the Galenist does not recognize a neutral state and therefore supposes that humans are in either pleasure or pain.

In accordance with the anti-hedonism of al-Rāzī's ethical writings, the above quotation of the *Doubts* goes on to demonstrate why the natural state rather than pleasure is the ideal condition, or 'good' (*ḫayr*), towards which humans should strive.[122] Al-Rāzī portrays the anonymous Galenic exegete

118 I wish to thank Peter Adamson for his help with interpreting this section of the *Doubts*.

119 I discuss in more detail Galen's treatment of pleasure in texts such as *Caus.Symp.* and *Plat. Tim.* in Chapter 4 (pp. 156–9).

120 See Kraus (1939), p. 37 ll. 9–10. On this passage, see Adamson (2008), 85–6.

121 See Adamson (2008), 85–7, who argues that Galen's concept of health as stasis may have influenced al-Rāzī's idea of the 'natural state'. See p. 118 above.

122 Cf. the claim of Goodman (1971) that al-Rāzī's thought, including his theory of pleasure, is Epicurean. Adamson (2008) argues that, while the late work *The Philosopher's Way of Life* considers

as a deviant in that his hedonism puts him at odds with Plato, mainstream philosophical opinion, and even Galen himself (specifically, the position of *On Character Traits*).[123] While the reference in the text to 'Plato's books' (*kutub Aflāṭun*) may denote the philosopher's discussions of pleasure in the *Gorgias* (491d–496e), *Republic* (558d–559d, 585a–c), and *Philebus* along with the *Timaeus*, al-Rāzī appears to know only the latter dialogue, as I mentioned above.[124] Thus, al-Rāzī may view this Galenist as contradicting the *Timaeus* in particular. The individual's strong hedonist reading of the *Timaeus*' theory, about which they probably learned from Galen's work, seems to assume that, as pain and pleasure are the only two conditions, pleasure must be the good of life. The *Doubts*, similar to *Spiritual Medicine* and *On Pleasure*, does not acknowledge the existence of intellectual pleasures, so al-Rāzī interprets the Galenist's theory to mean that the good is bodily pleasure.[125] Al-Rāzī's dialectical *coup de grâce* is to reveal the heretical consequences of this link between the experience of pleasure and the attainment of the good. He reasons that, if the highest good is the achievement of pleasure, then brute animals, who are ruled by their desires and pursue them without restraint, are superior creatures.[126] Thus, this Galenist's doctrine of pleasure demeans God, who is incapable of carnal desire, by ranking the deity below irrational beasts.

The *Doubts* turns Galen's Platonic notion of pleasure against him to disprove the contention in *UP* 3.10 that God was unable to create life without pain because of the constraints imposed by matter. The polemical point of the example of the Galenist's misunderstanding of the nature of pleasure is to underscore how Galen's weak grasp of the 'divine science' has caused his interpreters not only to replicate his mistakes but also to add to them. As a result of *UP*'s characterization of pain as an innate condition of the body, the Galenist has assumed that pleasure is a good and has

pleasure to be harmless if pursued in moderation, al-Rāzī was an anti-hedonist on the whole. Goodman (2015) responds to Adamson's criticisms of his Epicurean reading of al-Rāzī.

123 *On Character Traits* (Kraus 1937: 41=Davies 2013: 159), which survives in an Arabic summary by Ḥunayn, follows the *Timaeus* (69d2) in characterizing pleasure as a 'snare' (*miṣyada*; Gr. δέλεαρ).

124 For an overview of Plato's accounts of pleasure in these other dialogues, see Adamson (2008), 72–7.

125 On the absence of intellectual pleasures from al-Rāzī's theory of pleasure, see Adamson (2008), 88–92. Cf. Avicenna's identification of several classes of pleasure (Chapter 4, pp. 162–8).

126 This final argument in the *Doubts* parallels al-Rāzī's attack on those who imagine pleasure to be a good in *Spiritual Medicine* (Kraus 1939: p. 24 l. 8–p. 25 l. 11). In this text, al-Rāzī relates that, if gratifying carnal desires were noble, then the bull and ass would be superior to humans and God, who never lusts after anything. On this passage, see Adamson (2008), 92. Cf. *It Is Not Possible Even to Live Pleasantly according to Epicurus* (1091c, 1092a–b), where Plutarch accuses Epicurus of believing that irrational animals are more equipped to lead a good life because of their care-free indulgence in pleasure.

erroneously read Plato's doctrine in the light of this inference. In al-Rāzī's view, this position commits the Galenist to the theologically problematic belief that creatures governed by their appetites are better than God. Therefore, al-Rāzī insinuates that, while Galen himself may have reached the right conclusion about pleasure in texts such as *On Character Traits*, his failure to stress the importance of a thorough education in philosophy, including metaphysics, makes him responsible for this student's mistakes. He should have encouraged his readers to adopt the 'top-down' approach of the *Timaeus*, where metaphysics is used to elucidate corporeal phenomena.

Platonic and 'Anti-Platonic' Theories of the Soul

The final passage of the *Doubts* that I will discuss attacks *QAM*, whose titular thesis Galen finds support for in the *Timaeus*.[127] Dealing with the immortality of the soul, the critique attempts to refute the materialist message of *QAM*, which al-Rāzī understands to be that the soul is a corporeal mixture that dies with the body.[128] Al-Rāzī finds this supposed contention of *QAM* objectionable because it conflicts with his own recognition of the soul as one of the five eternals. Thus, unlike the foregoing quotations of the *Doubts*, this text is concerned as much with preserving the cosmological importance of the soul as with upholding God's omnibenevolence. Al-Rāzī employs the same polemical tactic as in his dispute about pleasure to discredit Galen's materialist stance, which *QAM* associates with Plato as well as Aristotle and Hippocrates: that is, to present himself as the better exegete of Plato.[129] Whereas al-Rāzī's rival, or 'anti-Platonic', positions on creation and pleasure reveal his engagement with Galenic readings of the *Timaeus* (especially *Com. Tim.*), he argues for a Neoplatonic view of the soul in what follows.

Al-Rāzī directs his criticism towards two passages in *QAM*, the first of which concerns the variation in the moral conduct of children, and the second the effects of bodily injuries on the soul.[130] He introduces his discussion of the latter issue, the focus of my analysis, by stressing Galen's conflict with Plato. He writes:

> وقال شبيها بالمناقض لأفلاطن: «ما بال النفس، إن كانت غير البدن، يضطرها خروج الدم الكثير وشرب الشوكران إلى مفارقته؟»، وامتد في هذا لكلام وتوهم أنّه يناقض من يقول :«إنّ النفس ذات قائمة على انفرادها». وأجاب نفسه عن أفلاطن وهو أنّ أفلاطن يقول :«إنّه ليس يصلح للحيوة

[127] See Chapter 1, pp. 51–3.
[128] Cf. Singer's (2013b: 340–59) interpretation of Galen's stance in *QAM*.
[129] See Chapter 1, p. 53.
[130] For the first passage, see Koetschet (2019), p. 218 l. 11–p. 220 l. 3. Cf. *QAM* 4.817–19K, where Galen hypothesizes that a child's moral character depends on their body's mixture.

بالنفس كل جسد، لكن الجسد الذي له أن ينفعل منها بقبول الحياة. فكما أنّك، إن أحدثت على مسكن بعض الحيوان حادثة لا يتهيأ له معها أن يسكنه، لم يسكنه بل زال عنه وخلاه، وكذلك تكون حال النفس عند هذه الأحوال التي تحدث في الجسد.»
ثم قال: «فقد أقر أفلاطن أنّ النفس مزاج حيث قال إنّ الإنسان تحدث له من تغير المزاج أمراض مختلفة كالماليخوليا وأنّ النفس تؤول إلى الشر والرداءة من قبل مزاج البدن»، وهذا مما أقر به أفلاطن يعلم بإقراره فيه، وجالينوس يحسب أنّه يجيء من هذه الأشياء أنّ النفس مزاج كما يحبه ويشتهيه، وليس يجيء من هذا ونحوه شيء مما يتمنى. فإن أفلاطن يقول له إنّ هذا الشر والرداءة لم يقع في جوهر النفس بل في الفعل الكائن بالآلة التي تستعملها النفس، كما أنّك إن أحدثت على عود العواد وزمر الزمار حادثة ردیئة، كان الإيقاع والزمر مختلطا متشوشا رديئا بحسب الحادث وإن كان الموسيقار سليما باقيا على حاله وحذقه.[131]

> He says something similar to Plato's opponent: 'Why is it that, if the soul is incorporeal, a voiding of much blood and drinking hemlock forces it to separate?' He expands on this argument and thinks that he contradicts the one who argues that the soul is an essence that subsists separately. He himself responds on Plato's behalf, namely that Plato would say: 'not every body is suited to be made alive by the soul, but only the body is capable of being affected by the soul in order to receive life. Just as you might cause something to happen to the dwelling of a certain animal that is not equipped to handle [the change or damage], but [the animal] does not dwell there but abandons and deserts it. Thus is the condition of the soul when these conditions happen to the body.'
>
> Then he says: 'Plato established that the soul is a mixture because he said that different diseases, like melancholy, happen to a person due to a change of mixture, and that the soul tends towards evil and wickedness on account of the mixture of the body.' This is what Plato acknowledged by acknowledging [the influence of mixture on the soul]. And, Galen reckons that it follows from these things that the soul is a mixture in proportion to its desires and appetites. But, nothing that he expects results from this [statement] or something similar. In fact, Plato says that this evil and wickedness do not occur to the substance of the soul but to the activity that arises in the instrument that the soul utilizes. It is just as whenever you damage the *ʿūd* [a type of lute] of an *ʿūdist* and the trumpet of a trumpeter, the rhythm and the blowing are mixed, distorted, and bad because of the accident, although the musician's condition and skill remains intact.

The passage responds to Galen's use of medical examples at *QAM* 4.774–7K to cast doubt on Plato's theory of an incorporeal, immortal soul. While al-Rāzī frames the text as a debate about the immortality of the entire soul, Galen seems to question the ability of only the rational soul (λογιστική ψυχή) to survive after the body's death, for

131 Koetschet (2019), p. 222 l. 1–p. 224 l. 4.

he takes the mortality of the desiderative and irascible parts as a given.[132] In the aforementioned section of *QAM*, however, Galen refers to both the 'rational soul' and the 'soul' more generally, so al-Rāzī may have thought that the Platonic thesis at stake in this Galenic text is the immortality of the soul as a whole, not just its rational part.[133] *QAM* focuses on challenging the imperishability of the rational soul, which out of the three parts of the soul has the best claim to immortality, to debunk the view of certain Platonists that the entire soul survives death.

Al-Rāzī notices that Galen's polemical strategy in *QAM* is to show how Plato contradicts himself on the question of the soul's immortality – a strategy that mirrors al-Rāzī's own critical treatment of Galen in the *Doubts*. He first reviews Galen's critique of the Platonic link between the soul's incorporeality and immortality, and then addresses the supposition that Plato's awareness of the impact of temperamental change on the soul supports his belief in the soul's corporeality and mortality. The passage begins with a citation from *QAM* (4.775K) that asks how the soul can be immortal when blood loss or poisoning, both of which greatly cool the body, cause it to separate.[134] Galen's reasoning is that, as the corporeal cannot affect the incorporeal, the soul must be a corporeal entity because bodily conditions prompt it to depart. Al-Rāzī counters Galen by pointing out that the soul influences the body, and not the other way around.

To illustrate the way in which the soul inhabits but is not part of the body, al-Rāzī uses the simile of an animal fleeing its den, which the *Doubts* presents as what Galen imagines Plato would have replied when confronted with his argument about the influence of blood loss and poisoning on the soul. The simile has no parallel in *QAM* but shares features with a comparison at *Loc.Aff.* 2.10.15 that Galen makes, and then rejects, between the logical soul and a person who remains unharmed when their house is damaged.[135] In dismissing the analogy at *Loc.Aff.*, Galen cites brain injuries as proof that the logical soul is in fact harmed when its house, the body, is impaired.[136] Thus, in the *Doubts*, al-Rāzī may be weaponizing against Galen the very analogy that he discards at *Loc.Aff.* to invalidate *QAM*'s thesis. Alternatively, because the image of the body as the soul's

[132] See *QAM* 4.782–3K.

[133] On the significance of Galen's change of expression, see Singer (2013a), p. 413, no. 4.15.

[134] Al-Rāzī's quotation omits 'raging fever' (πυρετὸς διακαής) from Galen's list of deadly afflictions.

[135] Gärtner (2015), p. 374, ll. 6–10.

[136] See Havrda (2017), 84.

habitation is hardly unique to Galen, it is possible that he is appropriating another source's argument.[137]

Al-Rāzī does not appear to dispute that temperamental imbalance can impair the functioning of the soul in the body; rather, he opposes the idea that it alters the soul's substance (Gr. οὐσία; Arab. *ǧawhar*).[138] In particular, the text of the *Doubts* takes issue with Galen's reading of Plato's account of the negative effect of melancholy – and by extension, all illnesses resulting from humoural excess – on the soul. While Galen refers to melancholy in *QAM* (4.777, 779 K) as an example of a disease that disturbs the rational faculty of the soul, he does not mention Plato when discussing it. Al-Rāzī's quotation of *QAM* seems to merge Galen's description of melancholy with his citations of *Ti.* 86e5–87a8 and 86c4–d6, which report that phlegmatic and bilious diseases injure all three parts of the soul and that wickedness arises due to poor health and education.[139] Galen invokes these passages from the dialogue to align Plato with his own notion of the relationship between the body and soul.[140] Against Galen's equation of his materialist psychology with Plato's, al-Rāzī attributes to the philosopher the view that diseases such as melancholy only render the body unsuitable for the soul's use. To explain how the soul remains unaffected by disease and even evil, he appeals to another analogy that likens the body to an instrument and the soul to a musician: just as a musician cannot produce a pleasant sound on a damaged instrument, so the soul is unable to realize fully its capacities for activities such as rational thought in an ill or wicked body.

This image of the body as the instrument of an independent (rational) soul broadly reflects a Neoplatonic conception of the body–soul relationship.[141]

[137] The analogy has roots in the Pythagorean notion that the body is a prison house, which is picked up by Plato at *Phaedo* 62b4. Cf. Lucretius, *DRN* 3.741–75; Plotinus, *Enn.* 6.7.35.

[138] Cf. al-Rāzī's note in the *Comprehensive Book* (al-Rāzī 1955–70: vol. I, p. 89 ll. 5–10) on Galen's explanation of the effect of moisture on the soul in his commentary on *Ti.* 44b1–6 in *Plat. Tim.*, book one, fr. 7–9 (on the passage, see Das 2014: 101–2). Perhaps following *QAM* 4.781K, al-Rāzī states that dryness makes the soul move more quickly and thus increases understanding. At *Secret of the Art of Medicine* 6.21 (Kuhne Brabant 1982: 385), al-Rāzī cites with apparent approval Galen's position that the soul follows the mixtures of the body. None of al-Rāzī's surviving works acknowledge this doctrinal inconsistency.

[139] See *QAM* 4.789–90K. The *Timaeus* (85a5–b2) mentions the harmful effect of black bile on the divine circuits in our heads but identifies the disorder that disrupts them as the 'sacred disease', or epilepsy.

[140] *QAM* 4.791K.

[141] Unlike the above quotation of the *Doubts*, Neoplatonic thinkers such as Plotinus and Proclus speak in terms of a tripartite soul and regard only the rational part as immortal. Arabic readers had access to an adapted discussion of Plotinus' account of the body–soul relationship at *Enn.* 4 via the famous

The comparison of the body to an instrument or tool (ὄργανον) is not, of course, a Neoplatonic innovation but has antecedents in Plato and Aristotle.[142] Both philosophers appear to advance an interactionist theory of the soul, where body and soul influence each other.[143] Therefore, al-Rāzī's position in the *Doubts* is more in line with the Neoplatonic distinction between the body and rational soul, according to which the former depends on the latter for its existence, or 'life' (*ḥayā*), but not vice versa.[144] The animal analogy indicates, however, that al-Rāzī departs from Neoplatonists such as Plotinus and Proclus in locating the entire soul, rather than just the appetitive and irascible parts, in the body.[145] Elsewhere in the *Doubts* he explains that, when in the body, the soul remains independent because it does not consist of the same substance as its corporeal seat, which is composed of elementary atoms.[146] Notwithstanding this doctrinal difference, the Neoplatonic scheme allows him to acknowledge that the body can enfeeble the soul's activities without damaging its very essence, whereas Galen's 'Platonic' doctrine supposes that evil as well as disease can affect the soul's substance.[147]

Al-Rāzī seems to find Galen's identification of soul with mixture in *QAM* unacceptable because it denies that all souls can achieve the ultimate aim of returning to the higher world – which his theory of the five eternals posits as the goal of human life.[148] The presumption is that those souls corrupted by evil would be unable to free themselves from the material world. This hypothesis seems to be in keeping with al-Rāzī's general characterization of Galen's system as lacking in the supervision of a benevolent deity. Again, then, he criticizes Galen on the basis of his perceived theological inadequacies, which have

pseudo-*Theology of Aristotle* (on which, see the Introduction, p. 23). For the text's depiction of the body as a tool of the rational soul, see, e.g., *TA* 9.12–13, 10.72; Badawī (1966), p. 122 ll. 5–12, p. 145 ll. 5–8. Moreover, an Arabic fragment of Proclus' commentary on *Ti.* 89e3–90c7 describes the body as the servant (*ḫaddām*) and organ (*āla*) of the soul's activities: see Arnzen (2013), p. 20 l. 6 [Arabic], 29 [English].

142 See Plato's *Tht.* 184c–d and *Alc.* 129c7–8, d4–e3 (I leave aside the question of this dialogue's authenticity); see, e.g., Aristotle *DA* 407b25–6, 415b18–20, 416b20–7, 433b19.

143 At least, Plato seems to do so in the *Timaeus*. On the interactionism in Plato and Aristotle's psychological theories, see Menn (2002), 86–90.

144 See Dörrie (1973), who surveys Neoplatonic theories of soul from Plotinus to Proclus. For a good introduction to the body–soul relationship in Plotinus, see Emilsson (1991).

145 At *Enn.* 4.9.4 Plotinus suggests that the body only contains an image of the soul. Proclus relates that the rational soul is housed in a luminous vehicle (ὄχημα αὐγοειδές), which is separate from the mortal body: see *El. Th.*, propositions 207–9 and *In Ti.* III 236.1–5.

146 See Koetschet (2019), 120–32.

147 Cf. *Enn.* 4.4.43=*TA* 6.43.3–7; Badawī (1966), p. 80 ll. 1–11.

148 See p. 110 above.

caused him to make incorrect inferences about the soul from his observations of melancholy and other bodily disorders.

A Different Disciplinary Model

I have argued that the aim of al-Rāzī's disputes with Galen over theories deriving from the *Timaeus* is to supplant him as the authority on Plato. The association of Galen with an eternalist cosmology in the *Doubts* is perhaps the most conspicuous example of al-Rāzī's push to undermine his predecessor's Platonic credentials. Al-Rāzī's writings show a profound engagement with the Galenic corpus, so his attempts to assert his superiority as a Platonic exegete may be his way of distinguishing himself from Galen, with whom he shares many affinities. The progressive view of science outlined at the beginning of the *Doubts* suggests that it is not enough for al-Rāzī to equal Galen – he ought to surpass him. Reclaiming Plato from Galen is integral to al-Rāzī's revision of Galenism, or disciplinary boundary work.

Concerned primarily with exposing the theoretical mistakes in Galen's thought, the *Doubts* offers only glimpses of al-Rāzī's alternative to Galenism. A different understanding of Plato and the *Timaeus* seems to be behind some of his major doctrinal shifts from Galen. For instance, my examination of al-Rāzī's critique of *QAM* uncovered how his separation of the body from the soul is more consistent with Neoplatonic psychologies than Galen's, which stresses the soul's reliance on its corporeal seat. I mentioned in passing that al-Rāzī also invokes Plato, specifically the account from the *Timaeus* (53d4–55b6) of the cubical and triangular structures of earth and fire, to endorse his atomistic conception of the elements.[149] While it is unclear whether this atomistic reading of Plato is original to al-Rāzī, his knowledge of the dialogue's depiction of the elements as geometrical solids may be based on Galen's *Com.Tim.*, which briefly summarizes the account.[150] Thus, al-Rāzī may have appealed to Galen's treatment of the *Timaeus* to attack Galen's theory of the elements, which supposedly goes back to the *Timaeus* too. This subversive use of Galen's exegeses of the *Timaeus* to discredit Galenic ideas that are inspired by the *Timaeus* is paralleled elsewhere in the *Doubts*, for I have demonstrated that the text juxtaposes two notions of pleasure which appear to stem from Galen's *Com.Tim.*

149 See p. 111 above. 150 Kraus and Walzer (1951), p. 15 ll. 2–5.

In his quarrels regarding creation, pleasure, and the soul, al-Rāzī connects Galen and his followers' shortcomings as Platonists, and as thinkers in general, to their failure to take sufficient account of the benevolence of God, the formative (*muṣawwir*) principle of the cosmos. He remarks that Galen may have achieved the rank of natural philosopher (*daraǧat al-ṭabīʿiyyīn*) but he would have benefited from discussions with metaphysicians (lit. 'experts in the divine science', *aṣḥāb al-ʿilm al-ilāhī*), whose goal is to acquire knowledge of God.[151] These comments about Galen's limited philosophical training do not necessarily imply that he was unsuccessful only as a philosopher and that his medical theories constitute the sole credible aspect of his thought. As my analysis of al-Rāzī's treatment of pleasure revealed, in his view Galen's lack of interest in theology debilitates his entire system: knowledge of God's nature enables one to reach the correct conclusions about corporeal experiences as well as broader cosmic questions. In placing God at the forefront of his investigations of the body and cosmos, al-Rāzī seems to advocate in the *Doubts* an epistemological approach that corresponds to the narrative structure of the *Timaeus*, which first establishes the Demiurge's goodness and then cites it as the ultimate cause of the heavens and the human body. This top-down model of explanation contrasts with Galen's use of the dialogue's discussion of the human body as an entry point into subjects beyond the body. Therefore, in the *Doubts* al-Rāzī has recourse to the authority of Plato to develop a more theologically oriented or metaphysical system of medicine and philosophy.

While al-Rāzī appears to fault Galen for his narrow focus on the physical, I highlighted at the start of this chapter how later Islamicate authors accuse al-Rāzī of disciplinary overreach for presuming that his medical expertise qualified him to write on metaphysics. As the next two chapters will relate, Avicenna and Maimonides censure Galen for placing questions belonging to physics within the province of medicine, so, in comparison, al-Rāzī's linking of medicine and metaphysics seems especially transgressive. In the passages at the start of this chapter, Avicenna and Maimonides target a single work by al-Rāzī, his *Metaphysics*, and do not pass judgement on his reformulation of the boundaries between medicine, philosophy, and theology in the *Doubts*.[152] Nonetheless, by attacking the *Metaphysics* as the work of a doctor rather than a philosopher, they reject

[151] See Koetschet (2019), p. 114 ll. 3–4 and p. 40 ll. 2–4. On the second passage, see Koetschet (2015), 195.

[152] Maimonides addresses al-Rāzī's critique of Galen in book twenty-five of his *Medical Aphorisms* (*Kitāb al-Fuṣūl fī l-ṭibb*); for this passage, see Chapter 5 (p. 189).

the disciplinary model that the *Doubts* puts forward in opposition to Galen's limited philosopher-doctor, the metaphysician-doctor. Despite this representation of al-Rāzī as an aberration, both thinkers also had dual careers as doctors and philosophers with specific interests in metaphysics and theology. Thus, in what follows I will examine how Avicenna and Maimonides perform their own boundary work to impose a more restrictive limit to what doctors can know but, at the same time, also justify their own professional identities as philosopher-doctors.

CHAPTER 4

Laying Down the Law: Avicenna and his Medical Project

Avicenna (*c.* 370–428/980–1037) claims that he was only sixteen when he taught himself medicine.[1] In his *Autobiography* (*Sīrat al-šayḫ al-ra ʾīs*), he writes:

> اشتغلت أنا بتحصيل الكتب من الفصوص والشروح[2] من الطبيعيات والإلهيات وصار أبواب العلم تنفتح عليّ. ثم رغبت في علم الطب وقرأت الكتب المصنفة فيه. وعلم الطب ليس هو من العلوم الصعبة، فلذلك برزت فيه أقل مدة حتى بدأ فضلاء الأطباء يقرؤون عليّ علم الطب.[3]
>
> I endeavoured to obtain books on physics (*ṭabīʿiyyāt*) and metaphysics (*ilāhiyyāt*) – both texts and commentaries. Various topics of knowledge began to open in front of me. Then I desired to study the science of medicine (*ʿilm al-ṭibb*), and I read books devoted to this subject. The science of medicine is not one of the difficult sciences (*al-ʿulūm al-ṣaʿba*). Therefore, I excelled in it after a very short period of time, so that excellent doctors began to read the science of medicine under me.[4]

Avicenna reports that he not only mastered but also began teaching medicine in his teenage years. Avicenna's description of his self-education in medicine is misleading, for Ullmann has shown that he studied the subject under at least two teachers.[5] Notwithstanding the veracity of the above account, Avicenna appears to have obtained his first job at eighteen as a court physician to the Sāmānid ruler Nūḥ b. Manṣūr, in the city of Buḫārā (now in Uzbekistan); he would later serve other Iranian

[1] Gutas (1987–8) argues that the date 370/980, which is given for Avicenna's birth in certain medieval sources, should be pushed back to 353/964.

[2] I have adopted the reading *šurūḥ* ('commentaries'), instead of Gohlman's *šurūʿ* ('beginning'), after Gutas (1988), 27nj=(2014), 16nj.

[3] Gohlman (1974), p. 24 l. 6–p. 26 l. 2.

[4] I follow with minor modifications the translation of Pormann (2013: 92), who has revised the translations of Gohlman (1974: 25, 27) and Gutas (1988: 27=2014: 16).

[5] Ullmann (1970: 147, 151) identifies Avicenna's medical instructors as Abū Manṣūr al-Ḥasan ibn Nūḥ al-Qumrī (d. after 380/990) and Abū Sahl ʿĪsā ibn Yaḥyā al-Masīḥī al-Ǧurǧānī (d. after 401/1010). See also Gutas (1988), 149–98=(2014), 170–225, who cautions that the *Autobiography* and *Biography* by Avicenna's student al-Ǧūzǧānī should be approached as literary rather than historical documents.

monarchs in this capacity.[6] While modern scholars have disputed the extent of Avicenna's clinical experience, he composed one of the most widely read pre-modern works on medical theory, the *Canon of Medicine* (*al-Qānūn fī l-ṭibb*).[7] Summarizing the learned traditions of Graeco-Arabic medicine, the *Canon of Medicine* circulated throughout the medieval Islamicate world, and its Latin version formed part of the medical curriculum in western European universities until the seventeenth century.[8]

In contrast to the brief attention that the *Autobiography* gives to Avicenna's medical studies, the text describes at length his pursuit of the philosophical sciences, or, to be more precise, his progression through the Aristotelian curriculum.[9] By the year 391/1000 Avicenna seems to have acquired a significant reputation for his philosophical learning, which spurred thinkers from Iran and elsewhere to test his expertise. Famously, the scientist Abū l-Rayḥān al-Bīrūnī (362–*c.* 442/973–*c.* 1050), who was from the region of Ḫwārazm (in present Uzbekistan and Turkmenistan), challenged Avicenna to defend the validity of Aristotelian natural philosophy.[10] Avicenna's conception of his own relationship to the Peripatetic tradition evolved throughout his life, but one of his most successful philosophical compositions, *The Cure* (*Kitāb al-Šifāʾ*), is a summa of the Aristotelian sciences.[11] Similar to the *Canon of Medicine*, *The Cure* had a significant impact on both Islamicate and European scholars, for it shaped later interpretations of Aristotelian doctrine and even the style of philosophical writing.[12]

6 In the *Biography* al-Ǧūzǧānī relates that the mother of the Būyid ruler Maǧd al-Dawla, who resided in Rayy, hired Avicenna as a court physician to cure her son of melancholy. See Gohlman (1974), p. 48 l. 9–p. 50 l. 1.

7 Based on her examinations of the *Canon of Medicine* and the *Autobiography*, Álvarez-Millán (2010) concludes that Avicenna had limited clinical experience. Cf. Pormann (2013), 96–102.

8 The extensive manuscript tradition of the *Canon of Medicine* testifies to its popularity in the Arabic-speaking world: see Anawātī (1950), 192–204; Ullmann (1970), 152n8. Gerard of Cremona (*c.* 1114–87) translated the *Canon of Medicine* from Arabic into Latin. On his translation and its circulation in medieval and early modern Europe, see Weisser (1983); Siraisi (1987); Jacquart (2005).

9 Gutas (1988), 149–59=(2014), 169–79.

10 Al-Bīrūnī's exchange with Avicenna, which consists of eighteen questions on theoretical astronomy, meteorology, and physics, has been edited by Naṣr and Muḥaqqiq (1995). For an overview of al-Bīrūnī's life and works, see Kennedy (1970); Bosworth (2010).

11 As Gutas (1988: 286–96=2014: 323–34) contends, although Avicenna saw himself as belonging to the Aristotelian tradition, in his mature years he expressed his ideological independence from past and contemporary Peripatetics. *The Cure*, which was composed over an eleven-year period (407–18/1016–27) covers logic, physics, mathematics, and metaphysics, and draws on texts from not only Aristotle but also Porphyry, Euclid, Ptolemy, and Nicomachus of Gerasa. On this composition, see Gutas (1988), 101–12=(2014), 103–15.

12 For surveys of the Islamic and Jewish receptions of *The Cure*, see respectively Wisnovsky (2013) and Freudenthal and Zonta (2013). On the medieval Latin translations and reception of *The Cure*, see, e.g., Hasse (2000); Bertolacci (2011, 2013b); Janssens (2007, 2011).

Although Avicenna was at least as eminent in medicine as in philosophy, he nonetheless writes dismissively about medicine as a 'science' (*ʿilm*). As I will explain, Avicenna developed a hierarchical classification of the sciences that ranks each science according to the abstraction of its object of enquiry from the material world.[13] Dealing with the human body, medicine holds an inferior status, which restricts the lines of investigation that its practitioners can pursue. Avicenna's demarcation of medicine from philosophy may partially account for the popularity of the *Canon of Medicine* and *The Cure*, in that both texts transmit more circumscribed versions of these disciplines which are easier to teach.[14] Even so, this chapter argues that Avicenna sets out to limit the domain of medicine, which Galen expanded through his engagements with Plato's *Timaeus*, to reassert philosophy's command over knowledge of the natural world. I will show that Avicenna's boundary work in the *Canon of Medicine* aims to weaken Galen's credibility in order to reduce the threat that Galenism (with its more sophisticated understanding of the body) posed to Aristotle's authority on natural philosophy.[15]

While Avicenna maintains a distinction between medicine and philosophy on a theoretical level, in practice it is not always easy to differentiate these two aspects of his output. This chapter also looks at the internal tension between Avicenna's restrictive boundary work and less exclusionary approach to knowledge, which is particularly evident in his discussions of topics that Galen, following the *Timaeus*, saw as pertaining to both body and soul. I will focus on Avicenna's response to Galen's interpretation of the *Timaeus*' accounts of the corporeal seat of the 'ruling' part of the soul and the nature of pleasure. After outlining in the first section of the chapter the boundary that Avicenna constructs between medicine and philosophy in the *Canon of Medicine*, my analysis will examine how he transgresses it in identifying the heart as the hegemonic organ. By attributing the faculties of sensation, voluntary motion, growth, and nutrition to the heart, Avicenna

[13] Avicenna is hardly unique in his hypothesis of a hierarchy of the sciences. Al-Kindī (*c.* 185–252/801–66), al-Fārābī (*c.* 259–339/872–950), the Iḫwān al-Ṣafāʾ ('Brethren of Purity', fourth/tenth century), and Ibn Ḥazm (d. 456/1064) – to name just a few – composed texts that enumerate and classify both the Greek ('foreign') and Arabic ('native') sciences. For an overview of this classificatory literature, see the Introduction (pp. 19–21).

[14] See Musallam (1987).

[15] See Musallam (1987). Avicenna stands in a long tradition of philosophers who have had to grapple with reconciling Aristotelian natural philosophy with Galenic medicine. For example, Greek thinkers such as John Philoponus (*c.* 490–575) show awareness of how Galen's research on the brain seems to disprove Aristotle's claim that the heart is the source of sensation. See Philoponus, *On Aristotle On the Soul* 1.1 (19.1): van der Eijk (2014), 34.

rejects the primacy that Galen (supporting *Ti.* 73c6–74a1) accords to the brain as the seat of the rational soul in his tripartite psychological scheme. As part of his polemic with Galen, Avicenna undermines his own disciplinary prescriptions to defend Aristotle's and his own conception of a unitary soul.

The next section draws attention to Avicenna's treatment of pleasure, a topic that is related to his championing of the heart as the source of sensation and the emotions. Avicenna offers distinct aetiologies of pleasure in the *Canon of Medicine*, the *Treatise on the Principles of Cardiac Drugs* (*Maqāla fī Aḥkām al-adwiya al-qalbiyya*), *Pointers and Reminders* (*Kitāb al-Išārāt wa l-tanbīhāt*), and *The Cure.*[16] In so doing, he appears to advance different disciplinary claims to the subject. I will demonstrate that the *Canon of Medicine* puts forward an explanation of pleasure that is based on Galen's interpretation of *Ti.* 64c8–d3 (which defines it as a return to a natural state), whereas *Cardiac Drugs* associates the sensation with the health of the pneuma in the heart. Both texts, however, largely define pleasure as a corporeal experience, and therefore suggest, in apparent opposition to *Pointers and Reminders* and *The Cure*, that the issue pertains to the doctor's domain, the body. While Avicenna's engagement with the Galenic–Timaean theory of pleasure highlights the negotiability of his definitions of medicine and philosophy, it also reveals how difficult it was to extricate the body from the soul after Galen.

As a preliminary to this chapter, I want to emphasize that Galen is not the only source that transmitted doctrines from Plato's *Timaeus* to Avicenna. For instance, D'Ancona has shown that Avicenna's theory of divine knowledge in the *Metaphysics* of *The Cure* traces back to Plotinus' exegesis of the *Timaeus* in *Enneads* 4–6, which was available to him via the *Theology of Aristotle.*[17] Furthermore, Avicenna appears to have learned (at least, in part) about Plato's theory of Forms, which does not receive extensive treatment in the *Timaeus*, from the works of Aristotle and his late antique commentators.[18] Aristotle's *Meteorology* (1.14, 351a10–353a25)

[16] Modern scholarship has largely neglected *Cardiac Drugs*. The collection of essays edited by Hameed (1983), which includes an English translation of the treatise, offers the most detailed study to date. Most of the essays in that volume are concerned with the efficacy of the drugs recommended by Avicenna and therefore are not written from a historical perspective.

[17] D'Ancona (2003b). Avicenna wrote a commentary on the *Theology of Aristotle* (now fragmentary), which formed part of a collection of Aristotelian exegeses called the *Fair Judgement* (*al-Inṣāf*). On this text, see Gutas (1988), 130–40=(2014), 144–55. For Avicenna's critical approach to the *Theology of Aristotle*, see Adamson (2004a).

[18] See Marmura (2006), 356n5; Arnzen (2011), 86–99. Plato's theory of Forms is mentioned at *Ti.* 50c–52d.

also provided Avicenna with such detailed information about the dialogue's discussion of cataclysmic events (*Ti.* 22c–23b) that his summary of the Aristotelian text circulated in Latin under the title *De Diluviis in Thimaeum Platonis* (*On Floods in Plato's Timaeus*).[19] While the Neoplatonic accents of Avicenna's philosophy have been noted, the impact of earlier iterations of Platonism on his thought has received relatively little attention.[20] Therefore, this chapter hopes to contribute to a more comprehensive understanding of Avicenna's relationship to Platonism.

Boundary Work in the *Canon of Medicine*

The standard English translation *Canon of Medicine* for *al-Qānūn fī l-ṭibb* does not convey the full significance of the title of Avicenna's medical opus. In religious and literary contexts a 'canon' often designates a body of texts that are deemed to be authoritative and worthy of study. While Avicenna's work incorporates material from earlier authors, whom he very rarely identifies by name, the Arabic term *qānūn* does not mean 'canon' in this sense.[21] A derivative of the Greek κανών, which first indicated a bar to straighten something, *qānūn* acquired the general meaning of '[secular] law' or 'principle'.[22] It is important to bear this sense of *qānūn* as 'law' in mind when referring to Avicenna's *al-Qānūn fī l-ṭibb*, as he stresses in the initial sections of the book what the doctor should and should not study. Avicenna seeks to regulate the body of knowledge that came to represent the field of medicine in his time.

At book one, subject one, lesson one, chapter two (1.1.1.2), Avicenna lists the subjects (*mawḍūʿāt*) that belong to medicine.[23] The text is largely negative in that it underscores the subjects that are outside the doctor's jurisdiction. While Avicenna acknowledges that medicine deals with the elements, humours, temperaments, pneumata, and faculties, he writes that it is the task of the physicist to work out what these things are:

[19] Bertolacci (2013a), 45n26.

[20] On some of the Neoplatonic elements of Avicenna's thought, especially his emanationist scheme of creation, see, e.g., Janssens (1987); Hasnawi (1990); Marmura (1992); D'Ancona (2003b).

[21] See van Gelder (2011).

[22] See *LSJ*, s.v. κανών I. For the various technical senses of the word in the fields of law and financial and public administration, see Linant de Bellefonds, Cahen, and İnalcık (2012).

[23] Hameed (1982), 34–6. Prepared by a group of scholars at Jamia Hamdard University under the direction of H. A. Hameed, the New Delhi edition of the *Canon of Medicine* provides a more critical text than the frequently cited Būlāq edition (1877). For the sake of brevity, I will hereafter refer to Avicenna's work as the *Canon*.

فبعض هذه الأمور إنّما يجب عليه من جهة ما هو طبيب أن يتصوره بالماهية فقط تصورا علميا، ويصدق بهليته تصديقا على أنّه وضع له، مقبول من صاحب العلم الطبيعي. وبعضها يلزمه أن يبرهن عليه من صناعته. فما كان من هذه كالمبادئ، فيلزمه أن يتقلد هليتها، فإنّ مبادئ العلوم الجزئية متسلمة. وتتبرهن في علوم أخرى أقدم منها، وكذلك حتى يرتقي مبادئ العلوم كلها إلى الفلسفة الأولى، التي يقال لها علم ما بعد الطبيعة. وإذا شرع بعض المتطببين وأخذ يتكلم في إثبات العناصر، والمزاج، وما يتلو ذلك، مما هو موضوع للعلم الطبيعي، فإنّه يغلط من حيث يورد في صناعة الطب ما ليس من صناعة الطب، ويغلط من حيث يظن أنّه يبين شيئا، ولا يكون قد بينه البتة . . . والذي يجب أن يتصوره، ويبرهن عليه الأمراض، وأسبابها الجزئية، وعلاماتها، وأنّه كيف يزال المرض، وتحفظ الصحة.[24]

It is necessary that the doctor, in his capacity as a doctor, acts as follows: for some medical matters he must form only cognitive concepts (*taṣawwur*) of their quiddity (*māhiyya*) and grant assent that they, in fact, exist, merely on the basis that they have been posited for his acceptance by the specialist of physics (*ṣāḥib al-ʿilm al-ṭabīʿī*), while for other medical matters he should provide demonstrative proofs in his art. He should accept on authority that whatever among the former set is like a first principle (*mabādiʾ*) exists, because the first principles of particular sciences (*ʿulūm ǧuzʾiyya*) are taken as granted and proven demonstratively only in other prior sciences. [This process continues] in this fashion until the first principles of all sciences are ultimately studied in the science of metaphysics. Were a doctor to begin discussing the proof of temperament, the elements, and so on – all of these things being posited for him in physics – he would be making a double error because, first, he would be introducing into medicine something which does not belong to it, and second, he would be thinking that he is explaining something while [in reality] he will not have explained it all . . . The things about which the doctor must form concepts and for which he must provide demonstrative proof are the following: diseases, their particular causes, and their symptoms; how to eliminate disease and preserve health.[25]

This passage offers implicit criticism of Galen's conception of medicine. The subjects that Avicenna declares to be off limits for the doctor – the nature of the elements, temperament, and so on – receive extensive treatment in Galen's writings.[26] Avicenna narrows down the area of knowledge that had defined the medical discipline for Galen. The text identifies disease as the appropriate subject of medicine, and it maintains, against Galen, that doctors can restore health without enquiring into the basic constituents of the body. Moreover, its characterization of physicists as the

[24] Hameed (1982), p. 36 ll. 3–17. [25] This translation is taken from Gutas (2003), 150–1.

[26] See, e.g., Galen's *On the Elements according to Hippocrates* (Περὶ τῶν καθ᾽ Ἱπποκράτην στοιχείων) and *On Temperaments* (Περὶ κράσεων). In the part of the text that I have not quoted (Hameed 1982: p. 36 ll. 12–14) Avicenna prohibits doctors from studying the nature of the humours, faculties, and pneumata – all subjects that Galen covers in his corpus.

rightful investigators of temperament, for instance, seems to challenge medicine's control over the realm of the body.

Avicenna subordinates medicine to physics in enjoining doctors to defer to physicists on questions about the principles of their science. He refers to his notion of a hierarchy of the sciences, which is discussed in *On the Divisions of the Intellectual Sciences* (*Fī Aqsām al-ʿulūm al-ʿaqliyya*), to establish philosophy's superior standing.[27] The epistle divides the sciences into two main categories, theoretical and practical; the former fall into a hierarchical order according to their subject's involvement with the material world.[28] Metaphysics ranks highest because it concerns entities (that is, intelligibles) that are immaterial and unchangeable, whereas physics ranks lowest because it has to do with material bodies that are subject to generation and corruption.[29] The work recounts that medicine – along with astrology, magic, and alchemy – belongs to a subcategory of sciences which derive their principles from physics.[30] Even though medicine stems from physics it is an inferior science, and as such its practitioners are barred from examining the subject matter of its 'parent' discipline.

This compartmentalization of the sciences does not seem to allow for polymaths, such as Avicenna himself, in that thinkers are confined to the epistemic domains of their respective disciplines. In the above quotation from the *Canon*, however, Avicenna defends his own wide-ranging knowledge by suggesting that personal expertise can be compartmentalized as well. The passage begins with a proviso which indicates that the subsequent regulations apply to the doctor acting 'in their capacity as a doctor' (*min ǧiha mā huwa ṭabīb*). The caveat implies that a doctor with expertise in multiple fields has the authority to examine non-medical topics, if they do so from the appropriate disciplinary perspective. As justification for his treatment of certain 'philosophical' subjects in the *Canon*, Avicenna flags these discussions by alleging that he is speaking in his capacity as

[27] For the Arabic text, see Avicenna (1908), 104–18.

[28] As Gutas (2003: 145–6) observes, this scheme derives from late antique classifications of Aristotle's books, according to which each work metonymically represents a field of study. The hierarchical epistemologies of third/ninth- and fourth/tenth-century Islamicate thinkers were especially informed by Paul the Persian's (*fl.* 567–80) introduction to the philosophy of Aristotle, on which see Gutas (1983) and the Introduction (pp. 19–21).

[29] Avicenna (1908), p. 105 l. 15–p. 107 l. 3. Cf. *Philosophy for ʿAlāʾ al-Dawla* (*Dānešnāme-ye ʿAlāʾī*: Morwedge 1973: 13), where Avicenna explains that physics is more comprehensible to humans because it deals with the material world, of which humans are a part. *Metaphysics* 1.2 of *The Cure* offers a similar hierarchy of the sciences.

[30] See Avicenna (1908), p. 101 l. 8–p. 111 l. 7. In his mature work *The Easterners* (*al-Mašriqiyyūn*), Avicenna further demotes medicine by assigning it to a category that is separate from the theoretical (or intellectual) sciences (see Gutas 2003: 147).

a physicist. For instance, before describing the four elements he writes: 'Let the doctor accept [the following information] from the physicist' (*li-yatasallam al-ṭabīb min al-ṭabīʿī*).[31] In other words, Avicenna directs the medical reader to learn from what he says qua physicist.

Avicenna attributes the subversion of medicine's boundaries, which the *Canon* aims to restore, to Galen's failure to approach philosophical subjects from a philosophical perspective. In his most explicit attack on Galen's expertise (I.I.I.2) he states that his predecessor erred in attempting to demonstrate the existence of the elements and other aspects of the natural world in his capacity as a doctor (*min ǧiha annahu ṭabīb*):

> وجالينوس إذا حاول إقامة البرهان على القسم الأول، فلا يجب أن يحاول ذلك من جهة أنّه طبيب، ولكن من جهة أنّه يجب أن يكون فيلسوفا، يتكلم في العلم الطبيعي كما أنّ الفقيه إذا حاول أن يثبت صحة وجوب متابعة الإجماع، فليس ذلك له من جهة ما هو فقيه، ولكن من جهة ما هو متكلم. ولكن الطبيب من جهة ما هو طبيب، والفقيه من جهة ما هو فقيه ليس يمكنه أن يبرهن على ذاك؛ وإلا وقع الدور.[32]

> Whenever Galen attempted to carry out a demonstration of the [matters pertaining to the] first division [i.e. the existence of the elements and their number etc.], he should have attempted this not in the capacity of a doctor, but in the capacity of a philosopher, [who] discusses physics. Just as a jurist (*faqīh*), if he were to attempt to justify the validity of obligatory compliance with the consensus of opinion (*wuǧūb mutābaʿat al-iǧmāʿ*), he [would do this] not in the capacity of a jurist, but in the capacity of a theologian (*mutakallim*). However, it is not possible for a doctor in the capacity of a doctor, and a jurist in the capacity of a jurist to demonstrate this – [if he tries to do so], he will argue in a circle.

Avicenna appeals to the hermeneutical hierarchy in Islamic law (*šarīʿa*), whereby a theologian (*mutakallim*) establishes the principles on which a jurist (*faqīh*) issues his opinions, to emphasize to the Muslim readers of the *Canon* that certain questions require certain expertise. Similar to the jurist exploring the theoretical basis on which he forms his judgements, Galen overstretched himself in examining subjects pertaining to physics. This classification of Galen as a mere doctor allows Avicenna to exclude him from the domain of natural knowledge and therefore weaken the credibility of his physical theories, with which he largely disagrees. As the next sections will show, Avicenna saw Galen's interpretation of the psychology of the *Timaeus* as a potent rival to his own understanding of the

[31] Hameed (1982), p. 37 ll. 1–2. Avicenna introduces his explanation of even and uneven temperament with a variation of this phrase at Hameed (1982), p. 38 ll. 14–18.
[32] Hameed (1982), p. 36 ll. 18–22.

soul, so the introduction to the *Canon* works to undercut Galen's authority to make Avicenna's theories seem all the more credible.

Rephrasing Old Debates: Cardiocentrism in the *Canon*

From an early phase of antiquity, study of the soul was not the exclusive concern of philosophy but rather a multidisciplinary enterprise. I explained in the first chapter that the physical location of the ruling part of the soul (ἡγεμονικόν), which was thought to govern sensation and voluntary movement, was one question that received attention from both philosophers and doctors.[33] Although the *Timaeus* does not identify the brain, but rather more vaguely the 'head' (κεφαλή, 44d5), as the seat of the rational soul, Plato was considered the chief proponent of encephalocentrism, whereas Aristotle championed cardiocentrism. As I discussed in Chapter 1, Galen asserts that he put this controversy to rest in *PHP*. There, he deploys his mastery of anatomy, obtained through study, clinical practice, and experimentation, in defence of not only Plato's encephalocentric position but also medicine's right to participate in this controversy.[34]

While Galen maintained that he settled the matter in Plato's favour, later Graeco-Roman and Islamicate thinkers continued to debate it.[35] Nonetheless, Avicenna and other thinkers with Peripatetic allegiances now had to address Galen's more refined anatomy when arguing for the primacy of the heart. Furthermore, philosophers had to prove that medicine does not offer the most reliable way to investigate the identity of the hegemonic organ, as Galen claims in *PHP*. Avicenna broaches the debate in the *Canon* in sections on the nature of the organs and the faculties – although he avoids framing it as a psychological controversy, perhaps so as not to be seen to be transgressing his own disciplinary laws. I will suggest that these passages' promotion of the heart as the centre of an organic network complements Avicenna's defence in his philosophical works of Aristotle's cardiocentric thesis as well as his own concept of a unitary soul.

Avicenna prefaces his description of the anatomy of the bones, muscles, nerves, and vascular system with a chapter 'on the quiddity of the part[s] of the body and their division' (*fī māhiyyat al-ʿuḍw wa l-aqsāmihi*, 1.1.5.1).[36]

[33] Chapter 1, pp. 42–6. [34] See pp. 45–6.

[35] Even Galen's contemporaries did not think that his arguments in *PHP* were definitive. Tieleman (1996: xxxvi–xxxvii; 1998: 315–18) points out that Alexander of Aphrodisias (*fl. c.* 200 CE) championed Aristotle's thesis of cardiocentrism, despite being aware of Galen's experiments. See Alexander, *De Anima*: Bruns (1887), p. 94 l. 7–p. 100 l. 17.

[36] Hameed (1982), p. 57 l. 5–p. 63 l. 19.

The text lists different groups of internal structures – for example, nerves, tendons, and arteries – and identifies their common features. One section of the chapter offers a more general classificatory scheme that divides the organs according to their ability to transmit their innate faculties, which are responsible for various processes, to other parts of the body. The scheme identifies four types of body parts: (1) a part (or organ) that both receives and donates a faculty (*ʿuḍw qābil muʿṭ*); (2) a part that donates but does not receive a faculty (*ʿuḍw muʿṭ ġayr qābil*); (3) a part that receives but does not donate a faculty (*ʿuḍw qābil ġayr muʿṭ*); and (4) a part that neither receives nor donates a faculty (*ʿuḍw lā qābil lā muʿṭ*).[37] The following passage, which is worth quoting in full, indicates that Avicenna introduces this classification as a way of commenting on the debate about the location of the ruling part of the soul:

أما العضو القابل المعطي فلم يشك في وجوده. لأنّ الدماغ والكبد اجمعوا على أنّ كل واحد منهما يقبل قوة الحياة، والحرارة الغريزية، والروح من القلب، وكل واحد منهما أيضا مبدأ قوة يعطيها غيره. أما الدماغ فمبدأ الحس عند قوم مطلقا، وعند قوم لا مطلقا. والكبد مبدأ التغذية <عند قوم> مطلقا، وعند قوم لا مطلقا. وأما العضو القابل غير المعطي فالشك في وجوده أبعد، مثل اللحم القابل قوة الحس والحياة، وليس هو مبدأ القوة، يعطيها غيره بوجه. وأما القسمان الآخران فاختلف في أحدهما الأطباء مع الكبير من الفلاسفة. فقال كبير الفلاسفة إنّ هذا العضو هو القلب، وهو الأصل الأول لكل قوة؛ وهو يعطي سائر الأعضاء كلها القوى التي تغذو، والتي تحيي، والتي تدرك وتحرك. وأما الأطباء وقوم من أوائل الفلاسفة فقد فرقوا هذه القوى في الأعضاء، ولم يقولوا بعضو معط غير قابل. وقوله عند التحقيق والتدقيق أصح؛ وقول الأطباء في بادي النظر أظهر. ثم اختلف في القسم الآخر الأطباء فيما بينهم والفلاسفة فيما بينهم: فذهبت طائفة إلى أنّ العظام واللحم الغير الحساس وما اشبههما، إنّما تبقي بقوى فيها <غريزية> تخصها. لم تأتها من مباد آخر؛ لكنها بتلك القوى إذا وصل إليها غذاؤها، كفت أنفسها. فلا هي تفيد شيئا آخر قوة فيها، ولا أيضا يفيدها عضو قوة أخرى. وذهبت طائفة إلى أنّ تلك القوى ليست تخصها، لكنها فائضة إليها من الكبد أو القلب في أول الكون ثم استقرت فيها.[38]

There is no doubt about the existence of the organ [that] receives and donates [a faculty]. There is agreement that the brain as well as the liver receives the vital faculty, innate heat, and pneuma from the heart. Each of them is also the source of the faculty which it donates to another organ, the brain being the absolute source of sensation according to some, and not absolutely according to others. The liver is the absolute source of nutrition according to some and not according to others. Nor is there much doubt about the existence of the organ that receives but does not donate [a faculty]; for example, the flesh receives the faculty of sensation and life, but it is not the principle of a faculty, and it gives [no faculty] to another [organ].

As for the other two divisions, the physicians differ from the great [one of the] philosophers [i.e. Aristotle] about one of [the divisions, sc. the organ that donates but does not receive a faculty]. For, the great [one of] the

[37] Hameed (1982), p. 59 l. 5. [38] Hameed (1982), p. 59 ll. 6–22.

> philosophers says that the heart is such an organ. It is the primary source of all the faculties. It gives all the parts of the body the faculties of nutrition, vitality, perception, and movement. On the other hand, doctors and some of the ancient philosophers attribute these faculties to various organs and do not believe in an organ which might donate but not receive. A careful enquiry and scrutiny uphold his view, while on the face of it, the doctors' view appears plausible.
>
> Next, there is a disagreement about the other division [i.e. the organ that neither receives nor donates a faculty] among doctors and philosophers. Some hold the view that bone, insensitive flesh, and the like only continue [to live] by means of the natural faculty that resides in them. Therefore, they do not receive it from another principle. But they possess this faculty whenever their nutriment is conveyed to them, and it suffices them. Therefore, they do not furnish another thing with the faculty that they contain, nor does a part of the body furnish them with another faculty. Some hold the view that that faculty does not reside in them but flows to them from the liver or the heart during the first part of its existence then settles in them.

Avicenna relates that doctors and philosophers agree on the existence of organ types (1) and (3) but are in conflict about the existence of types (2) and (4). While the disagreement about organ types (2) and (4) ostensibly concerns distinct controversies, there is actually one thesis at stake: the notion that every faculty in the body originates from one source, the hegemonic organ. For, those who deny the existence of organ type (2) reject the notion that the faculties come from a common repository and hold instead that each faculty has its own organic seat. Similarly, those who acknowledge the existence of organ type (4) dismiss the idea of a shared origin of the faculties, but they do so on the premise that every part of the body possesses an innate faculty. Avicenna may have in mind here Galen's attractive faculty, which is inherent in every part of the body.[39] As I will explain in more detail below, this passage sets Aristotle's physiology of the soul, which recognizes the heart as the source of all faculties, in opposition to Galen's Platonic scheme, which distributes the soul into three main organs.

It is important to note that Avicenna advances a different understanding of the hegemonic organ from that of his ancient predecessors. In the above passage he characterizes it as the source of not just sensation and voluntary movement – the definitive activities of the ἡγεμονικόν for thinkers such as Galen – but all other faculties as well. On these terms, organ type (2)

[39] See *Nat.Fac.* 1.14 and Chapter 1, pp. 61–2.

qualifies as the hegemonic part. This broadening of the definition of the ruling organ appears to be part of a tactic to minimize the significance of Galen's findings about the sensory role of the brain. Building on the work of prior anatomists, including Herophilus and Erasistratus, Galen demonstrated, contra Aristotle, that the source (ἀρχή) of the nerves is in the brain instead of the heart. As a student of Galenic medicine, therefore, Avicenna cannot defend the cardiocentric position on the basis that the heart is the seat of sensation and voluntary movement. On the other hand, by contending that the heart donates the faculty of sensation (*quwwat al-ḥiss*) to the brain, Avicenna can establish the heart's primacy over the brain while maintaining the brain's involvement in sensation.[40] Accordingly, the heart is the source of the sensitive faculty but not the seat of its activities.[41] This conclusion also exposes the theoretical limitations of medicine, for the anatomical experiments that Galen cites as demonstrative proof of encephalocentrism do not invalidate cardiocentrism. That is to say, the cessation of sensation following a brain injury may indicate, as Galen interprets, that the organ is the source of sensation, but it does not exclude the possibility that the animal has become insensate because its brain is no longer capable of receiving the sensory power from the heart.

The above quotation from the *Canon* endorses the Aristotelian depiction of the heart as the hub of an organic network of faculties. Avicenna does not name the camp opposing 'the great [one] of the philosophers' (*al-kabīr min al-falāsifa*), but the unspecified 'doctors' (*aṭibbāʾ*) and ancient philosophers (*qawm min awāʾil al-falāsifa*) undoubtedly refer to followers of Galen and Plato.[42] This passage, I will now argue, champions

40 Avicenna takes a different approach to defending Aristotle's cardiocentrism at 8.3.1 (Muntaṣir, Zāyid, and Ismāʿīl 1980: 39–45) of the *Book of Animals* (*Kitāb al-Ḥayawān*) of *The Cure*, for the text argues that the nerves originate in the heart. Even so, as in the *Canon*, he concludes that the brain is where the activities of sensation and voluntary movement take place, while the heart is the source of all faculties. Cf. al-Fārābī's defence of cardiocentrism in *On the Perfect State* (*Mabādiʾ ārāʾ ahl al-madīna al-fāḍila*): Walzer (1985), 174–80. Al-Fārābī places the roots of the nerves in the brain but does not attribute a sensory capacity to the organ. Instead, he maintains that the cooler temperature of the brain allows the nerves, which derive their sensory power from the heart, to function without drying up owing to the heart's heat. In emphasizing the brain's cooling function, al-Fārābī follows Aristotle (see *PA* 652b2–35) more closely than Avicenna.

41 This claim, that the source of a faculty is not necessarily its seat, may have been inspired by Alexander of Aphrodisias. In *De Anima* (Bruns 1887: 98–100), Alexander argues that, while the faculties have their origin (ἀρχή) in the heart, their activities (ἐνεργεῖαι) occur in 'subordinate' (sing. ὑπηρετικόν) organs. On the now-lost Arabic translation of Alexander's text, see Peters (1968), 43. Cf. Plotinus, *Enn.* 4.3.23, who seems to understand ἀρχή in a similar sense. On this passage from the *Enneads* and the possible influence of Alexander on Plotinus, see Tieleman (1998).

42 Avicenna also refers to Aristotle by the honorific titles 'the philosopher' (*al-faylasūf*) and 'the first teacher' (*al-muʿallim al-awwal*); see, e.g., *al-Aǧwiba ʿan masāʾil Abī l-Rayḥān al-Bīrūnī* (Naṣr and Muḥaqqiq 1995: p. 41 l. 6) and *Kitāb al-Naǧāt* (*Book of Salvation*: Fakhry 1985: p. 302 l. 16).

cardiocentrism over encephalocentrism as a way of criticizing Galen's tripartite psychology, which builds on *Ti.* 69c5–72b5. Avicenna brings up this psychological theory in his discussion of organ type (1). In keeping with Galen's interpretation of the *Timaeus* in works such as *PHP*, he lists the brain, heart, and liver as the chief organs. Whereas the dialogue declares that these organs house the logical, irascible, and desiderative parts of the soul, Avicenna describes them as the seats of the vital, sensitive, and nutritive faculties. Similar to Galen, who claims to switch his psychological terminology when addressing readers from different disciplinary and sectarian backgrounds, the medical context of the *Canon* accounts for Avicenna's use of 'faculty' *(quwwa)* instead of 'soul'.[43] Because Avicenna allocates psychology to physics, he needs to rephrase both Plato and Galen's theories – at least as he expresses it in works that speak in terms of either three 'souls' (ψυχαί) or psychic parts – to minimize their philosophical significance and therefore render them suitable for discussion in his medical compilation. Moreover, to avoid the suggestion that doctors are just as qualified as philosophers to participate in this controversy, the above quotation points out that doctors have only offered plausible rather than true explanations of the location of the hegemonic organ.

Avicenna does not object to the identification of the brain, heart, and liver as the three chief organs, but he does have a problem with Plato and Galen's strict separation of the faculties, or parts of the soul. The first paragraph of the text reports that there are differing views about whether the brain and liver are the 'absolute' (*muṭlaq*) sources of the sensitive and nutritive faculties or not. Plato and Galen hold the affirmative side in this controversy, for their psychological schemes regard the brain, heart, and liver as distinct ἀρχαί (meaning both 'source' and 'seat'), though they allow for communication between the faculties or souls housed in them.[44] This position precludes the heart from donating its sensory power to the brain, let alone constituting the ultimate source of all the faculties. Avicenna's hypothesis of organ type (2) contravenes the vision of a tripartite soul and body put forward in the *Timaeus* because it unites all the parts of the body in their dependence on the heart.

[43] See *Prop.Plac.* 3.6; LG, p. 70 ll. 1–9. Cf. *Plat.Tim.* 3.2 (Schröder 1934: p. 12 ll. 17–21), where Galen says that it makes no difference whether one refers to 'souls' (ψυχαί) as 'faculties' (δυνάμεις).

[44] See Tieleman (1998), 312, for Galen's understanding of ἀρχή. For an example of this psychic exchange, see *Ti.* 70a2–c1 and *PHP* 7.3.2 (De Lacy 2005: p. 438 l. 28–p. 440 l. 3), where Plato and Galen explain how reason rouses the heart to anger. On Galen's notion that the nerves act as a communication system between the organs, see Gill (2009), 420–3.

Avicenna's support of a unified network of faculties in the *Canon* dovetails with his stress on the oneness of the soul in his psychological works. Notwithstanding his support of Aristotle's cardiocentrism, Avicenna does not ascribe to his hylomorphic psychology (*DA* 412a19–22), which contends that the soul is inseparable from the body and thus perishes with it. As Adamson observes, Avicenna keeps to a middle ground between radical dualism, where soul and body are separate substances, and hylomorphism: he asserts that a human soul consists of two aspects, one of which is immaterial and separable (the rational soul) and the other (the animal soul) mortal.[45] Texts such as the *Salvation* and the *De Anima* of *The Cure* maintain that these aspects are not independent but stand in a hierarchical relation, with the lower faculties of the animal soul making the activities of the rational soul possible.[46] In the latter work, Avicenna points to the common origin of the animal soul's faculties in the heart as proof of this aspect's unity.[47] He recounts that the faculties 'emanate' (*tafīḍu*) from the heart into the brain, liver, and other parts of the body.[48] By employing language that features in his emanationist account of creation, Avicenna draws a parallel between the systems of the body and the cosmos.[49] Both the body and cosmos are unified structures in that the diverse powers at work in them derive from a single source – respectively, the heart and the necessary existent, God. Nonetheless, unlike Galen and al-Rāzī, Avicenna does not interpret this correspondence between the body and cosmos to mean that the study of anatomy can lead to theological truths.

Pneuma and the Hegemony of the Heart

I want to conclude this discussion of cardiocentrism in the *Canon* by considering how Avicenna adapts Galen's pneumatic theory to specify in what sense the heart 'donates' (*yuʿṭī*) the sensitive faculty to the brain. Pneuma (Gr. πνεῦμα; Arab. *rūḥ*) plays a key role in Avicenna's explanation of pleasure in *Cardiac Drugs*, so the following analysis serves as a preface to the second half of this chapter as well. Galen did not invent the concept of

[45] Adamson (2004b), 61. At *DA* 1.1 of *The Cure* (Rahman 1959: p. 8 ll. 4–8), Avicenna defines the soul as a double perfection (*kamāl*): the rational soul is the first perfection and the animal soul is the second perfection. See Wisnovsky (2003), 112–41, on how a soul can comprise two perfections yet be unified.

[46] See *Salvation* 2.6.15 (Fakhry 1985: 228–30=Rahman 1952: 64–8) and *DA* 5.7 (Rahman 1959: 250–62).

[47] *DA* 5.8: Rahman (1959), 264–7. [48] *DA* 5.8: Rahman (1959), p. 264 ll. 8–11.

[49] For his emanationist account of creation, see, e.g., *Metaphysics* of *The Cure* 9.3–4: Anawātī and Zāyed (1960), p. 401 l. 9–p. 407 l. 8.

pneuma – an invisible, vaporous substance in the body – but his formulation of it, which I will now summarize, had an enduring legacy.[50] He identifies a number of types of pneuma, the most physiologically important of which is 'psychic pneuma' (πνεῦμα ψυχικόν). I noted in Chapters 1 and 2 that, according to Galen, the brain is the repository of this pneuma, and the soul uses it as an instrument (ὄργανον) to perform the activities of sensation and voluntary movement.[51] Galen proposes initially that psychic pneuma arises from 'vital' (ζωτικόν) pneuma, which is generated from inspired air that passes into the left ventricle of the heart via the lungs. This pneuma then travels through the arteries to the retiform plexus and choroid plexuses of the brain, where it is refined into psychic pneuma.[52] Galen's experiments with ligating the carotid arteries of animals compelled him to find another aetiology for psychic pneuma, for he observed that interrupting arterial flow from the heart did not deprive his test subjects of sensation.[53] At *On the Use of Breathing* 4.501–5K he hypothesizes that psychic pneuma can also arise from air that travels through the nostrils into the anterior ventricles of the brain. Therefore, the brain does not require the heart to produce pneuma.

Avicenna uses Galen's pneumatic theory in the *Canon* to explain how sensation happens in the body. While Galen's conception of the pneumatic system serves to support his (and Plato's) encephalocentric model of sensation, Avicenna selects elements from this previous scheme to articulate a version that is more in line with his own cardiocentric physiology. Most significantly, he omits Galen's second aetiology, which allows the brain to create its own supply of pneuma, and instead highlights the heart's contribution to the pneumatic system. At *Canon* 1.1.6.1, which reviews the functions of the various faculties in the body, Avicenna states that the vital faculty (*quwwa ḥayawāniyya*) controls pneuma, the 'vehicle of sensation and movement' (*markab fī l-ḥiss wa l-ḥaraka*).[54] Even if he does not explicitly disclose in this section that pneuma originates in the heart, he brings it under the heart's dominion because the organ governs the faculty that governs this substance.[55] Unlike the two Galenic aetiologies outlined above, Avicenna does not spell out whether pneuma experiences any qualitative change when it collects in the brain. He remarks that the vital

[50] For a survey of pneumatic theories before Galen, see Rocca (2003), 59–64.
[51] See *PHP* 7.3.30: De Lacy (2005), p. 446 ll. 11–33. See pp. 46, 85 above.
[52] See *UP* 7.8: Helmreich (1907), p. 393 l. 23–p. 394 l. 6=May (1968), vol. I, p. 347. See also Rocca (2003), 64–5.
[53] See Rocca (2003), 224–37.
[54] Hameed (1982), p. 123 ll. 1–4.
[55] See Hameed (1982), p. 126 ll. 24–5, where Avicenna attributes pneuma's origin to the heart.

faculty 'prepares' (*tuhayyi'u*), in some unspecified way, the pneuma in the brain to receive the faculties of sensation and voluntary movement. This vague comment describes a two-step, unidirectional exchange between the heart and brain, where the former organ first donates to the latter the vital faculty, which primes its pneuma to accept the second donation of the sensitive faculty. *Canon* 1.1.6.1 appears to repeat the suggestion made earlier in the text (1.1.5.1) that the brain only provides the site where the faculties involved in sensation interact.

In his discussion of the vital faculty at 1.1.6.4, Avicenna further emphasizes the brain's passive participation in sensation by omitting Galen's notion that the organ's temperament has the ability to alter pneuma.[56] Rather, he elaborates that pneuma becomes a vehicle of sensation in the brain when the substance originates from 'refined humours' (*laṭāfat al-amšāǧ*) and, in keeping with 1.1.6.1, takes on the vital faculty.[57] Here, Avicenna departs from Galen in alleging that humours, instead of inspired air, are the basic materials from which pneuma is generated. Furthermore, Avicenna qualifies that pneuma's derivation from 'fine' (sing. *laṭīf*) humours endows it with a particular temperament (*mizāǧ*), which, if altered, renders the substance incapable of receiving the vital and therefore sensitive faculty.[58] The *Canon* gives the impression that the brain, apart from its spatial contribution, is superfluous in this system, because pneuma possesses an innate temperament that enables it to assume the vital and sensitive faculties. Contrary to Galen's contention, it is the heart instead of the brain that has the more significant interventionist role through its donation of the vital faculty.

Avicenna's pneumatic scheme does not posit a special relationship between the brain and pneuma. It does not make a hard distinction between vital and psychic pneumata, and so deprives the brain of its unique status as the repository of the soul's first instrument. To underline his doctrinal independence from Galen, Avicenna places at 1.1.6.4 his own theory of pneuma in opposition to that of his predecessor.[59] The passage neither identifies Galen as the proponent of the argument that the temperament of the brain transforms (vital) pneuma into psychic pneuma (*rūḥ*

[56] Galen asserts that an organ's temperament determines its physiological function; see *PHP* 7.5.13–14 (De Lacy 2005: p. 456 ll. 5–15) and Rocca (2003), 216. For the Arabic text of 1.1.6.4, see Hameed (1982), p. 126 l. 17–p. 128 l. 7. Cf. *Cardiac Drugs*: Hameed (1983), p. 222 l. 18–p. 223 l. 3, where Avicenna admits that the brain's temperament modifies the vital pneuma coming from the heart. Nonetheless, this temperamental change does not generate psychic pneuma, but rather allows the brain to receive the sensitive faculty from the heart.

[57] Hameed (1982), p. 127 ll. 8–9. [58] Hameed (1982), p. 126 ll. 26–7.

[59] Hameed (1982), p. 127 ll. 10–25.

nafsānī), which is attributed to unnamed 'doctors', nor openly polemicizes against this view. In aligning his own position with 'the philosopher Aristotle's' (*al-faylasūf Arisṭūṭālīs*), Avicenna calls attention to the theoretical inadequacy of the 'medical' account. As I demonstrated, *Canon* 1.1.1.2 locates the subject of pneuma in physics' limits, and thus insists that doctors such as Galen lack the conceptual framework to produce reliable claims about it. Be that as it may, Avicenna never addresses Galen's most persuasive evidence for the primary role of the brain in his pneumatic system: namely, his experiments on the carotid arteries. He may have overlooked this evidence as a way of preserving not only his own cardiocentric vision of pneuma but also philosophy's epistemic authority over the hegemonic organ controversy.[60]

Platonic Pleasures in the *Canon*

Besides the sensitive faculty, *Canon* 1.1.6.4 also places the 'moving faculty' (*quwwat al-ḥaraka*), which regulates the emotions, under the governance of the vital faculty. Following Aristotle (*DA* 408b9–10), who revises Plato's description of the irascible soul (θυμός) at *Ti.* 70a2–d6 and *Resp.* 441d–e, Avicenna lists anger (*ġaḍab*) and fear (*ḫawf*) as paradigmatic movements (or emotions) of this heart-centred faculty.[61] The *De Anima* (1.5) of *The Cure* and the *Salvation* (2.4.2) include desire (*šahwa*), which provokes movement towards what is useful or necessary in the search for pleasure (*laḏḏa*), as another exemplary emotion of the moving faculty.[62] Avicenna may have omitted the 'movement' of desire from *Canon* 1.1.6.4 to avoid delving into a subject with considerable philosophical baggage in a medical context – even if this concern does not always inhibit him. Ancient philosophers, especially Platonists and Peripatetics, debated whether desire involves sensation in some form. Chapter 1 noted how Plato attributes desire to the lowest soul, which is only capable of a lesser kind of sensation, whereas Aristotle connects it with imagination (φαντασία), which cannot arise without sensation.[63] The passages from *The Cure* and the *Salvation* more or less endorse Aristotle's position. While the *Canon* does not broach the topic of desire, it does treat its object, pleasure (*laḏḏa*). I will now argue that, in apparent contradiction to his Aristotelian conception of desire,

60 For how a cardiocentrist might respond to Galen's experiments, see Rocca (2003), 231n99.
61 Hameed (1982), p. 126 ll. 20–1.
62 See Rahman (1959), p. 41 ll. 4–11; Fakhry (1985), p. 197 ll. 16–23=Rahman (1952), 26.
63 See *Ti.* 70d7–72b5 and *DA* 414a30–b17, 428b12–19. As I showed in Chapter 1 (p. 58), Galen interprets Plato's position very differently.

Avicenna presents an aetiology of the sensation of pleasure that appears to expand on a Galenic interpretation of Plato's *Timaeus*. Furthermore, as will be shown, Avicenna's decision to cover pleasure – a subject which he discusses in several of his philosophical works – in the *Canon* shows how authoritative Galen's map of medical knowledge was. Avicenna cannot draw it afresh.

At *Canon* 1.2.2.23, Avicenna brings up pleasure as part of a broader enquiry into the causes and symptoms of different diseases.[64] This characterization of pleasure as a medical topic has its roots in Galen, who examined the sensation in his nosological texts *Differences of Symptoms* (7.44K) and *Causes of Symptoms* (7.115–27K).[65] The grouping of pleasure in the *Canon* with affections that alter, but do not necessarily harm, the body conforms to Galen's description of it as a πάθημα and a πάθος in the aforementioned treatises.[66] In *Caus.Symp.*, Galen acknowledges that his conception of pleasure as an affection is based on Plato's *Timaeus* (64c7–65b3).[67] Avicenna's short discussion adopts aspects of Galen's Timaean explanation of the sensation:

> هذه أيضا محصورة في جنسين: أحدهما جنس ما يغير المزاج الغير الطبيعي دفعة، ليقع به الإحساس. والثاني جنس ما يرد الإتصال الطبيعي دفعة. وكل ما يقع لا دفعة؛ فأنّه لا يحس، فلا يلذ. واللذة حس بالملائم؛ وكل حس فهو بقوة حساسة، ويكون الإحساس بانفعالها. فإذا كان بملائم أو بمناف، كان لذة أو ألما بحسب ما يتأثر.[68]

> These [i.e. the causes of pleasure] are limited to two genera: (1) when an imbalanced temperament suddenly changes so that it [i.e. the change] is perceived; (2) when the natural continuity suddenly returns. As for every [change that] does not happen suddenly, because it is not perceived, it is not felt as pleasure. Pleasure is the perception of what is agreeable, and every sensation comes from the sensitive faculty and arises from the reaction of [that faculty]. Whenever [the reaction] is agreeable or contrary, there is pleasure or pain according to what is affected.

[64] Hameed (1982), p. 182 ll. 6–13.

[65] According to Ḥunayn's *Epistle* (Bergsträsser 1925: p. 11 l. 11–p. 12 l. 10=Lamoreaux 2016: p. 25 l. 8–p. 27 l. 5), Ḥubayš translated from Syriac into Arabic both *Symp.Diff.* and *Caus.Symp.*, which circulated together under the title *Book of Diseases and Symptoms* (*Kitāb al-ʿIlal wa l-aʿrāḍ*).

[66] Johnston (2006: 137n21) observes that Galen uses the terms πάθημα and πάθος interchangeably. At *Symp.Diff.* 7.44–7K, Galen stresses that a πάθος/πάθημα is not the same thing as a νόσος ('disease'): the former is a change or alteration, whereas the latter is a condition that persists over a period of time.

[67] At *Caus.Symp.* 7.118K, Galen also refers to Plato's *Philebus*. For an overview of the theory of pleasure in the *Philebus*, see Tuozzo (1996); van Riel (2000), 17–29; Harte (2004).

[68] Hameed (1982), p. 182 ll. 7–10.

Avicenna writes that the body experiences the sensation (*ḥiss*) of pleasure when either its natural temperament (*mizāǧ*) or continuity (*ittiṣāl*) – that is, internal cohesion – is suddenly altered, or restored, after some disruption. The passage leaves unexplained why the body's temperament or continuity has been disturbed in the first place. With regard to continuity, however, Avicenna reports in an earlier chapter on its dissolution that wounds, ulcers, and inflammations damage the body's structural unity.[69] Avicenna's association of pleasure with an immediate change, which his second aetiology specifies as the body's 'return' (*yaruddu*) to its prior unaffected state, reflects the description of the sensation at *Ti.* 64d1–2 as 'a sudden return to a natural condition' (τὸ δ' εἰς φύσιν ἀπιὸν πάλιν ἀθρόον ἡδύ). As in the *Timaeus* (64d3–5), the *Canon* emphasizes that pleasure is imperceptible if the return is gentle and gradual. The correlation of the intensity of pleasure with the speed of the body's return to its natural state is distinctive to the *Timaeus*; it does not appear in Plato's earlier treatments of the sensation.[70]

I have suggested above that Galen's *Caus.Symp.* and, to a lesser extent, *Symp.Diff.* may have shaped Avicenna's idea of pleasure as a corporeal affection; nonetheless, the two aetiologies in the *Canon* do not exactly reproduce these treatises' accounts of the sensation. While *Caus.Symp.* (7.115K) may quote *Ti.* 64c8–d3, the tract only mentions how a restoration of continuity (συνέχεια) gives rise to pleasure (7.116–18K).[71] It does not connect pleasure with a rebalancing of temperament. Galen expresses Plato's notion of pleasure somewhat differently in other works, so Avicenna may have taken his aetiologies from another Galenic source besides, or perhaps in addition to, *Caus.Symp.*[72] For instance, book two of *Plat.Tim.* offers a twofold aetiology of pleasure that is more consistent with what Avicenna says in the *Canon*: it relates that pleasure occurs when either the temperament (κρᾶσις) or continuity (συνέχεια) of the body is brought back to its natural state (πρὸς τὸ κατὰ φύσιν) after some disturbance.[73] Unlike *Caus.Symp.*, the surviving material from Galen's commentary does not relate the strength of the sensation to the suddenness of the body's restoration – although a lost passage probably made this

[69] See Hameed (1982), p. 134 ll. 3–29.

[70] See Adamson (2008), 72–8, who surveys Plato's evolving views about pleasure in the *Gorgias*, *Republic*, *Philebus*, and *Timaeus*.

[71] On the concept of continuity in Galen, see De Lacy (1979).

[72] E.g., *Com.Tim.* § 14 (Kraus and Walzer 1951: p. 19 ll. 10–14), *PHP* 7.6.32–6 (De Lacy 2005: p. 468 l. 16–p. 470 l. 2), and below.

[73] *Plat.Tim.* fr. 30: Larrain (1991), 29=Larrain (1992), 170.

point.[74] Avicenna's silence regarding his source texts makes any precise identification of them difficult, but this brief exercise in *Quellenforschung* has established that the *Canon* promotes a Platonic theory of pleasure which is articulated in Galenic terms.

Avicenna also makes his own modifications to Galen's Timaean aetiology of pleasure. He seems to disagree with the suggestion that pleasure is only a physical response to a change in the body, for he adds in the above quotation that it results from a reaction of the sensitive faculty (*quwwat al-ḥiss*). The text implies that pleasure is not a rudimentary kind of sensation that even the lowest forms of life, which lack a sensitive faculty (such as plants), can experience; rather, it is akin to all other sensations in that it involves this higher power. Thus, in accordance with Aristotelian thought, Avicenna appears to strip Plato and Galen's desiderative soul of the capacity to feel pleasure by attributing this capacity to the sensitive faculty, which belongs to the vital faculty (or animal soul, in his philosophical works). The *Canon* does not clarify how the sensitive faculty perceives the body's return to a natural condition as 'agreeable' (*mulāʾim*); in this respect, its description of pleasure seems underdeveloped. Although Avicenna may include pleasure in the *Canon*, he hints here that only those who have the right to comment on the vital faculty – namely, philosophers – should pursue the topic in detail. Even so, despite this attempt to curtail doctors' enquiry into pleasure to safeguard philosophy's jurisdictional control over it, the fact that Avicenna introduces the subject in the *Canon* captures his inability to erase all the more expansive epistemic claims that Galen makes for medicine. The next section looks at Avicenna's rejection of the Platonic–Galenic conception of pleasure in *Cardiac Drugs*, which a number of medieval sources classify as a medical work. As I will explain, when setting out his alternative to the Timaean notion of pleasure in this small book, Avicenna seems to attenuate further the restrictive line of demarcation that the *Canon* places between medicine and philosophy.

Redrawing Boundaries: Pleasure in *Cardiac Drugs*

Similar to the *Canon*, the *Treatise on the Principles of Cardiac Drugs* (*Maqāla fī Aḥkām al-adwiya al-qalbiyya*; Lat. *De Medicinis Cordialibus*)

[74] Cf. *Plat. Tim.* fr. 32: Larrain (1991), 29=Larrain (1992), 173. There, Galen reports that pain results from a violent, sudden affection (βίαιον ἀθρόον πάθος) in the body, and he adds that the sensation is imperceptible (ἀναίσθητος), if the affection occurs gradually.

discusses pleasure with reference to the body.[75] The text details how an individual's emotional state depends on the quality and quantity of the vital pneuma in their heart. It also advises how to use certain drugs to modify the condition of a patient's vital pneuma to improve their emotional well-being. Before turning to the chapter on pleasure in *Cardiac Drugs*, I want to consider how Avicenna defines this work, as it takes a different approach to the sensation from that of the *Canon*. Avicenna composed *Cardiac Drugs* around 406/1015, a couple of years after he began writing the *Canon*, for al-Saʿīd Abū l-Ḥusayn ʿAlī ibn al-Ḥusayn ibn al-Ḥasanī, a Shiite official in Hamaḏān (western Iran).[76] In an insertion in book four, section four of the *DA* of *The Cure*, al-Ǧūzǧānī quotes several passages from *Cardiac Drugs* and remarks that Avicenna produced the text for a friend who was a beginner (*baʿd al-mubtadiʾīn min aṣdiqāʾihi*). Al-Ǧūzǧānī does not specify in which subject this friend was a novice, but he presumably means philosophy (his own area of expertise). Al-Ǧūzǧānī's comment implies that Avicenna wrote *Cardiac Drugs* for a philosophically inclined lay audience – although al-Ǧūzǧānī may be downplaying al-Ḥasanī's level of learning to assert his own intellectual superiority.[77]

Notwithstanding the philosophical interests of al-Ḥasanī, Avicenna appears to regard *Cardiac Drugs* as a medical treatise. In *DA* 4.4 of *The Cure*, which covers the moving faculty, Avicenna relates that he discussed in his 'medical books' (*fī kutubinā al-ṭibbiyya*) the reason that different individuals are inclined towards emotions such as joy (*faraḥ*), grief (*ġamm*), and hatred (*ḥiqd*).[78] Avicenna's text breaks off at this point in *DA* 4.4, but al-Ǧūzǧānī's aforementioned insertion of passages from *Cardiac Drugs* suggests that his teacher may have been referring to it. With chapters on joy, grief, and other emotions, the contents of *Cardiac Drugs* lend support to al-Ǧūzǧānī's reading that the vague 'medical books' at *DA* 4.4 encompasses this tract. *Cardiac Drugs* is a 'medical' book in a very different sense from the *Canon*, which gives cursory attention to the emotions, for it deals with topics that are supposedly exclusive to the physicist's expertise: the nature of pneuma (*rūḥ*), the elements (*ʿanāṣir*), and both active (*fāʿil*) and

[75] The physician Arnald of Villanova (*c.* 1238–1311), who taught medicine at Montpellier, translated *Cardiac Drugs* into Latin; on his translation, see Dulieu (1955), 93.

[76] See al-Ǧūzǧānī's *Biography*: Gohlman (1974), p. 60 ll. 6–8. See also Mahdavī (1954), 23–4; Gutas (2014), 514. The dedicatory inscription relates that al-Ḥasanī asked Avicenna to write a brief tract on cardiac drugs for his court (*maǧlis*): see al-Bābā (1984), p. 221 ll. 8–9.

[77] Al-Ǧūzǧānī was concerned to present himself as Avicenna's most important pupil. As Gutas (1988: 101–2=2014: 103–4) observes, al-Ǧūzǧānī takes all the credit in his *Biography* for prompting Avicenna to write *The Cure*, and he omits that he made the request along with a number of other disciples.

[78] Rahman (1959), p. 201 ll. 13–15.

passive (*infiʿāl*) potentialities.[79] *Cardiac Drugs* reveals that Avicenna appears to configure his map of medical knowledge to achieve different rhetorical effects: he narrows down medicine's epistemic space in the *Canon* as part of a polemical tactic to weaken Galen's authority, whereas in *Cardiac Drugs* he expands it, perhaps to suit the philosophical tastes of his patron.

Furthermore, the definition of pneuma in the second chapter of *Cardiac Drugs* gives the impression that Avicenna composed this text with an ethical agenda in mind. It describes pneuma as a corporeal substance that arises from an elemental blend which constitutively resembles the basic mixture of the heavenly bodies.[80] Consequently, if pneuma retains its original condition, humans (as rational creatures) have the capacity to reach 'perfection' (*istikmāl*), here defined as existing in a state similar to what the heavenly bodies enjoy.[81] The point of administering cardiac drugs is to restore a person's heavenly element to its innate disposition, which enables them to experience joy as opposed to hatred and anger.[82] Avicenna counsels al-Ḥasanī and his retinue to aim for the heavenly life by caring for their pneumatic health and thus emotional well-being. In warning against extreme emotional states, *Cardiac Drugs* appears to follow in the tradition of 'spiritual medicines', except that it advises the reader to take drugs rather than philosophical lessons to cure them of their passions. Avicenna seems to place emotional health within medicine's boundaries. For the author of the *Canon*, this allocation has an uncomfortable repercussion: it appears to endorse Galen's argument, expounded in texts such as *QAM*, that doctors are equipped to intervene in ethical matters relating to personal conduct.[83] This boundary work, however, may serve the pragmatic end of enhancing Avicenna's intellectual capital, and therefore social standing, in Hamaḏān, where he had recently won favour from the Būyid ruler Šams al-Dawla (r. 387–412/997–1021) for curing him of a bout of colic. *Cardiac Drugs* signals that, as a doctor, Avicenna has more to offer his wealthy patrons than treatments for intestinal obstructions.[84]

79 al-Bābā (1984), 221–7. Avicenna also touches on the emotions at *Canon* 1.2.1.14, which investigates the influence of 'psychological movements' (*al-ḥarakāt al-nafsāniyya*) on the body. The passage summarizes Galen's explanation at *Ars Med.* 24.8 (Boudon-Millot 2002a: p. 351 ll. 2–6) of how the affections of the soul (anger, grief, etc.) – one of the six non-naturals – influence the condition of the body. For an overview of Avicenna's discussion of the emotions, see Knuuttila (2004), 218–26.

80 al-Bābā (1984), p. 226 ll. 5–6. 81 al-Bābā (1984), p. 226 ll. 2–3.

82 al-Bābā (1984), 234–6. This idea that a balanced life for humans involves preserving their divine element seems to have its roots in the Platonic definition of the good life as the life most like that of the gods. See *Resp.* 613a8–b3, *Tht.* 176b1–2, *Ti.* 90c–d, and *Phdr.* 248a.

83 See Chapter 1, p. 54.

84 For Avicenna's employment under Šams al-Dawla, see Reisman (2013), 18.

The text's more inclusive figuration of medicine is particularly conspicuous in its chapter on pleasure.[85] As I will now show, *Cardiac Drugs* draws on the theory of perception outlined in the *DA* of *The Cure* to offer a definition of pleasure, which it then sets against the Platonic–Galenic understanding of the sensation. Avicenna comments on pleasure in connection to joy, characterizing it as follows:

> الفرح لذة ما. وكل لذة فهي إدراك لحصول الكمال الخاص بالقوة المدركة، مثل الإحساس بالحلو والعرف الطيب <للقوة> الحاسة، والشعور بالانتقام للقوة الغضبية، والشعور بالمتوقع النافع – وهو الأمل – للقوة الظانة أو المتوهمة. وكل كمال فهو أمر طبيعي ومنعكس، وكل شعور بأمر طبيعي لقوة ما فهو التذاذ لها.[86]

> Joy is a [kind of] pleasure. Every pleasure is the perception (*idrāk*) of the attainment of a perfection (*kamāl*) that is specific to the faculty perceiving it: for example, the sensation of sweetness and the acquaintance with a pleasant smell [is a perfection specific] to the sensitive faculty (*li-l-quwwa al-ḥāssa*); the awareness (*šuʿūr*) of revenge [is a perfection specific] to the irascible faculty (*li-l-quwwa al-ġaḍabiyya*); and the awareness of a beneficial expectation – namely hope – [is a perfection specific] to the opinative or estimative faculty (*li-l-quwwa al-ẓānna aw al-mutawahhima*). Every perfection is a natural entity and a reflex, and every awareness of a natural entity by a faculty is pleasing to it [i.e. the faculty].

The passage identifies pleasure as a 'perfection' (*kamāl*) of the faculties. It dismisses the Platonic–Galenic view, put forward at *Canon* 1.2.2.23, that pleasure is a sensation resulting from a change in either the body's temperament or continuity – a view that he proceeds to refute, as I will discuss below. Instead, Avicenna argues that, as each faculty has its own distinctive perfection, there is a corresponding diversity of pleasures. This notion of pleasure seems to take inspiration from Aristotle's *Nicomachean Ethics* (1152b–1154b, 1172a20–1175b35), which proposes that there are different pleasures related to different activities.[87] There, Aristotle explains that pleasure is the 'perfection' or 'completion' (τελέωσις) of an 'activity' (πρᾶξις or ἐνέργεια), and rejects the Timaean idea that it involves a process of change.[88]

Although Avicenna's theory of pleasure in *Cardiac Drugs* features strong Aristotelian accents, it still shows signs of engagement with the Platonic–Galenic conception that it seeks to replace. Avicenna departs from Aristotle

85 al-Bābā (1984), p. 226 l. 10–p. 230 l. 5. 86 al-Bābā (1984), p. 227 ll. 11–15.

87 On Aristotle's understanding of pleasure, see Wolfsdorf (2013), 103–43. Isḥāq ibn Ḥunayn rendered Aristotle's *EN* into Arabic; on his translation, see Dunlop, Akasoy, and Fidora (2005), 26–8. Cf. also *Resp.* 580d–587a, where Plato acknowledges that each part of the soul has its own pleasure and desire.

88 For Aristotle's criticism of the Platonic notion that pleasure is a return (or movement), see *EN* 10.3–4.

by stressing that pleasure is not just the attainment of some perfection but also the perception (*idrāk*) of that attainment.[89] This emphasis on perception is paralleled in the *Canon*, which follows the *Timaeus* in explaining that a person only experiences pleasure if they sense (n. *ḥiss*) the change in their body's condition. It is important to observe the difference in the terms that Avicenna uses in these two passages: *idrāk* covers various kinds of perceptions, of which *ḥiss* ('sensation') is only one. At *DA* 2.2 of *The Cure*, Avicenna ranks *ḥiss* as an inferior kind of *idrāk* based on its reliance on the five 'external' senses (sight, touch, etc.), which prevents it from 'abstracting' (*ǧarrada*) the form (*ṣūra*) of a material object from matter (*mādda*).[90] On the other hand, the imagination (*ḫayāl*), a higher kind of *idrāk*, can more fully abstract the object's form from matter, as it does not require the object to be present to perceive it.[91] By referring to perception as *idrāk*, therefore, Avicenna indicates in *Cardiac Drugs* that pleasure does not necessarily depend on the body: one can experience it without using the sensory organs. While the faculties mentioned in the above quotation all require a corporeal instrument (namely, pneuma) to perceive, Avicenna wants to leave room for a class of pleasures that have no relation to the body: intellectual pleasures.[92] His hierarchy of pleasures introduces a category that transcends the purely physical idea of pleasure set out by Galen in his exegeses of the *Timaeus*.

Avicenna appears to be concerned that this stress on perception brings his own theory of pleasure too close to the position of Plato and Galen. Because certain kinds of perception follow a change in the body, his reader might be led to infer along Platonic–Galenic lines that pleasure results from a change in the body's condition. He attempts to distance himself from the view that 'pleasure is the departure from an abnormal condition' (*al-laḏḏa ḫurūǧ ʿan al-ḥāla al-ġayr al-ṭabīʿiyya*).[93] Although he does not mention its supporters by name, this is the idea developed in the *Timaeus* and summarized in the *Canon*. It is a mistake, Avicenna writes, to suppose that the shedding of the

[89] Perception does figure in Aristotle's theory of pleasure, for the *EN* argues that we derive pleasure not only from 'completing' some activity but also from enjoying the sensations consequent on that activity. On the extent to which the enjoyment of an activity can be separated from the enjoyment of the sensations associated with it, see Urmson (1967); Taylor (2008). Although sensation is closely linked with pleasure, Aristotle states at *EN* 10.5.7 that 'we must not regard pleasure as a thought or sensation – this is absurd' (οὐ μὴν ἔοικέ γε ἡ ἡδονὴ διάνοια εἶναι οὐδ' αἴσθησις – ἄτοπον γάρ).

[90] Rahman (1959), p. 59 ll. 11–14, p. 61 l. 18–p. 64 l. 7. In what follows, I offer a very brief account of Avicenna's theory of perception; for a more detailed discussion of it, I refer the reader to Naǧātī (1985), Black (2008), and McGinnis (2010), 97–116.

[91] On how the imagination (or imaginative faculty) can produce an image of an object based on stored sensory data, see Rahman (1959), p. 171 l. 17–p. 175 l. 8.

[92] See pp. 165–8 below.

[93] al-Bābā (1984), p. 228 l. 1.

'abnormal condition' is the essential cause (*bi-l-ḏāt*) of pleasure when it is only incidental (*bi-l-ʿaraḍ*) to the experience.[94] In his view, then, pleasure does not necessarily depend on changes in bodily states, but these changes can affect the real cause of pleasure, which is perception. He gives the example of a fever, which raises the temperature of the body, and thus makes it difficult to perceive the heat of sensible objects.[95] When the fever passes, the body returns to its natural temperament. Only with the body in this ideal state can the various perceptive faculties attain the perfection that brings pleasure.

The distinction between Avicenna and Galen here seems to be minimal. In the case of the fever patient, Avicenna argues that this individual's pleasure derives from the perfect functioning of their perceptive faculties, which ensues from a restoration of temperament, whereas Galen would contend that their pleasure comes from perceiving that restoration of temperament. As I explained above, by describing perception as *idrāk*, which encompasses both corporeal and incorporeal perception, Avicenna proposes that pleasure is not contingent on the body. Even so, his association of pleasure with health – in particular, a balance in pneumatic temperament, which can be restored by drugs – appears to tie the experience to the body.[96] Admittedly, Avicenna focuses on bodily perception in *Cardiac Drugs*, but he relates in the *De Anima* of *The Cure* and the *Salvation* that illness can impede incorporeal powers too.[97]

Combining lists of *materia medica* with concepts from psychology and physics, *Cardiac Drugs* redraws the boundary between medicine and philosophy that the *Canon* is so determined to fix and maintain. While *Cardiac Drugs* utilizes philosophical language to express its theory of pleasure and the emotions, it nonetheless places their therapy in the hands of the doctor, as seems to have been Galen's ambition in *QAM*. Avicenna devotes most of the work to providing recipes of simple and compound drugs that can alter the emotions by changing the temperament of the pneuma in the heart. For instance, chapter ten highlights a class of drugs called 'exhilarants' (*al-adwiya allatī tufarriḥu*), including substances

94 al-Bābā (1984), p. 228 ll. 3–4.

95 al-Bābā (1984), p. 228 ll. 9–13. Avicenna may have adopted this example of a fever altering a person's perception of hot objects from *EN* 10.5.9. Whereas Avicenna employs the example to stress how illness can impede the perception of pleasure, Aristotle uses it to illustrate the diverse nature of pleasure: what is pleasant to a fever patient is unpleasant to a healthy person.

96 al-Bābā (1984), p. 229 l. 4–p. 230 l. 5.

97 At *DA* 1.5 of *The Cure* (Rahman 1959: p. 47 ll. 11–17) Avicenna explains how bodily states can affect the practical intellect (or 'practical power', *quwwa ʿamaliyya*). He reiterates this position at *Salvation* 2.6.10 (Fakhry 1985: p. 219 l. 16–p. 220 l. 20=Rahman 1952: 53–4).

such as pearl and chebulic myrobalan, that enables a patient to feel joy by restoring their vital pneuma to its natural luminosity.[98] Because knowledge of the emotions requires a grounding in philosophy, *Cardiac Drugs* appears to suggest that their ideal therapist is the Galenic doctor – a model criticized in the *Canon* for subverting the separation of the disciplines that Avicenna's scientific hierarchy demands.

Putting Pleasure beyond the Body

The *Canon* and *Cardiac Drugs* present pleasure as a largely corporeal phenomenon, and only gesture towards the possibility of experiencing it independently of the body. In this last section I will look at how Avicenna brings up the incorporeal pleasures of the intellect in the *Metaphysics* of *The Cure* and *Pointers and Reminders* (*Kitāb al-Išārāt wa l-tanbīhāt*), a late summa composed between 421/1030 and 426/1034, to encourage his readers to pursue a philosophical life.[99] Concerned with the fate of the soul after death, both texts renounce bodily pleasures, towards which Avicenna remains impartial in his medical writings, in favour of intellectual pleasures, which are felt more fully in the hereafter. Their devaluing of the body and its experiences serves to demote medicine as a source of knowledge, for the discipline, according to *On the Divisions of the Intellectual Sciences* (Avicenna's 'blueprint' to *The Cure*), can only derive facts about natural reality through its study of this material entity, unlike philosophy.[100] The two compositions also associate the attainment of pleasure with psychic rather than corporeal health, perhaps with the aim of weakening medicine's relevance to the subject. Although Avicenna does not mention the Platonic–Galenic notion of pleasure as a restoration in either work, he rehashes with minor variations his theory from *Cardiac Drugs*, elements of which, as I have argued, trace back to the *Timaeus*. As I will show, by characterizing corporeal pleasures as false in the *Metaphysics* of *The Cure* and *Pointers and Reminders*, Avicenna is able to adapt his doctrine of pleasure from *Cardiac Drugs* to elevate philosophy as the indispensable discipline for human well-being.

The *Metaphysics* of *The Cure* and the metaphysical section of *Pointers and Reminders* comment on pleasure in connection with the soul's separation from the body. In particular, these works examine pleasure in chapters

98 See al-Bābā (1984), p. 242 l. 6–p. 245 l. 3.
99 On the dating of *Pointers and Reminders*, see Gutas (1988), 145=(2014), 155–7.
100 I borrow the characterization of Avicenna's epistle on the sciences as a 'blueprint' to his larger philosophical composition from Biesterfeldt (2000), 93.

on 'the return' (*al-maʿād*) – that is, the afterlife – and on beauty (*bahǧa*) and happiness (*saʿāda*).[101] They both allege that true happiness comes from the perfection (*kamāl*) of the intellect (*ʿaql*), or rational soul (*nafs nāṭiqa*), which is achieved by grasping the form (*ṣūra*) of everything through philosophical reflection.[102] Becoming aware of its own perfection after the body's death, the perfected soul experiences intense pleasure during its return to God, in contrast to the imperfect soul, which feels distress (*šaqāwa*).[103] The two texts single out philosophy as the surest path to real pleasure and happiness.

The *Metaphysics* and *Pointers and Reminders* preface this account of incorporeal pleasures with a brief explanation of the nature of pleasure. Apart from mentioning the intellect, the latter text closely follows the definition of pleasure in *Cardiac Drugs*. It reports that 'pleasure is the perception and the attainment of the perfection and good of that which perceives'.[104] The text lists food and dress, victory, and truth and beauty as the respective perfections of the appetite (*šahwa*), spirit (*ġaḍab*), and intellect (*ʿaql*). As in *Cardiac Drugs*, *Pointers and Reminders* identifies 'perception' (*idrāk*) as a key element of pleasure, but it develops its theory with reference to the parts of the soul, which is divided according to the Platonic scheme of tripartition rather than by faculties. Avicenna wants to make clear that he is speaking about the soul in this chapter, not the body.[105] The *Metaphysics*, however, describes pleasure as the 'awareness' (*šuʿūr*) of the attainment of a perfection – a term which also appears in *Cardiac Drugs*.[106] Although Avicenna famously uses *šuʿūr* (specifically, the phrase *šuʿūr bi-l-ḏāt*) to denote the soul's awareness of itself, it can also signify the soul's awareness of other objects.[107] Thus, its meaning

[101] *Metaphysics* 9.7 (Anawātī and Zāyed 1960: 423–32=Marmura 2005: 347–57) and *Pointers and Reminders* 2.8 (Forget 1892: p. 190 l. 1–p. 198 l. 13=Goichon 1951: 467–501 [in French]). In his *Epistle on the Afterlife for the Feast of the Sacrifice* (*al-Risāla al-Aḍḥawiyya fī l-maʿād*), Avicenna emphasizes that the soul alone returns to the hereafter to be judged by God: see Lucchetta (1969), p. 139 ll. 4–6.

[102] *Metaphysics* 9.7.14 (Anawātī and Zāyed 1960: p. 428 ll. 3–8=Marmura 2005: 351) and *Pointers and Reminders* 2.8 (Forget 1892: p. 194 ll. 5–16=Goichon 1951: 472).

[103] *Metaphysics* 9.7.17–18 (Anawātī and Zāyed 1960: p. 428 l. 9–p. 429 l. 4=Marmura 2005: 352–3) and *Pointers and Reminders* 2.8 (Forget 1892: p. 195 l. 7–p. 197 l. 3=Goichon 1951: 474–8).

[104] Forget (1892), p. 191 l. 15–p. 192 l. 2=Goichon (1951), 469.

[105] The *Metaphysics* (9.7.4) also develops its account of pleasure with explicit reference to the powers of the soul: see Anawātī and Zāyed (1960), p. 423 l. 13–p. 434 l. 3=Marmura (2005), 348.

[106] *Metaphysics* 9.7.4; Anawātī and Zāyed (1960), p. 424 ll. 1–2=Marmura (2005), 348.

[107] For the latter sense of the term, see Avicenna's *Notes* (*Taʿlīqāt*): Badawī (1973), p. 30 ll. 16–23 and p. 148 ll. 1–11. Avicenna's conception of self-awareness (*šuʿūr bi-l-ḏāt*) has received a lot of scholarly attention: see, e.g., Pines (1954); Marmura (1986); Black (2008); Adamson (2012); Kaukua (2015).

in the passage on pleasure in the *Metaphysics* appears to be equivalent to *idrāk*.[108]

With some minor terminological changes, Avicenna reformulates his 'medical' discussion of pleasure as a philosophical enquiry. He furthers philosophy's claim to the subject of pleasure when elaborating on the sensation's link with health. As I have argued above, *Cardiac Drugs* and the *Canon* assert the relevance of medicine to the investigation of pleasure by emphasizing, albeit in different ways, that illness impedes the perception of it. The *Metaphysics* and *Pointers and Reminders*, on the other hand, introduce this same point about illness and the perception of pleasure to explain how the soul can be hindered from obtaining pleasure in the hereafter.[109] Employing language with medical resonances, Avicenna writes in the *Metaphysics* that, as disease occludes the perception of bodily pleasure, a soul's excessive preoccupation with the body – such as its pleasures – numbs (n. *ḫadar*) its perception of the intellectual pleasures in this world and prevents it from attaining happiness in the next.[110] With the exception of a small number of more attuned souls, this numbness lasts as long as the body and soul are joined; once separated, the soul experiences intense pleasure or pain depending on whether we are able to 'slip off the noose of appetite and anger' (*ḫalaʿanā ribqat al-šahwa wa l-ġaḍab*).[111] Psychological health, then, comes from studying philosophy, which enables one to perceive a modicum of the incorporeal pleasures that await the perfected soul in the afterlife.

In relaying that the pleasures associated with the mortal aspect of the soul injure the well-being of the immortal soul, the *Metaphysics* and *Pointers and Reminders* imply that the pleasures discussed in *Cardiac Drugs* and the *Canon* are in fact forms of pain. Drugs can only achieve an illusory form of pleasure, whereas philosophy gives rise to real pleasures that endure even after the loss of the body. This depiction of bodily pleasure as a kind of ailment recalls Avicenna's grouping of pleasure with diseases in the *Canon*, although the classification there follows a Galenic nosological tradition. Thus, through the suggestion that corporeal pleasures are actually pains, *Metaphysics* and *Pointers and Reminders* seem to

108 See Black (2008), 83n5.

109 Both texts use the example of an ill person's aversion to sweet tastes to illustrate how disease can prevent a faculty (or part of the soul) from attaining and perceiving their perfection. Cf. *Metaphysics* 9.7.8 (Anawātī and Zāyed 1960: p. 425 ll. 3–6=Marmura 2005: 349) and *Pointers and Reminders* 2.8 (Forget 1892: p. 192 ll. 14–17=Goichon 1951: 470).

110 *Metaphysics* 9.7.15–16: Anawātī and Zāyed (1960), p. 427 l. 5–p. 428 l. 3=Marmura (2005), 351–2. Cf. *Pointers and Reminders* 2.8: Forget (1892), p. 194 l. 17–p. 196 l. 11=Goichon (1951), 473–7.

111 *Metaphysics* 9.7.14: Anawātī and Zāyed (1960), p. 426 l. 17=Marmura (2005), 351.

invalidate doctors' contribution to the subject of pleasure, of which they remain ignorant on account of their preoccupation with the body, as well as to downgrade the importance of medicine to human life.

Although the theory of pleasure in the *Canon*, *Cardiac Drugs*, *Metaphysics*, and *Pointers and Reminders* shares elements with the doctrine in Plato's *Timaeus*, each of these tracts offers distinct formulations of it to perform different kinds of boundary work. Avicenna portrays pleasure as primarily a physical phenomenon in the *Canon* to confine Galen's expertise to the corporeal, whereas *Cardiac Drugs* and the two philosophical treatises introduce the soul into their accounts either to expand or narrow down the doctor's purview. Regardless of whether Avicenna presents himself as a doctor or a philosopher, the various boundaries that these four texts construct between medicine and philosophy all serve to increase the prestige and authority of their creator.

Conclusions: Breaking the *Qānūn*

This chapter has demonstrated that Avicenna's work offers two opposing conceptions of the relationship between medicine and philosophy. I have argued that his *Canon of Medicine* constitutes a recuperative project, whose aim is to reinstate the parameters of the two disciplines that Galen and subsequent doctor-philosophers such as al-Rāzī had muddled. While Avicenna outlines at the beginning of the *Canon* a number of disciplinary 'laws' that restrict the doctor's knowledge, he goes on to undermine these very laws by disputing Galenic doctrines that are informed by Plato's *Timaeus*, such as the identification of the brain as the hegemonic organ. As an apology for these disciplinary infractions, Avicenna invokes his expertise as a physicist to emphasize his own capacity to range beyond the confines of medicine, or he alters the terms of his disputes to downplay their philosophical connotations.

My analysis of the sections on pleasure in the *Canon* and *Cardiac Drugs* made clear that, notwithstanding his own apologetic rhetoric and criticism of Galen's 'philosophization' of medicine, Avicenna contributes to a more expansive figuration of the discipline by introducing material that doctors supposedly lack the epistemic framework to examine. In both texts he mentions the Platonic–Galenic characterization of pleasure as a physical reaction (*Ti.* 64c7–65b3), with which he seems to find fault for not stating that the experience requires a level of psychic complexity – the possession of perceptive faculties. Moreover, in *Cardiac Drugs* Avicenna underscores the relevance of pleasure to the study of the soul by drawing on Aristotle's definition of it as a perfection (Arab. *kamāl*) and by using the word *idrāk* to indicate that the experience is not dependent on the body. These passages seem to call for the reader to transgress the limits of medicine to acquire the psychological context to comprehend Avicenna's remarks. Thus, the limitations imposed on medicine in the *Canon* appear to have more rhetorical than epistemological force. Avicenna appeals to these laws as a way of critiquing Galen's contribution to the field. In this way, he can present his system of thought as superior to that of Galen.

Avicenna's subversion of his own disciplinary rules can also be interpreted as a sign of his affiliation with the Galenic tradition. Although Avicenna's Aristotelian commitments may have compelled him to address certain subjects in the *Canon*, Galen's discussions of, for example, the hegemonic organ showed generations of doctors that they had a right to comment on this issue too. To defend his own excursion into 'philosophical' territory, Galen, as Chapter 1 explained, called upon the authority of Plato's *Timaeus*, whose entangling of the body and cosmos seemed to license the venture. Gained through study and praxis, a doctor's knowledge of the human body, according to Galen, gives them insight into issues relating to the powers of the soul (if perhaps not its nature), the elements, and the causes that govern the actions and reactions of all things. After Galen, the human body, soul, and cosmos arguably became even harder to disentangle from each other, and this ambiguity afforded opportunities for boundary work. The legacy of Galen's reading of the *Timaeus* can thus be seen in Avicenna's drawing and redrawing of the boundaries of medicine and philosophy.

CHAPTER 5

Uprooting the Timaeus: *Maimonides and the Re-medicalization of Galenism*

In a letter to his favourite student, Joseph b. Judah (d. 623/1226), Moses Maimonides (532–600/1138–1204) complains about how his medical activities consume most of his day.[1] The missive seems to boast of the success of Maimonides' practice in Ayyūbid Cairo and the spread of his reputation as a doctor, but it also reveals an unease about his association with the discipline. He reports:

> ואעלמך אן קד חצלת לי שהרה̈ ע̇טימה̈ גדא פי אלטב ענד אלכברא . . . פכאן הד̇א דאעיא
> לתלאף אלנהאר דאימא פי אלקאהרה̈ פי זיארה̈ אלמרצ̇א, ואד̇א ג̇ית מצר פגאיתי אן אקדר
> פי בקיה̈ אלנהאר מע אלליל אן אטאלע מן כתב אלטב מא אחתאג̇ אליה . . . וכאן הד̇א
> דאעיא אן לא אג̇ד סאעה̈ לנט̇ר שי מן אמר אלשריעה̈ ולא אקרא אלא יום סבת פקט. ואמא
> סאיר אלעלום פלא נג̇ד וקת לנט̇ר שי מנהא. וקד תאד̇ית כת̇יר גדא מן הד̇א אלבאב.[2]

> And I hereby inform you that I have achieved great renown in medicine among the great ones [of the realm] . . . This is the reason that my day is always consumed in Cairo visiting patients, and when I return to Fusṭāṭ [a suburb of Cairo], in what is left of the day and during the night, I am able at most to read what is necessary in my medical books (*kutub al-ṭibb*) . . . And as a result, I am unable to find an hour to reflect on any issue of the religious law (*amr al-šarīʿa*) and I do not read [the Bible] except on the Sabbath. As for the rest of the sciences (*sāʾir al-ʿulūm*), I cannot find time to reflect on any of them. I am sorely vexed by this state of affairs.[3]

Maimonides portrays his medical obligations, which sometimes took him to the royal court, as a distraction from his study of Jewish law and

[1] On the life and writings of Joseph b. Judah as well as his correspondence with Maimonides, see Munk (1842). This letter to Joseph has been dated to either 583–6/1187–90 (Lewis 1993: 184) or 586–7/1190–1 (Lieber 1979: 280).

[2] Baneth (1946), p. 69 l. 11–p. 70 l. 11. This and many of the other texts discussed in this chapter are composed in Judaeo-Arabic (a form of Arabic in Hebrew lettering), which was used by Arabic-speaking Jewish scholars in the medieval period. On the distinguishing features of Judaeo-Arabic, see Blau (1981). For a survey of the various languages that Maimonides knew and how he employed them, see Hopkins (2005).

[3] The translation is taken from Lieber (1979), 279–80 [with minor modifications].

philosophy, to which the unnamed 'sciences' seem to refer collectively. The letter's prioritization of the latter fields of learning over medicine may stem, in part, from the fact that the medical profession was not Maimonides' first career choice. While Maimonides trained in medicine, among other subjects, as a young man in Morocco, where his family had initially fled in their attempt to escape religious persecution from the Almohad caliphate (524–668/1130–1269) in al-Andalus (southern Iberia), financial hardship prompted him to start practising when he settled in Cairo.[4] After his younger brother David, a gem merchant in the India trade, perished in a shipwreck in the Indian Ocean sometime between 564–5/1169–70, Maimonides had to find a way to pay off the debts owed to investors and to recoup his family's fortune.[5]

Maimonides taught Joseph philosophy, and dedicated his philosophical masterpiece *The Guide for the Perplexed* (*Dalālat al-ḥāʾirīn*) to him, so this letter may reflect his attitude as a philosopher towards medicine: he views it as a separate and inferior discipline.[6] Perhaps influenced by Maimonides' own presentation of himself as a philosopher first and a doctor second, subsequent readers, from the medieval period onwards, have placed emphasis on his philosophical rather than medical accomplishments; he is often ranked as the most important medieval 'Jewish philosopher'.[7] Maimonides is recognized for his harmonization of philosophy with Jewish Scripture.[8] Although there is debate as to whether Maimonides

[4] Infamously, the Almohads (or al-Muwaḥḥidūn, 'those who proclaim God's unity') did not view their Christian and Jewish subjects as 'protected people' (*dimmī*), and thus pressured them to convert to Islam or emigrate. See Viguera Molins (2014) for an overview of and bibliography on Almohad rule and culture in southern Iberia. Maimonides and his family were forced to convert to Islam while living in the Maghreb. On their conversion, see Mazor (2007); Kraemer (2008), 116–24.

[5] On David and Maimonides' involvement in the India trade, see Goitein and Friedman (2007) *passim*. It is unclear how soon after David's death Maimonides started to practise medicine: Stroumsa (2009: 9) and Cohen (2017: 95) suggest that he embarked on his medical career immediately after his brother's passing, whereas Lieber (1979: 277) and Lewis (1993: 184) argue that he entered the profession years later, after 1185. Regardless of the timing of his career change, as Goitein (1980: 163) observes, Maimonides was still investing in the India trade as late as the 580s/1190s.

[6] *The Guide for the Perplexed* (hereafter, *Guide*) was published in 586/1190, either a few years after or around the same time as the composition of the letter to Joseph (see n. 1 above). Goitein (1980: 163) reports that Maimonides taught medicine in addition to philosophy; on the evidence for this claim, see Friedman (2007).

[7] See Frank (1997), 2–6, and Leaman (2003), 5–15, on the problems with the label 'Jewish philosopher'. For Maimonides' pre-modern and modern reception, see, e.g., Silver (1965); Septimus (1975); Kohler (2012); Diamond (2012, 2014). Maimonides' medical texts have, until very recently, been poorly served by modern editors. Gerrit Bos and several collaborators are currently editing and translating into English all of Maimonides' surviving medical output through Brigham Young University's Middle Eastern Text Initiative and Brill.

[8] Stroumsa (2009), 38. Cf. Leaman (2003), 6, who describes Maimonides' contribution as the 'import[ation] of philosophical ideas into Judaism'.

should be regarded as a rationalistic theologian (*mutakallim*) instead of a philosopher working on theological subjects, his project, which seeks to establish new 'roots' (or 'principles', *uṣūl*) for Jewish belief, collapses the distinction between religion and philosophy.[9] For instance, in the first book of his *Mishneh Torah*, a work in Hebrew on Jewish law (*halakha*), Maimonides not only imposes a catechism of Aristotelian doctrines about God's nature but also includes physics and metaphysics within Talmud, which he defines as the study of the principles underlying the Torah.[10] As a legal text, the *Mishneh Torah* determines what is acceptable belief or action; so, by incorporating Aristotelian philosophy within his code, Maimonides makes it a part of Jewish faith.[11]

This chapter investigates how Maimonides' devaluing of his own medical pursuits in the above letter may serve his broader polemic with medicine, which aims to neutralize the danger that Galen's theories posed to the 'roots' of his philosophical–religious system. Similar to Avicenna, Maimonides perceived Galen's defence of the *Timaeus*' account of the body, soul, and cosmos as threatening Aristotle's credibility on these matters, but he held that it had the potential to disrupt Jewish belief as well. The chapter will examine three strategies that Maimonides employs to undermine the authority of Galen and the Timaean 'roots' of Galenism. First, I will look at two mature works, the *Guide* and the *Medical Aphorisms* (*Kitāb al-Fuṣūl fī l-ṭibb*), to show that Maimonides regarded the *Timaeus* – especially Galen's interpretation of it – as a heterodox text because it seems to deny the notion of creation *ex nihilo* and thus the oneness and omnipotence of God. In a manner reminiscent of al-Rāzī in the *Doubts*, Maimonides in the *Medical Aphorisms* characterizes Galen as a heretic, a term with a very specific sense in his writings, to argue for the need to reform Galenism.

As the second half of the chapter will explain, Maimonides carries out this reformist project by narrowing down the domain of medicine and by

9 This debate about Maimonides' status as a *mutakallim* is encapsulated in the opposing positions of Strauss (1952: 40–1) and Harvey (1991). My interpretation of Maimonides' philosophical–religious 'project' is indebted to Stroumsa (2009: 53–83), who reads his 'fundamentalism' – that is, his concern to reform the basic roots of Jewish belief – in light of the revivalist approach of the Almohads to Islam.

10 See Hyamson (1962), 34a–40a. Cf. the introduction to the *Guide*; M–J, p. 3 ll. 7–9=Pines (1963), 6. See also Berman (1974), 164n31, who regards the equation of physics and metaphysics with Talmud as a 'classic example of revolution by redefinition within Rabbinic Judaism'.

11 As Kellner (1987) explains, Maimonides understands faith as the acceptance of certain propositions, so the rejection of any of the precepts set out in the *Mishneh Torah* and other works (such as the famous thirteen principles in the *Commentary on the Mishnah*, *Sanhedrin*: Twersky 1972: 417–23) is heretical.

're-medicalizing' Galenism. My analysis of Maimonides' boundary work in *On Asthma* (*Maqāla fī l-Rabw*), *Regimen of Health* (*Fī Tadbīr al-ṣiḥḥa*), and the *Commentary on Hippocrates' Aphorisms* (*Šarḥ fuṣūl Abuqrāṭ*) will demonstrate that, in putting the soul beyond the scope of doctors, he limits medicine to the strictly corporeal – namely, knowledge of the treatment of bodily diseases and the maintenance of bodily health. While Maimonides' boundary work in the two treatises parallels Avicenna's in the *Canon*, he demotes medicine further than his Muslim forerunner by questioning the discipline's reliability and therefore utility. In so doing, he constructs medicine in such a way that it cannot usurp philosophy's claim to epistemic authority.

Finally, I will draw attention once again to the *Medical Aphorisms* to assess how Maimonides suppresses, edits, and attacks Galen's doctrines that are inspired by Plato's *Timaeus*, such as his tripartite psychology and encephalocentrism, to 'de-philosophize' Galenic medicine. Echoing the title of the famous Hippocratic *Aphorisms*, Maimonides' collection of medical sayings endeavours to bring medicine back to a 'pre-Galenic' time when the discipline was not tainted by Galen's intellectual overreach. The *Medical Aphorisms*, however, consist mostly of extracts from the Galenic corpus; thus, I will propose that the aforementioned interventions are a way for Maimonides to work within Galenism to reform this system of medicine.

The Heresy of the *Timaeus*

Maimonides does not have much time for Plato, or so his oft-cited letter to the Hebrew translator Samuel ibn Tibbon suggests.[12] He dismisses Plato as an author of incomprehensible parables and praises Aristotle both for having an intellect second only to the prophets and for establishing the 'roots and principles' (*ha-shorashim ve-ha-ʿiqqarim*) of all the sciences.[13] Because of Maimonides' own recognition of the expediency of parabolic discourse, Leo Strauss famously argued that the medieval thinker was in fact a crypto-Platonist.[14] There has been considerable pushback in recent scholarship against Strauss' interpretation, which emphasizes the esoteric and political aspects of both Plato and Maimonides' works; the tendency now is to situate Maimonides in relation to the intellectual culture of

[12] On this letter, see p. 105n5 above.
[13] Marx (1935), 379–80; for an English translation of this passage, see Pines (1963), lix.
[14] See Strauss (1935, 1936, 1937); Pines (1963), lxxvi. For the role of parables in Maimonides' writings, see the introduction to the *Guide* (M–J: 2–9=Pines 1963: 5–14); Stern (2013), 18–63.

Muslim Spain, where Aristotelianism dominated.[15] While Maimonides' admiration of Aristotle in his exchange with Ibn Tibbon is probably sincere, the short shrift that he gives to Plato belies a deeper anxiety about the challenge that the *Timaeus* presented to his conception of Jewish belief.

Before discussing why Maimonides saw the dialogue as religiously problematic, I will consider briefly the sources that may have shaped his reading of it.[16] In the few instances where Maimonides cites the *Timaeus* by name (instead of just referring to Plato), he appears to be drawing on either Aristotle, an Aristotelian exegete, or Galen. For example, *Guide* II,13 mentions the Platonic text in connection to Aristotle's literal interpretation of the dialogue's cosmogony at *Phys.* 251b19–20, and the *Medical Aphorisms* contain six excerpts from Galen's *Plat. Tim* (*Tafsīr Ǧālīnūs li-Kitāb Ṭīmāwus*, or *Šarḥuhu li-Ṭīmāwus*).[17] If the Platonic lemmata still accompanied Galen's exegesis in the sixth/twelfth century, *Plat. Tim.* would have given Maimonides access to a significant portion of the *Timaeus*; the six quotations in the *Medical Aphorisms*, however, do not provide enough evidence to determine whether he knew this Galenic work directly or through an intermediary.[18] Moreover, while Maimonides shows familiarity with Galen's synopses of Plato's *Laws* and the *Republic*, it is unclear if he made use of *Com. Tim.*, which also takes the dialogue's cosmogony literally.[19]

These sources contributed to Maimonides' perception of the *Timaeus* as a text that espouses temporal creation and encourages the crossing of

[15] See Gutas (2002), 19–24, who strongly criticizes Strauss' approach to Maimonides and Islamicate philosophy in general. For a response to Gutas' critique, see Harvey (2018), 233–9. The widely read Aristotelian commentators Ibn Bāǧǧa (Lat. Avempace, d. 533/1139) and Ibn Rušd (Lat. Averroes, 520–95/1126–98) were also born in Spain; in his letter to Ibn Tibbon, Maimonides indicates that he was familiar with their exegeses (Marx 1935: 379=Pines 1963: lix–lx).

[16] Cf. Pines (1963: lxxv–lxxvi) and Seeskin (2005: 35), who stress Maimonides' reliance on paraphrases and doxographical writings.

[17] For the passage from the *Guide*, see M–J, p. 198 ll. 3–5=Pines (1963), 283. *Phys.* 251b19–20 does not cite the *Timaeus* by name, so Maimonides may have added this reference himself or possibly taken it from another Aristotelian source, such as a commentary or summary. For the citations of *Plat. Tim.*, see aph. 6.95 (Schröder 1934: 8–9=Bos 2007: 22), 23.6, 23.61, 22.109, 24.58, 25.51 (Schröder 1934: 3–5, 7–9, 26=Bos 2017: 26, 52, 72, 102, 156). Maimonides also cites *Plat. Tim.* in his *Commentary on Hippocrates' Aphorisms* (Schliwski 2004: p. 10, § 11), which dates to around 1195 (Schliwski 2004: xxii).

[18] Only one of Maimonides' excerpts of *Plat. Tim.* (that is, aph. 6.95, on which see Das 2014: 99–100) is cited in an earlier Islamicate source. His quotation of unique passages lends credence to the idea that he was working directly with the commentary.

[19] Maimonides quotes from Galen's synopsis of the *Laws* in his *Commentary on Hippocrates' Aphorisms* (see Schliwski 2004: p. 6, § 11). Kraemer (1984: 112n9) maintains that Maimonides had access to the same Platonic summary underlying Averroes' *Commentary on Plato's 'Republic'*, namely Galen's synopsis of the *Republic*.

disciplinary boundaries.[20] As I will explain below, Maimonides finds Plato's cosmogony threatening because it shares features with the creation account in Jewish Scripture. His engagement with this theory of the dialogue in the *Guide* and other treatises also reveals a heightened sensitivity to its theological implications. Maimonides' reading of the *Timaeus* as a theological work may be a legacy of another of his Platonic sources, al-Fārābī (d. 339/950) – although a range of thinkers, going back to Aristotle, have examined Plato's conception of God through his position on creation. It is from al-Fārābī's commentary on Aristotle's *Sophistical Refutations* that Maimonides learns about the Platonic doctrine of the receptacle of becoming (*Ti.* 49a1–53a7).[21] A keen student of al-Fārābī, Maimonides may have derived his general understanding of the major themes of the Platonic dialogues, including the *Timaeus*, from *The Philosophy of Plato* (*Falsafat Aflāṭūn*).[22] Whereas his contemporary al-Masʿūdī (d. 345/956) associates the *Timaeus* with physics, al-Fārābī writes in his tract that it deals with metaphysics, the part of philosophy that studies intelligibles: '[Plato] presented in the *Timaeus* an account of the divine and natural being as they are perceived by the intellect and known by means of that science.'[23] Metaphysics' ultimate subject of enquiry is God, so al-Fārābī depicts the *Timaeus* as Plato's explanation of the divine.[24]

Book two of the *Guide* sets out how Plato's cosmogony contravenes what Maimonides elsewhere calls 'the basic principle of all basic principles and the pillar of the sciences' (*yesod ha-yesodot ve-ʿammud ha-ḥokhmot*): the tenet that God alone is primordial.[25] The rejection of this diseased 'root' (*aṣl*), which entails that God created the cosmos out of nothing, constitutes 'radical unbelief' and 'heresy'.[26] At *Guide* II,13, Maimonides evaluates the

[20] At *Guide* II,6 (M–J, p. 183 ll. 3–4=Pines 1963: 263), Maimonides ascribes to Plato an emanationist account of creation with Plotinian echoes, but he does not interpret this view as conflicting with the belief in temporal creation.

[21] See Robinson (2003). [22] On al-Fārābī's influence on Maimonides, see Berman (1974).

[23] Mahdi (2001), p. 15, § 9. Cf. the *Book of Notification and Review* (*Kitāb al-Tanbīh wa-l-išrāf*, translation in Zimmermann 1986: 150), where al-Masʿūdī reports that the dialogue covers 'the genesis of the physical world and what it contains' (*kawn al-ʿālam al-ṭabīʿī wa-mā fīhi*). Connelly (2016) speculates that al-Fārābī's description of the dialogues may come from the same Middle Platonic source that underlies the Platonic catalogue in the *Compendiosa Expositio*, which is attributed to Apuleius of Madaura (*c.* 124–70 CE).

[24] Cf. Albinus (second century CE), *Introduction to Plato's Dialogues* 5.25: 'Since it is also necessary to have knowledge of divine matters, so that one who has acquired virtue can become assimilated to them, we will delve into the *Timaeus*. By reading this investigation into nature – and so-called theology and structure of the universe – we will get a direct and clear look at the divine' (Fowler 2016: 49–50 [slightly modified]).

[25] See the *Book of Knowledge* of the *Mishneh Torah*: Hyamson (1962), 34a.

[26] See the *Letter on Astrology*: Twersky (1972), 468.

cosmogonies of Moses, Plato, and Aristotle, and finds fault with the philosophers' positions for proposing that matter is eternal and thus coexistent with God. He describes Plato's opinion, which is listed second, as follows:

> אלת̇אני הו ראי כל מן סמענא כ̇ברה וראינא כלאמה מן אלפלאספה̈ וד̇לך אנהם יקולון אן מן אלמחאל אן יוג̇ד אללה שיא מן לא שי . . . ווצף אללה ענדהם באנה קאדר עלי הד̇א כוצפה באנה קאדר עלי אלג̇מע בין אלצ̇דין פי אן ואחד . . . ואלמפהום מן כלאמהם אנהם יקולון כמא אנה לא עג̇ז פי חקה לכונה לא יוג̇ד אלממתנעאת אד̇ ללממתנע טביעה̈ ת̇אבתה̈ ליס הי מן פעל פאעל פלד̇לך לא ימכן תג̇ירהא כד̇לך לא עג̇ז פי אד̇א לם יקדר אן יוג̇ד שיא מן לא שי אד̇ הד̇א מן קביל אלממתנעאת כלהא פלד̇לך יעתקדון אן ת̇ם מאדה̈ מא מוג̇ודה̈ קדימה̈ כקדם אלאלאה לא יוג̇ד דונהא ולא תוג̇ד דונה. . .
>
> ואפלטון איצ̇א הד̇א אעתקאדה אנת תג̇ד ארסטו יחכי ענה פי אלסמאע אנה יעתקד אעני אפלאטון אן אלסמא כאינה̈ פאסדה̈ והכד̇א תג̇ד מד̇הבה מצרחא פי כתאבה לטימאוס לכנה לא יעתקד אעתקאדנא כמא יט̇ן מן לא יעתבר אלארא ולא ידקק אלנט̇ר ויתכ̇יל אן ראינא וראיה סוא וליס אלאמר כד̇לך לאן נחן נעתקד כון אלסמא לא מן שי אלא בעד אלעדם אלמטלק והו יעתקד אנהא מוג̇ודה̈ מכינה̈ מן שי.[27]

> The second opinion is that of all the philosophers of whom we have heard reports and whose discourses we have seen. They say that it is impossible that God would bring a thing into existence out of nothing . . . To predicate of God that He is able to do this is, according to them, like predicating of Him that He is able to bring together two contraries in one instance . . . What may be understood from their discourse is that they say that just as His not bringing impossible things into existence does not argue a lack of power on His part – since what is impossible has a firmly established nature that is not produced by an agent and that consequently cannot be changed – it likewise is not due to lack of power on His part that He is not able to bring into existence a thing out of nothing, for this belongs to the class of impossible things. Hence, they believe that there exists a certain matter that is eternal as the deity is eternal; and that He does not exist without it, nor does it exist without Him . . .
>
> This is also the belief of Plato. For you will find that Aristotle in the *Akroasis* [i.e. *Physics*] relates of him that he, I mean Plato, believed that the heaven is subject to generation and passing-away. And you likewise will find his doctrine plainly set forth in his book to Timaeus. But he does not believe what we believe, as is thought by him who does not examine opinions and is not precise in his speculation; he [the interpreter] imagines that our opinion and his [Plato's] opinion are identical. But this is not so. For as for us, we believe that the heaven was generated out of nothing after a state of absolute nonexistence, whereas he believes that it has come into existence and has been generated from some other thing.[28]

[27] M–J, p. 197 l. 10–p. 198 l. 8. [28] Pines (1963), 282–4.

According to Maimonides, Plato's cosmogony in the *Timaeus* is unacceptable to Jewish belief on the grounds that it denies the uniqueness of God in alleging that the world came into being from pre-existing, eternal matter.[29] Moreover, while Plato and other proponents of the 'second opinion' may allege that their thesis of creation out of pre-cosmic material does not diminish God's agency, Maimonides indicates at the end of II,13 that it undermines God's omnipotence and even free will.[30] The supreme God of the *Timaeus* is unable to create whatever they wish because eternal matter imposes certain limitations on and therefore determines what they can make.[31]

Aristotle's doctrine of an eternal cosmos also conflicts with the foundation of Judaism and the sciences for similar reasons, but Maimonides excuses his 'heresy' by suggesting that the philosopher never claimed demonstrative status for his arguments.[32] Maimonides' commitment to Aristotelianism notwithstanding, the *Guide*'s generous treatment of Aristotle may have to do with how unlikely eternalism is to be taken as true belief: leaving no room for divine intervention, Aristotle's opinion stands in stark opposition to scriptural accounts, whereas the creation story in the *Timaeus* comes uncomfortably close.[33] In the passage quoted above, Maimonides warns that the dialogue's recognition of God's direct causal role in the world's creation could lead one to confuse Plato's opinion with his own.[34] In another section of the *Guide* (II,25) Maimonides admits that numerous 'obscure passages' (*šubah*) of the Torah also appear to support the Platonic thesis of creation out of pre-existing matter, but he is quick to point out that Plato's cosmogonic claim has not been logically demonstrated.[35]

Although the *Guide* does not explicitly identify Galen as a champion of the *Timaeus*' cosmogony, it does highlight his deviation from Aristotle's stance. At *Guide* II,15 Maimonides portrays the theory of an eternal world as logically preferable – or, in his words, 'nearer to correctness' (*aqrab ilā al-ṣiḥḥa*) – to the theories of Aristotle's opponents, which are based on weaker inferences about the nature of the

[29] M–J, 196–9=Pines (1963), 281–5. Seeskin (2005: 56) calls the Platonic theory 'creation *ex novo*'.

[30] See M–J, p. 199 ll. 7–9=Pines (1963), 285, where Maimonides contrasts this view with the Mosaic idea that it is incumbent on God to create out of non-existence.

[31] See Seeskin (2005), 58. See also Langermann (1992), who argues that Maimonides' rejection of astrology is connected to his concern to preserve God's free will.

[32] M–J, p. 203 ll. 19–25=Pines (1963), 292. [33] See Pines (1963), lxxv.

[34] See Davidson (1979), Ivry (1986), and Samuelson (1991), who hold that Maimonides actually followed the cosmogony of the *Timaeus*.

[35] *Guide* II,25: M–J, p. 229 l. 29–p. 230 l. 1=Pines (1963), 328–9.

cosmos.[36] In the context of this apology for Aristotle, Maimonides relays al-Fārābī's 'contempt' (*istaḫaffa*) for Galen's contention that the eternity of world cannot be demonstrated.[37] The report frames Galen's aporia concerning the origin of the world as a doubt only about Aristotelian eternalism, even though his remarks in the extant text of *DD* 4 and works such as *Prop.Plac.* (2) indicate that his uncertainty applies as well to Plato's account.[38] Maimonides does not comment on al-Fārābī's criticism; by his silence, he seems to condone his predecessor's judgement. Therefore, Maimonides may regard Aristotle as intellectually honest for (supposedly) realizing that his arguments for eternalism are not demonstrative, but he does not express the same admiration for Galen's hesitance to take a definite position on this cosmological debate.[39]

Book twenty-five of the *Medical Aphorisms*, which was completed at the end of Maimonides' life, attributes to Galen a Platonic view of creation and condemns him for misrepresenting Jewish belief on the issue.[40] In the light of this later attack, Maimonides seems to use al-Fārābī in the *Guide* to call into question Galen's competence to engage in cosmological speculation. The final book of the *Medical Aphorisms* professes to contain only Maimonides' doubts (*šukūk*) about Galenic medical ideas, although aph. 62–72 treat not only the subject of creation but also the dispute over the identity of the hegemonic organ.[41] I will investigate Maimonides' possible reasons for labelling Galenic theories with philosophical import as 'medical' later in this chapter; however, it is worth noting here that he appears to criticize Galen's medical concepts (aph. 2–56) in the first half of book twenty-five to emphasize how unqualified his predecessor is to range beyond the discipline of which he is a putative expert.[42]

The text that prompts Maimonides to refute Galen's notion of creation is *UP* 11.14, which compares the hypothetical answers that Epicurus and Moses might give as to why the eyelashes and eyebrows do not grow, but

36 M–J, p. 203 ll. 15–16=Pines (1963), 292. 37 M–J, p. 203 l. 29–p. 204 l. 1=Pines (1963), 292.

38 As Maimonides' Farabian source has not been identified, it is unclear which Galenic treatise(s) al-Fārābī is targeting (see Pines 1963: 292n13).

39 According to Maimonides' reading of *DC* 279b4–12, Aristotle admits that his argument in favour of the world's eternity is non-demonstrative.

40 On the dating of the *Medical Aphorisms*, see Bos (2004), xx.

41 See Bos (2017), p. 107 [English], p. 108 ll. 3–5 [Arabic]. In this introduction, Maimonides separates his project from al-Rāzī's *Doubts about Galen*, which deals with 'issues that have no relationship at all to the medical art' (*umūr lā madḫal lihā fī ṣināʿat al-ṭibb aṣlan*: Bos 2017: p. 105 [English], p. 106 ll. 7–8 [Arabic]). On the relationship between al-Rāzī's and Maimonides' doubts, see p. 189 below.

42 Langermann (1993), 186.

stay at a constant length: the former would allege that it is due to random interactions of atoms, whereas the latter would point to the will of God.[43] While Moses seems to come off better than Epicurus for acknowledging God's role in the creation of the body and cosmos, Galen dismisses the prophet's doctrine as causally defective because it ignores the constraints that matter places on God's agency.[44] God is responsible for keeping the even length and number of the eyelashes and eyebrows in the sense that the deity chose, out of the material available to them, to implant this kind of hair in cartilage, which renders it hard, small, and incapable of growth. With its stress on God's benevolence, which is the reason for the divinity's selection of the best possible material for their creation, the passage promotes the cosmological scheme of the *Timaeus* – or, as Galen calls it, 'our own opinion, and that of Plato and the other Greeks who follow the right method [in the study] of nature' (ἥ θ' ἡμετέρα καὶ ἡ Πλάτωνος καὶ ἡ τῶν ἄλλων τῶν παρ' Ἕλλησιν ὀρθῶς μεταχειρισαμένων τοὺς περὶ φύσεως λόγους).[45] I am not going to delve into Maimonides' response to Galen's critique of Moses, as he uses many of the same arguments that the *Guide* employs to discredit Plato's cosmogony.[46] I will look, however, at how Maimonides depicts Galen as a heretic not only to justify his polemic against him but also to show the need for a reformation of Galenism, which the *Medical Aphorisms* aims to achieve.

Prior to the excerpt of *UP* 11.14, Maimonides asks the reader to keep in mind that 'he who quotes the words of an unbeliever is not an unbeliever [himself]' (*ḥākī al-kufr laysa bi-kāfir*).[47] This caveat flags that the ensuing material is offensive to Jewish belief. Maimonides rescues himself from the charge of heresy on the grounds that he is merely reporting another's opinions, but he goes on to exempt Galen as well in view of the fact that he is a religious outsider.[48] The text, then, defines a heretic as someone who deviates from the established norms of their own religious community. Be

43 See aph. 25.62–8: Bos (2017), 177–93. For the Greek text of the passage, see Helmreich (1909), p. 158 l. 2–p. 160 l. 6. Maimonides generally seems to have a favourable impression of *UP*, for he cites the work's teleological conception of the body at *Guide* III,32 (M–J, p. 384 l. 5=Pines 1963: 525) to defend his theodicy.

44 See Tieleman (2005) for a fuller treatment of Galen's criticism of the Mosaic account of creation.

45 Helmreich (1909), p. 158 ll. 20–2. Cf. aph. 25.62 (Bos 2017: p. 179 [English], p. 180 l. 7 [Arabic]), which omits the relative clause qualifying the 'other Greeks', perhaps to make this position seem less epistemologically secure.

46 Namely, Maimonides counters that the hypothesis of creation out of pre-existing matter denies free will to God (Bos 2017: p. 189 [English], p. 190 ll. 6–9 [Arabic]). On the passage, see Schacht and Meyerhof (1937), 60–2.

47 Bos (2017), p. 177 [English], p. 178 l. 1 [Arabic].

48 Bos (2017), p. 177 [English], p. 178 ll. 2–3 [Arabic].

that as it may, Maimonides' description of Galen in the foregoing aphorisms (25.59–61) suggests that his predecessor deserves the designation 'heretic' inasmuch as he is guilty of the same missteps for which a Jew would earn the label. Earlier writings such as the *Commentary on the Mishnah* connect heresy with intellectual overreach, and aph. 25.59 singles out this 'human disease' (*al-maraḍ al-insānī*) as the reason for Galen's repudiation of Moses.[49] In contrast to the heretic, who vilifies the religious law in the belief that they know more than the prophets, Galen's insolence stems from a disciplinary infraction: he contends that his medical expertise allows him to discuss physics and metaphysics. In identifying Galen's venture into philosophy as an intellectual transgression, Maimonides signals that the philosophical aspects of Galenism violate disciplinary norms and therefore need to be removed.

Maimonides' final polemical blow is his comparison of Galen to a false prophet at aph. 25.61. He alleges that Galen's overestimation of medicine's relevance to philosophy propelled him to stake a claim to divine knowledge:

وما وقف عند هذا الحد بل من شدة التذاذه بما ظهر من بعض منافع الأعضاء ادعى النبوة وقال إنّ جاءه ملك من عند الله وعلمه كذا وأمره بكذا.

> He did not stop at this limit [i.e. stating that medicine is similar to the theoretical sciences], but because of the excessive pleasure he took in what became evident to him about some of the uses of the organs, he pretended to be a prophet [lit. laid claim to prophecy, *iddaʿā al-nubūwa*] and said that an angel came to him from God and taught him such and such and ordered him such and such.[50]

Perhaps as a result of Ḥunayn and his circle's adaptation of the pagan content of the Galenic corpus, the above passage seems to interpret Galen's report at *UP* 10.11 of a dream that he had which censured him for neglecting the anatomy of the eyes as an angelic encounter.[51] Maimonides' accusation of false prophecy would have resonated very deeply with his contemporary Jewish readers, because just before and during their lifetimes messianic claimants had appeared in Jewish communities in the Maghreb and Yemen.[52] For subverting the Torah and leading the faithful astray,

[49] See Bos (2017), p. 167 [English], p. 168 ll. 3–8 [Arabic], p. 169 [English], p. 170 ll. 8–16 [Arabic]. On this passage from the *Commentary on the Mishnah*, see Stroumsa (2009), 39–51, who writes that the equation of heresy with intellectual overreach is a topos in Maimonides' corpus.

[50] Bos (2017), p. 175 [English], p. 176 ll. 10–11 [Arabic].

[51] I examine Galen's dream account in Chapter 2 (p. 82).

[52] In this letter, Maimonides advises the Yemeni Jewish community on how to deal with their false prophet and lists four other false messiahs who preceded this individual. See Twersky (1972), 428–62.

Maimonides had declared in his *Epistle to Yemen* (1172) that these pretenders deserve to be put to death.[53]

Maimonides leaves unsaid whether Galen warranted this punishment (especially as he was non-Jewish), but he compels the reader, nonetheless, to reject the Galenic system as debased by falsehoods. When confronted with heresy and false sciences (such as astrology), Maimonides commands the faithful in the *Letter on Astrology* to '"hew down the tree and cut off its branches" (Dan. 4:11)' and 'plant in its stead "the tree of knowledge of good and evil" (Gen. 2:9)'.[54] As I have argued above, Maimonides regards Galen's support of the doctrine of creation in the *Timaeus*, which contradicts the foundation of the Torah (God's omnipotence), as a diseased 'root' (*aṣl*) of Galenism. I will show in the latter part of this chapter that Maimonides attempts to cut out, or at the very least minimize, the Timaean elements of Galenism to produce a system of medicine which is more compatible with the roots of his own thought, Judaism and Aristotelianism. However, before doing so, I will consider how Maimonides weakens medicine's claim to epistemic authority through his attempts at redrawing its disciplinary boundaries in a more limiting way. In narrowing down medicine's scope and questioning its trustworthiness, Maimonides, I will suggest, seeks to undermine Galen's efforts to bolster the credibility of his more philosophically charged ideas on the basis of his medical knowledge; in this way, Maimonides can also challenge the soundness of the Platonic theories that Galen supports.

Turning Medicine Inwards

As his definition of 'Talmud' illustrates, one way in which Maimonides performs his disciplinary boundary work is by investing new meaning into a key term.[55] Whereas he reformulates 'Talmud' to expand the domain of Jewish faith to include philosophical studies, the semantic tactic serves an exclusionary purpose in his meta-disciplinary discussions of medicine, which are scattered throughout his medical writings. There, Maimonides fixes more specialized senses to a range of words that are common to both medicine and philosophy so as to separate the two areas of learning. Paradigmatic in this respect is Maimonides' definition of the first part of

[53] See the *Letter on Astrology* (Twersky 1972: 473) and Kraemer (1984), 135–40.

[54] See the *Letter on Astrology*; Twersky (1972), 473. See Berman (1974), 165, who observes how Maimonides invokes the image of Abraham tearing out the roots of idolatry to characterize his own reformist project in the *Guide*.

[55] See p. 172 above.

medicine – the subject of the doctor's craft (*mawḍūʿ ṣināʿatihi*) – in the *Commentary on Hippocrates' Aphorisms*: 'the science of anatomy' (*ʿilm al-tašrīḥ*), or knowledge of the human body.[56] While this equation of medicine's core with anatomy may indicate that Maimonides wants to keep doctors focused inwards on the body, it is actually his definition of the components of this science that reveals a move to prevent disciplinary straying. In addition to comprising an understanding of the uses, mixtures, and locations of the parts of the body, anatomy covers 'the state of their substance' (*ḥāl ǧawharihi*), which is qualified as their relative softness, hardness, thickness, and thinness.[57] Maimonides gives the philosophically loaded word *ǧawhar*, which often designates a thing's substance (similar to the Greek οὐσία), or fundamental aspect, literally a superficial meaning.[58] In *Hipp.Elem.*, Galen cites the constituents of the organs, which he progressively breaks down into their homoeomerous parts (for example, bone and cartilage), humours, and then the four elements, to justify his treatment of the latter, the building blocks of the natural world.[59] Through his redefinition of *ǧawhar*, Maimonides forestalls doctors from using the organs as a stepping stone to physics by suggesting that, for them, the most basic information about these parts relates to their appearance.

Compared to Avicenna's *Canon*, which advises doctors to leave the subject of the four elements to physicists, the above example of Maimonides' boundary work is subtler.[60] Both authors, however, employ particular expressions to demarcate the doctor's knowledge from the philosopher's in their discussions of the soul and its relevance to medicine. The two place the soul under philosophy's jurisdiction and steer their medical readers to refer to the power that is in charge of the body as either a set of faculties, which reside in various organs, or nature, respectively.[61] Recognizing that 'nature' is a polysemous word, Maimonides argues in *Regimen of Health* (*Fī Tadbīr al-ṣiḥḥa*), which was composed in 1198 on behalf of the Ayyūbid sultan Malik al-Afḍal (the son of Saladin), for a medical usage that restricts this power to the realm of the body:

وأكثر الأطباء يغلطون جدا في ذلك، ويظن أنّه يعاضد القوة في ذلك وهو يهدها أو يعيقها أو
يشوش طريقها. ولذلك يقول أرسطوطاليس في كتاب الحس والمحسوس إنّ أكثر من يموت إنّما

[56] Schliwski (2004), p. 8 § 3. [57] Schliwski (2004), p. 8 § 3.

[58] Schwarz (1992: 162–4) notes that, in his description of the opinions of the *mutakallimūn* in the *Guide*, Maimonides utilizes *ǧawhar* to denote 'atom'.

[59] See De Lacy (1996), 126–8. [60] See pp. 144–6 above.

[61] As I remarked above (p. 152), Galen maintains that he alters the terms of his psychological discussions in consideration of the disciplinary backgrounds (medical or philosophical) and sectarian affiliations (Platonic or Stoic) of his readers.

يموت من الطب لجهل أكثر الأطباء بالطبيعة. والأطباء يعنون بقولهم طبيعة في هذا الغرض القوة المدبرة لبدن الحيوان.[62]

> Most doctors err greatly in this, supposing that they are aiding the faculty, yet they destroy it, hinder it, or confuse its ways. Accordingly, Aristotle says in his book on *Sense and Sensibles* that the majority of those who die only die from treatment because of the ignorance of most doctors about nature. Doctors mean by 'nature', in this connection, the faculty which governs the bodies of living creatures.[63]

While the passage insinuates that the concept of 'nature' in medicine differs from the 'philosophical sciences', it does not articulate precisely how they are distinct. It is not clear whether Maimonides is using 'nature' as a terminological stand-in for 'soul' to adapt his discussion to a medical context, as Avicenna, following Galenic precedent, does with 'faculties' in the *Canon*. Alternatively, the medical sense of 'nature' may designate an innate power that is responsible for the most rudimentary activities of life (that is, growth and nutrition) – similar to Galen's concept of φύσις at *Nat. Fac.* 1.1, which is, nonetheless, identified with the soul later at *Prop.Plac.* 3.6.[64] The term's ambiguity notwithstanding, Maimonides narrows down doctors' field of enquiry by establishing that the highest power with which they should concern themselves is something closely tied to, if not inseparable from, the body. The above passage can also be understood as limiting in that it only authorizes doctors' study of the nature of the body and not the world at large, which would require training in physics, as Galen, Ḥunayn, and al-Rāzī encouraged their medical readers to pursue. Maimonides' disparaging comment about most doctors' ignorance (*ǧahl*) of even this more circumscribed notion of nature serves to validate the very restrictions that he imposes on their research by underscoring their struggle to gain mastery over the domain allotted to them.

In line with Galen's *Ars Med.* 23.8, *Regimen of Health* and the earlier tract *On Asthma* accept that the emotions (lit. 'the movements of the soul', *ḥarakāt al-nafs*) affect the body's health.[65] Even so, they put the practical philosopher, the theoretical philosopher (lit. the one trained in 'theoretical considerations', *al-iʿtibārāt al-ʿilmiyya*), and expert in the 'disciplines and

[62] *Regimen of Health* 2: Kroner (1923), p. 296 ll. 2–6.

[63] Bar-Sela, Hoff, and Faris (1964), 21 [modified]. Cf. aph. 6.94; Bos (2007), p. 20 l. 15–16: 'You should know that the term nature is a homonym (*ism muštarak*) which has many meanings. One of all these meanings is the faculty which governs the body of living beings (*al-quwwa al-mudabbira li-badan al-ḥayawān*), for the doctors also call this faculty "nature".'

[64] See LG, p. 70 ll. 1–9.

[65] For the chronological relationship between *Regimen of Health* and *On Asthma*, see Bos (2002), xxxiii.

admonitions of the Law' (*al-ādāb wa-l-mawā ʿiẓ al-šarʿiyya*) in charge of these psychic movements instead of the doctor.[66] This allocation of the soul's care to adepts of philosophy and Jewish Scripture, or religion more generally, reinforces the point that medicine deals strictly with the corporeal and curtails the therapeutic purview, and thus pertinence, of doctors. Maimonides goes further in minimizing the agency of doctors by alleging that a patient's recovery often has to do with the strength of their nature rather than their practitioner's intervention.[67] For example, chapter thirteen of *On Asthma* relegates doctors to the position of auxiliaries of nature and regards even good practitioners as dispensable: 'one can do without a physician more than one needs him, even when he is excellent and knows how to support nature and does not confuse it and divert it from its proper way'.[68] In denying medicine a monopoly on health as well as questioning its capacity to effect it, Maimonides weakens the basis of the discipline's prestige.

Maimonides credits al-Fārābī with the observation that a patient's outcome is more dependent on their nature than the skill of their doctor.[69] Al-Fārābī's emphasis on medicine's contingency also seems to underlie Maimonides' attack on the discipline's epistemic authority in texts such as the *Commentary on Hippocrates' Aphorisms*. For al-Fārābī medicine was not a 'science' (*ʿilm*) but a 'practical art' (*ṣināʿa fāʿila*) because the many particulars that have to be taken into consideration – for example, a patient's age, their location, and the weather – make it difficult (or even impossible) for doctors to derive universal principles, or roots, for their practice.[70] In the introduction to his Hippocratic exegesis, Maimonides adds that the particulars of medicine are not just numerous but in flux (for instance, people age and the weather changes), so a practitioner can only develop an 'aptitude' (*malaka*) for interpreting what a patient's symptoms reveal about their condition and chance of recovery.[71] As the commentary implies, the absence of certainty in medicine disqualifies it from being a

[66] See Boudon-Millot (2002a), p. 347 l. 1. Cf. *Regimen of Health* 3 (Kroner 1924: p. 67 ll. 18–21=Bar-Sela, Hoff, and Faris 1964: 25) and *On Asthma* 8.3 (Bos 2002: p. 38 ll. 10–13).

[67] *On Asthma* 13.6: Bos (2002), p. 84 ll. 4–5.

[68] *On Asthma* 13.6; Bos (2002), p. 85 ll. 3–4.

[69] *On Asthma* 13.6; Bos (2002), p. 84 l. 1. He also cites an aphorism from al-Rāzī's *Guide* (Bos 2002: p. 84 ll. 16–19) that advises doctors to assess the strength of a patient's nature before deciding whether to intervene.

[70] See Zimmermann (1976), 402–3, who demonstrates al-Fārābī's engagement with Aristotle's comparison of medicine with rhetoric at *Rhet.* 1355b8–31. On the parallels between al-Fārābī and Maimonides' conceptions of medicine, see Stroumsa (1993, 2009: 134).

[71] See Schliwski (2004), p. 10 § 10, p. 11 § 14. Galen admits that medicine has certain 'stochastic', or unpredictable, elements, but maintains that it is not stochastic per se; for the relevant Galenic references, see Hankinson (1998a), 238; for Galen's notion of the role of conjecture in medicine, see Boudon-Millot (2003), 288–96.

source of demonstrative knowledge.[72] By lowering the epistemological status of medicine, Maimonides is able to demolish Galen's assertion that he 'demonstrated' controversial theories such as Plato's encephalocentrism. Galen built his arguments on observations of human and animal bodies, which, owing to their own mutability and many particulars, are unable to provide a path to general truths.

While medicine's reliance on conjecture means that it cannot discover universally true principles for itself or any other field, Maimonides, following al-Fārābī, holds that it is nonetheless composed of rules, as is every *ṣināʿa* ('art').[73] The medical works discussed above all contain remarks setting limits on the doctor's areas of expertise, but the *Medical Aphorisms* appears to take a more comprehensive approach to what constitutes the 'art' of medicine: the text serves a fundamentally prescriptive function. One of its books details the 'general laws' (*qawānīn ʿāmmiyya*) and 'principles' (or 'roots', *uṣūl*) of medicine, which are to be understood as such in a lesser sense because of the discipline's contingency.[74] Furthermore, the title of the composition consciously recalls the Hippocratic *Aphorisms*, which aims to define and thus demarcate the boundaries of medicine.[75] The Greek tract encapsulates medicine in fixed and memorizable statements; it omits what its author regards as extraneous to the discipline and, through this epitomatory process, establishes what doctors should and should not know. Just as the Hippocratic writer shapes the field of medical knowledge by selecting its essential components, so Maimonides, I shall argue, aims to reconfigure it by creating his own aphorisms.

Notwithstanding Maimonides' attempt to connect himself to Hippocrates through his own aphoristic project, the elite medical culture in which he situated himself was dominated by Galen – for example, his Hippocrates was mediated through Galen, as was the case with most Islamicate authors.[76] The previous section maintained that Maimonides viewed Galenic medicine as a flawed system because Galen espouses Plato's cosmogony and other theories from the *Timaeus*. Although Maimonides was unable to expunge Galen from the medicine of his day, I will examine in what follows how he works to edit out the *Timaeus* from Galenism in the

[72] Cf. *Regimen of Health* 2: 'Yet there is not a tenet in the doctrines of medicine that is an absolute one, but for anything allowable there are necessary reservations' (Kroner 1923: p. 298 ll. 19–20=Bar-Sela, Hoff, and Faris 1964: 22).

[73] See Stroumsa (2009), 134. [74] See Bos (2004), 34–60.

[75] See Grant (2016), 6, who explains the purpose of the Hippocratic *Aphorisms* in light of the etymology of 'aphorism': ἀπό ('off') and ὁρίζειν ('to set bounds').

[76] See, e.g., p. 117n72 above.

Medical Aphorisms. My analysis will show that he deploys some of the same tactics that feature in his boundary work across his diverse corpus, such as the redefinition of terms and concepts, to achieve this end. At the start of the *Medical Aphorisms* Maimonides admits that his aphorisms, similar to Hippocrates', cannot encompass all of medicine but only the matters that 'should always be retained, or are neglected, or are beneficial for what one needs in most cases'.[77] This text is concerned, therefore, with the very foundations of medicine. I will suggest that, by removing the Timaean roots of Galenism, Maimonides neutralizes the threat that the system poses to his philosophical and religious beliefs by 're-medicalizing' it.

Eradicating the *Timaeus*

Most of the approximately 1,500 aphorisms that make up the twenty-five books of the *Medical Aphorisms* come from Galen or tracts attributed to him.[78] Maimonides seems to have had access to a large portion of the Galenic corpus, including works that are now lost or fragmentary in Greek.[79] There is only a small number of references in the *Medical Aphorisms* to the group of Timaean writings that I treated in Chapter 1: Maimonides quotes from *PHP* eight times, *Plat.Tim.* six times, both *QAM* and *Prop.Plac.* once, and *Com.Tim.* not at all.[80] Apart from reproducing the title of *Plat.Tim.* (*Tafsīr Ǧālīnūs li-Kitāb Ṭīmāwus*; *Šarḥuhu li-Ṭīmāwus*), Maimonides does not mention the *Timaeus* by name, but instead refers to Plato when discussing the dialogue's doctrines, as will be shown below. In view of his extensive familiarity with Galen in Arabic, it seems probable that Maimonides' minimal quotation from the aforementioned Galenic texts has little to do with the resources at his disposal but rather may represent a polemical strategy to suppress the Timaean aspects of Galen's oeuvre. He makes his hostility towards at least *PHP* and *Prop.*

77 Bos (2004), p. 2 ll. 7–9. 78 Bos (2004), xxiv.

79 For instance, he cites genuine material from Galen's *Commentary on Hippocrates' Humours* (e.g. aph. 24.19: Bos 2017: p. 82 ll. 1–2), the extant Greek text of which is considered to be a Renaissance forgery (Manetti and Roselli 1994: 1540), and *On Problematical Movements* (e.g. aph. 24.20: Bos 2017: p. 82 ll. 3–5), which survives in a medieval Arabic translation and two Latin renditions (see Nutton and Bos 2011). Prior to the publication of the *Medical Aphorisms*, Maimonides composed a collection of verbatim extracts of different Galenic works under the title *Epitomes* (*al-Muḫtaṣarāt*) (see Bos 2004, p. 2 ll. 15–16). Baneth (1960–1) calculates that Maimonides' library held at least thirty-seven Galenic volumes.

80 For the citations to *PHP*, see aph. 1.10–12 (Bos 2004: p. 9 l. 8–p. 10 l. 3), aph. 24.55–7, aph. 25.59, and aph. 25.71 (Bos 2017: p. 100 ll. 6–16, p. 102 ll. 1–6, p. 172 l. 2, and p. 196 ll. 5–13); for the citations to *Plat.Tim.*, see p. 174n17 above; for the citation to *QAM*, see aph. 6.16 (Bos 2007: p. 4 ll. 16–17); for the citation to *Prop.Plac.*, see aph. 25.59 (Bos 2017: p. 172 l. 2).

Plac. (as well as *Sem.*) clear at aph. 25.59, where he targets them for both dealing with physics and metaphysics and containing 'refutations of Aristotle' (*al-rudūd 'alā Arisṭū*).[81] Thus, Maimonides' two aims of de-philosophizing medicine and preserving Aristotle's authority appear to be behind his near neglect of Galen's output on the *Timaeus*.

Maimonides also seems to downplay the philosophical contents of these Galenic works, for the passages he extracts from them give the impression that they are primarily of lexical or antiquarian interest. For instance, the sole quotation of *QAM* is a gloss on the term 'melancholy', which the *Medical Aphorisms* understands to mean 'fearfulness' (*tafazzu'*) in Greek; furthermore, three of the six excerpts from *Plat. Tim.* consider medical definitions, a few of which had become obsolete by Galen's lifetime.[82] Maimonides does address, in his composition, Galen's defence of arguably the most important theory to him from the *Timaeus*: Plato's encephalocentric thesis. The way in which Maimonides frames those aphorisms dealing with Galen's interpretation of the theory seems designed either to undercut the credibility of their material or to curb their disciplinary reach.

For example, at the end of book twenty-four, whose subject is medical curiosities (*nawādir*) and rarities (*umūr šāḏḏa qalīla*), Maimonides summarizes Galen's description at *PHP* 1.6 of his vivisection of an animal's heart and treatment of a patient's skull fracture.[83] The Galenic passage contrasts the absence of any discernible disruption to the animal's sensory abilities when its heart was crushed during the vivisection with the patient's total loss of sensation when Galen pressed down on their brain with the meningophylax ('meninges protector') tool while extracting pieces of broken skull.[84] Although Galen adduces this experiment and clinical case as demonstrative proof of Plato's encephalocentric position, Maimonides weakens the narrative's claim to truthfulness by grouping it with fantastical accounts. The initial aphorism of book twenty-four seems to signal that all the ensuing information is suspect, for it reproduces a passage from pseudo (?)-Galen's *Commentary on Hippocrates' Diseases of Women* that relates how a solar eclipse in Sicily caused a number of women to menstruate from their mouths or give birth to babies with two heads.[85] Moreover, after reporting

[81] Bos (2017), p. 172 ll. 1–3.

[82] See aph. 6.16, 23.6, 61, and 109. Galen does discuss melancholy in *QAM* (see pp. 52, 135 above), but he does not comment on the etymology of the term there (see Bos 2007: 100n29). The text's Arabic translator, Ḥubayš or perhaps Abū Ǧa'far (who revised Ḥubayš's version in the light of the Greek), may have added the gloss. On the tract's translation into Arabic, see Ḥunayn, *Epistle* § 134: Bergsträsser (1925), p. 50 ll. 8–12=Lamoreaux (2016), p. 125 ll. 5–8.

[83] See aph. 24.55. [84] See *PHP* 1.6.6–10: De Lacy (2005), p. 78 l. 33–p. 80 l. 13.

[85] Aph. 24.1: Bos (2017), p. 74 ll. 6–10.

Galen's anatomical observations at *PHP* 1.6, Maimonides quotes from *PHP* 6.8.79–83 an internal reference to Homer's *Odyssey* (9.576–8) that recounts how in Hades two vultures perpetually consume the giant Tityus' liver as punishment for his attempted rape of the goddess Leto.[86] Whereas Galen cites this myth as poetic evidence for his location of the desiderative soul in the liver, Maimonides uses it to further question the veracity of *PHP*.[87]

As I explained in Chapter 1, Galen appeals to the tripartite psychology of Plato's *Timaeus* and *Republic* in his polemics with philosophers to contest their monopoly on psychological knowledge; his defence of the Platonic idea affords him the opportunity to illustrate medicine's capacity to generate reliable information about the soul.[88] Perhaps in response to the boundary work that this theory does for Galen in service of his expansion of medicine, Maimonides redefines it at aph. 6.94 so as to strip it of its psychological significance. He writes:

> قد علمت قول الأطباء: قوى نفسانية وقوى حيوانية وقوى طبيعية. ولنسم الآن في هذا الإصطلاح جميع أفعال بدن الإنسان الأفعال البدنية. فأقول إنّ أشرف الأفعال البدنية التنفس وبعده النبض وبعده الإحساس وأشرف الحواس البصر ثم السمع وبعد الإحساس شهوة الطعام والشراب وبعد ذلك الكلام وبعد ذلك التمييز أعني به التخيل والفكر وبعد ذلك حركة سائر الأعضاء على معتادها وهذه الرتبة في الشرف إنّما هي بحسب ضرورية الحياة أو صلاحية إستمرارها.

> It is well known that the doctors speak about psychic faculties, animal faculties, and natural faculties. Now, according to this convention, let us call all the activities of the human body 'corporeal activities'. I say that the most eminent of the corporeal activities is respiration, followed by the pulse, and after that sensation. The most eminent sense is vision, followed by hearing. After sensation comes the desire for food and drink, then speech, and then discernment – namely, imagination and thought. Then comes the movement of the other parts of the body according to their habit. This gradation in eminence pertains only to the requirements for life or its proper continuation.[89]

While the faculties listed in the first sentence correspond to the Platonic logical, irascible, and appetitive parts of the soul, the passage omits the philosopher's name and instead attributes the tripartite scheme to 'doctors' in general, possibly to erase its philosophical associations. Maimonides'

86 See aph. 24.57. Cf. De Lacy (2005), p. 425 ll. 18–33.

87 Although arguing from poetic testimony may rank second to last in Galen's methodological hierarchy (on which, see De Lacy 1966: 263–4), Rosen (2013) shows how it still plays an important part in Galen's 'rhetoric of science'.

88 See pp. 42–7 above.

89 Bos (2007), p. 20 ll. 9–14 [Arabic], ll. 14–23 [English, slightly modified].

classification of these powers as 'corporeal activities' (*af'āl badaniyya*) also appears to minimize their relevance to the soul.

The aphorism revises the hierarchy that Plato and Galen establish between the three faculties, or parts of the soul, by ranking their actions according to how essential they are to the maintenance of life. Whereas speech and rational thought (which belong to the rational soul) are the 'most eminent' (*ašraf*) activities in the Platonic–Galenic model of tripartition, Maimonides demotes them and puts respiration first. The desire for nourishment, which is an impulse of the appetitive soul, even comes before these cognitive processes. Maimonides' elevation of respiration may not represent a complete reversal of the Platonic–Galenic ordering of faculties/psychic parts, for he does not specify here whether he rejects Galen's identification of the activity as a psychic as opposed to vital faculty, which later authors such as Themistius and Qusṭā ibn Lūqā (d. *c.* 300/912–13) held.[90] Nonetheless, Maimonides' downgrading of the importance of speech, imagination, and thought may serve to discourage the medical readers of the *Medical Aphorisms* from investigating them. He creates a new hierarchy, with respiration and the pulse at its top, that accentuates the disjunct between the principal concern of doctors, who are to maintain these basic functions to safeguard the life of the body, and philosophers, who oversee those functions contributing to the life of the soul.

Book twenty-five, Maimonides' *Doubts about Galen*, offers more explicit criticism of the psychology outlined in *PHP* – especially its contention that sensation originates in the brain – than the preceding examples. I mentioned earlier that, at the start of the book, Maimonides tries to distance his own critical project from al-Rāzī's, who, he says, refuted Galen on philosophical rather than medical topics.[91] The extended attack on Galen's reading of the *Timaeus*' cosmology (introduced above) and encephalocentrism in the latter half of book twenty-five reveals that Maimonides does the very thing for which he admonishes al-Rāzī. Similar to Avicenna, he may have found Galen's discussions of these subjects to be too authoritative, too threatening, to leave undisputed. Furthermore, the aphorisms cited below will reveal that Maimonides' polemical strategy mirrors al-Rāzī's in a number of respects: he pairs quotations from different texts to highlight inconsistencies in Galen's positions, calls attention to his logical

[90] For Galen's classification of respiration as an activity of the psychic faculty, see *Us.Puls.* 5.162K. Cf. Themistius, *Letter to Julian* (Swain 2013: 155) and Qusṭā ibn Lūqā, *On the Difference between the Soul and the Spirit* (*Fī l-Farq bayna l-nafs wal-rūḥ*: Cheikho 1911: p. 108 l. 21), who place respiration under the vital faculty.

[91] See p. 178n41 above.

missteps, and teases out the troublesome theological implications of his views.[92] Maimonides' claim in the opening of book twenty-five that the subsequent doubts only pertain to medical matters may be rhetorically loaded as well. First, the statement seems to limit the scope of Galen's expertise to medicine alone by discounting the philosophical import of the ideas that follow – even if this significance is precisely what prompts Maimonides to bring them up. Second, in applying the label 'medical' to all the Galenic contents of book twenty-five, Maimonides weakens their argumentative strength, because medicine, as the *Commentary on Hippocrates' Aphorisms* declares, cannot produce epistemologically certain facts.

Aph. 70–2, which conclude book twenty-five, comprise a three-pronged attack against Galen's encephalocentric stance in *PHP*: the texts issue charges against his consistency, the soundness of his reasoning, and even his honesty. Maimonides begins by setting his predecessor's opinion in opposition to Aristotle's; in so doing, he makes clear that what is at risk in the ensuing controversy is the validity of a definitive 'root' of Aristotelianism, cardiocentrism. As at aph. 6.94, he avoids mentioning the soul, and reformulates Galen's tripartite psychology, which distributes the soul's part or faculties into three organic seats, as a tripartite physiology, where the brain, heart, and liver are discrete sources (*mabādiʾ*) of certain powers. In contrast, Aristotle identifies only one major organ, the heart, which endows the other parts of the body with their powers.[93] Therefore, on Maimonides' retelling, Galen holds that the brain alone is responsible for sensation, whereas Aristotle contends that the heart 'sends out' (*yabʿaṯu*) the power of sensation to the former organ, which then performs sensory tasks.[94]

This summary seems to oversimplify Galen's understanding of sensation to create a more pronounced difference between his and Aristotle's positions. Contrary to Maimonides' account, Galen's tripartite scheme does not isolate the three principal organs by denying any exchange between them, for it proposes that the heart participates in sensation through its supply of vital pneuma to the brain – although the brain is the place in which this substance becomes a vehicle of sensation.[95] Maimonides' report of 'Aristotle's' view bears a close resemblance to the explanations of prior Aristotelians such as Avicenna, who accept that the brain has a sensory

[92] According to Maimonides, al-Rāzī's agenda is to point out Galen's logical deficiencies; see Bos (2017), p. 106 l. 9.

[93] See Bos (2007), p. 194 ll. 13–16.

[94] Bos (2007), p. 194 l. 17–p. 196 l. 1.

[95] See pp. 154–5 above.

rather than refrigeratory role, perhaps in the light of Galen's experiments.[96] These interpretations, which acknowledge the brain's involvement in sensation yet preserve the heart's physiological (and psychic) hegemony, enable Maimonides to combat Galen's critique of Aristotelian cardiocentrism on the basis of its ignorance of the brain's function. On the other hand, the strict division of the brain, heart, and liver that Maimonides reads into Galenic encephalocentrism, where 'none of these fundamental organs derive its particular powers from another organ in whatever way', makes this opposing opinion more vulnerable to rebuke for its apparent dismissal of the heart's contribution to sensation.[97]

Aph. 71 and 72 juxtapose extracts from *PHP* (2.4.43–6) and *Loc.Aff.* (5.2) to demonstrate how Galen undercuts himself on the question of the heart's physiological importance.[98] Maimonides misrepresents Galen's investigative goal in *PHP* as the search for the part of the body that is most indispensable to life instead of the corporeal seat of the faculties of sensation, voluntary motion, and rational thought – the defining activities of the hegemonic organ – to create a false tension between the two Galenic texts. The citation of *PHP* furnishes as autoptic evidence against cardiocentrism Galen's observation of animal sacrifices, where the victims, despite having had their hearts removed (without damage to their thoracic cavity), did not perish immediately but ran around until they bled out. Maimonides gives the impression that Galen utilizes this example because it shows the ability of animals to survive without the heart. Galen never makes such a radical claim about the heart's insignificance in *PHP* or elsewhere; in fact, he refers to this phenomenon from animal sacrifices because the animals' flight from the altar proves that the organ is not responsible for voluntary motion.[99] This tendentious reading of *PHP* allows Maimonides to accuse Galen of self-contradiction in *Loc.Aff.*, which states that an extreme temperamental imbalance (dyscrasia) of the heart occasions a swift death.[100] The point of conflict is that the former work depicts the heart as being so inessential that the body can continue to function without it, while the latter alleges that life ceases when the organ is imbalanced, let alone removed.

[96] While Maimonides does not appear to have had direct familiarity with Avicenna's summaries of Aristotelian philosophy (Zonta 2005), he used the *Canon* extensively (Bos 2015: 171n117). Therefore, Maimonides' reading of Aristotle's cardiocentric thesis may be informed by Avicenna's discussion of it in book one of the *Canon*, on which see pp. 148–56 above. Avicenna is not the originator of this interpretation of Aristotelian cardiocentrism, so Maimonides could, of course, be drawing on a much earlier, possibly Greek, source.

[97] Bos (2017), p. 194 l. 14. [98] See Bos (2017), p. 196 ll. 5–18.

[99] See De Lacy (2005), p. 126 ll. 19–25. [100] See 8.303K.

Maimonides deploys a *reductio ad absurdum* argument to rebut Galen's conclusion that his observations of animal sacrifices disprove Aristotle's cardiocentric thesis. He reasons that the heart cannot be a trivial organ as Galen assumes, otherwise these sacrificial animals could be kept alive, if the haemorrhaging was staunched. Aph. 72 brings out this impossibility from Galen's supposed line of thinking at *PHP* 2.4.43–6:

> والقول الآخر وهو أنّ القلب يعصر أو يشق أو يقتلع ويرمى في موضع آخر والحيوان حي يصيح ويجري ويتنفس حتى يقتله كثرة خروج الدم كما ذكر في هذا القول الآخر. ولعل نقول له أيضا إذ وموته إنّما يتبع إجحاف خروج الدم لعلنا لو مسكنا أطراف تلك العروق التي يخرج منها الدم بأيدينا مدة طويلة لدام الحيوان حيا وهو لا قلب له. وهذا عجيب.
>
> The second statement [sc. aphorism] is that the heart can be squeezed, cut open, or removed and thrown into a different place, yet the animal lives, bellows, runs and breathes until it is killed by an excessive loss of blood, as he mentions in this other statement. Perhaps, we could also say to him that, because [the animal's] death only results from the harm caused by the loss of blood, if we were to grasp the edges of the vessels from which the blood is flowing with our hands for a long time, the animal would remain alive even though it has no heart. This is astonishing![101]

Maimonides' selective quotation of *PHP* distorts the role that the heart plays in Galen's physiology. Read in isolation, *PHP* 2.4.43–6 suggests that Galen identifies the heart as a vital organ only because of its vascular connections, which, if severed, cause fatal blood loss. Maimonides fails to mention that immediately following the passage (2.4.49) Galen recognizes that the heart is the source of the movement of the pulse; additionally, the text states elsewhere (for example, at 6.8.76) that the organ helps to keep the body alive through its contribution of not only vital pneuma but also innate heat, which is critical to the processes of generation, digestion, and growth.[102] Therefore, by suppressing this information about the heart's function, Maimonides can propose that Galen's encephalocentric position commits him to the above inference about the survival of the sacrificial animals.

Maimonides appears to accept that his defence of Aristotle requires him not only to expose the error of Galen's logic but also to explain the phenomenon Galen observed in such a way as to protect a cardiocentric physiology. In response, he conjectures that, while the root (*al-aṣl*) of sensation and motion may have been removed from the bodies of the

[101] Bos (2017), p. 198 ll. 3–7 [Arabic], p. 197 [English].

[102] See De Lacy (2005), p. 128 ll. 3–4, p. 424 ll. 3–4. On the importance of innate heat in Galen's physiology, see Durling (1988).

sacrificial animals, these powers remain active for a short time until they fade away.[103] To illustrate his theory, he has recourse to an analogy that compares the hearts of these creatures to an overflowing artesian well (*'ayn*) and the powers to the excess water that flows into irrigation channels until the overspill stops. The agricultural (and thus economic) prosperity of Egypt depended on a system of irrigation canals and reservoirs, which funnelled water from the Nile and oases, so this analogy would have enabled Maimonides' Egyptian readers to visualize in a particularly clear manner the invisible process occurring in the bodies of sacrificial animals.[104] Maimonides finds additional support for his contention that the powers of the heart do not cease along with the heart itself from his experience of dealing with the corpses of recently deceased persons, which sometimes stay warm for around an hour. In these cases, the innate heat that emanated from the heart before it stopped eventually dissipates because it can no longer be replenished.[105]

Maimonides' explanation does not demolish encephalocentrism, but rather shows that Galen's 'demonstration' of this theory from the *Timaeus* in *PHP* is not conclusive. Targeting this stance more directly, he responds with his own observation of instances where decapitated animals were still able to move parts of their bodies.[106] The continued activity of these animals should preclude the brain from being the hegemonic organ according to Galen's logic (or rather, Maimonides' understanding of it). This example may also serve an additional argumentative purpose. Just after the passage of *PHP* (2.4.43–6) quoted at aph. 25.71, Galen refers to the sudden loss of sensation, motion, and breath in sacrificial cattle whose spinal cords have been cut at the first vertebra in support of the brain's primary role.[107] Maimonides does not address this evidence in his own text, but he expects that some of the readers of the *Medical Aphorisms* will consult the original Galenic sources.[108] His own experience of seeing movement in decapitated animals troubles the causal connection that Galen draws between brain injuries and the complete disruption of sensory and motor functions

[103] See Bos (2017), p. 198 ll. 8–11.

[104] On the management of Nile water for irrigation in the Fayyūm (Middle Egypt) about a half century after Maimonides' death, see Rapoport and Shahar (2012). I wish to thank my colleague Brendan Haug for his helpful discussion of this analogy with me.

[105] See Bos (2017), p. 198 ll. 12–14. [106] Bos (2017), p. 198 ll. 14–15.

[107] See *PHP* 2.4.47: De Lacy (2005), p. 126 ll. 28–31.

[108] In the preface to the *Medical Aphorisms*, Maimonides explains that he added references at the end of each aphorism so readers can check the original source texts, if they have questions about his interpretations of them (see Bos 2004: p. 3 ll. 4–7).

based on the above phenomenon. Maimonides' example makes Galen's seem less decisive.

Maimonides is aware that Galen's epistemic authority comes from his expertise in anatomy, encompassing not only knowledge of the parts of the body but also the skill to bring these structures to view.[109] His polemic against the Platonic physiology of *PHP* largely focuses on its logical deficiencies, but he concludes by going for this linchpin of Galen's credibility. Book twenty-five of the *Medical Aphorisms* closes with the charge that Galen lied about seeing the hearts of the sacrificial animals being removed without damage occurring to the thoracic cavity. Because Galen asserts at *PHP* 2.4.43–6 that he himself has performed this type of vivisection, Maimonides appears to criticize his predecessor for exaggerating his technical proficiency as well.[110] He asks:

> وأما كيف يخرج القلب ولا ينثقب أحد تجويفي الصدر فهو أن يشق من المنحر في آخر العنق ويتلطف من هناك في إخراج القلب من غلافه ويترك غلاف القلب كما هو متصل بالظهر والصدر. وهذا في غاية العسر إذا فعلته بعد موت الحيوان وأما في حال حياته كما ذكر فهو أمر في غاية البعد. وإنّما هذا فرض فرض لنصر الرأي لاغير. ولله أعلم.

> But how can one take out the heart without puncturing one of the two cavities of the chest? This can only be done by splitting the site of the throat at the back of the neck and by gently extracting the heart from its membrane. The membrane of the heart is left as it is, connected to the back and the chest. [Such an operation] is very difficult if one attempts to do it after the death of the animal. However, when the animal is alive as [Galen] mentions, it is something that is most improbable. He only made this assumption to support his opinion, nothing else. God is all-knowing![111]

The level of detail in the instructions in this passage indicates that Maimonides may have personally performed this operation on a dead animal.[112] He seems to extrapolate from his own difficulty in pulling out the heart from the carcass that both the priests conducting the sacrifice and

[109] At aph. 25.59 (Bos 2017: p. 170 ll. 13–15), Maimonides admits that Galen had a clearer understanding of human anatomy than Aristotle.

[110] See *PHP* 2.4.43–4: De Lacy (2005), p. 126 ll. 18–22.

[111] Bos (2017), p. 198 l. 18–p. 200 l. 3 [Arabic], p. 199 [English, slightly modified].

[112] While there were no prohibitions against the dissection of either human or animal bodies in the medieval Islamicate world, the evidence for them actually being performed is scant and often dubious (see Savage-Smith 1995). Ebrahimnejad (2008) speculates that Islamicate anatomists did not widely practise animal dissections for an epistemological reason: they believed that the bodies of these creatures were fundamentally different from those of humans, and so could reveal little about the inner workings of the latter. However, cf. Ibn Ṭufayl's (d. 581/1185–6) philosophical novella *Ḥayy ibn Yaqẓān* (Goodman 1972: 112–15), where the titular character dissects various animals in his endeavour to understand the world around him, including himself.

Galen himself could not have done this manoeuvre on a living creature. The text leaves the reader, then, with the thought that Galen fabricated evidence to make his logically weak defence of Plato's encephalocentric thesis from the *Timaeus* appear stronger.

Throughout *PHP* (and other writings) Galen invokes his 'hands-on' anatomical demonstrations to compel opponents, both living and long dead, to assent to the truth of the theories from Plato's *Timaeus*, including encephalocentrism, that form the roots of his system.[113] In disputing the veracity of a number of Galen's anatomical observations and demonstrations, Maimonides casts doubt onto the trustworthiness of the rest of them. He undermines a key element of Galen's argumentative approach in *PHP* and therefore reduces the formidable challenge that it presents to followers of Aristotle. Maimonides' identification of Galen's anatomical 'lie' works also to establish his medical prowess over Galen. Unlike previous critics with Aristotelian allegiances such as Avicenna, Maimonides puts on display his ability not only to out-philosophize Galen but also to outdo him on his own turf, the body. Considering the near-universal acclaim that Galen received in the Islamicate world for his knowledge of medicine (as opposed to philosophy), this medical one-upmanship provides the most cogent justification for Maimonides' revision of Galenism, the culmination of which was the toppling of the Timaean physiology of the soul.

From Hippocrates to Moses

Soon after Maimonides' death, there circulated a Hebrew saying comparing him to the biblical Moses, 'From Moses to Moses, there arose none like unto Moses' (*mi-Moshe le-Moshe lo qam ke-Moshe*).[114] The phrase reveals Maimonides' success in shaping subsequent perceptions of his authorial persona, for it identifies him with his own paradigm of intellectual perfection: Moses, the philosopher-prophet-king.[115] In works such as the *Guide for the Perplexed*, Maimonides cultivates this connection to the distant Jewish past through his 'revivalist' project, which presents itself as recovering the lost philosophy endemic to Judaism. Incorporating Aristotelian doctrine, the philosophical–religious system that Maimonides builds in his corpus remakes, rather than recuperates, Jewish belief so that it dovetails with his own philosophical leanings. Even in this act of revision,

113 On Galen's anatomical demonstrations as acts of coercion, see Gleason (2009), 94 and *passim*.

114 In what follows, I draw on Stroumsa (2009), 185–7.

115 Stroumsa (2009: 186) traces Maimonides' model of intellectual perfection to al-Fārābī's philosopher-king-*imām*.

Maimonides implies his own affinity with Moses in casting himself as a giver of *uṣūl*, meaning roots, laws, or fundaments of belief.

Not everyone, Maimonides declares, has the disposition required for philosophy – unlike medicine.[116] In the light of this assessment, the irritation that Maimonides gives vent to in his letter to Joseph b. Judah (discussed at the start of this chapter) regarding his medical commitments has been read as an expression of his intellectual elitism: as a discipline of the few, philosophy provides the arena in which he can prove the distinctiveness of his expertise.[117] Be that as it may, I have proposed that Maimonides' subordination of medicine to philosophy – as seen, for example, in his devaluing of his own medical activities – is polemically charged. By minimizing the prestige as well as the scope of medicine, Maimonides aims to curtail the influence of Galen, whose defence of Plato's *Timaeus* posed a powerful challenge to the credibility of the Aristotelian and Jewish roots of his system. While Galen turned to the *Timaeus* to justify his philosophical interests, Maimonides' polemic relies on identifying him exclusively as a medical authority. As I explained, Maimonides implies in the *Medical Aphorisms* that Galen's insufficient comprehension of philosophy led him to adopt the dialogue's cosmogony, which he finds heretical, and encephalocentric stance, which contravenes Aristotle's cardiocentrism. With his superior grasp of philosophy and own medical experience, Maimonides positions himself as the candidate to reform the theologically and philosophically flawed system of Galenism by re-medicalizing it.

This reformist project parallels his 'revival' of Judaism in that it endeavours to reinstate the supposed *uṣūl* of medicine that Galen subverted. Maimonides' boundary work in texts such as *On Asthma*, *Regimen of Health*, and the *Commentary on Hippocrates' Aphorisms* imposes a set of norms for medical enquiry that steer doctors away from the corporeally indeterminate – for instance, the soul and emotions – and therefore throws into relief Galen's disciplinary deviancy. These treatises also deprive medicine of epistemological certainty, perhaps as a way of denying that Galen 'demonstrated' Plato's tripartite psychology from the *Timaeus* and *Republic*. Through a process of suppressing, redefining, and assailing the Timaean roots of Galen's thought, the *Medical Aphorisms* – one of the last, if not the last, of Maimonides' compositions to be published – seems to realize the improved Galenism that he seeks to formulate throughout his medical writings.

[116] See Stern (2013), 126. [117] See Lieber (1979), 285.

Maimonides' decision to call his medical *magnum opus* after the Hippocratic *Aphorisms* signals a desire to link himself to 'the greatest of the excellent doctors' (*aʿẓam fuḍalāʾ al-aṭibbāʾ*).[118] While Hippocrates is not faultless in Maimonides' eyes, his error was neither of the kind nor of the magnitude of Galen's.[119] I noted that Maimonides read his Hippocrates through a Galenic filter, so his separation of philosophy from Galenism may be an attempt to make medicine more Hippocratic. Thus, Maimonides' medical and philosophical–religious projects both invoke the past to authorize their re-creation of their respective epistemic realms. Fashioning himself as the true successor of Hippocrates, Maimonides overshadows Galen's intellectual achievements as well as those of his Islamicate predecessors by laying claim to the title of not just doctor-philosopher but doctor-philosopher-prophet-king.

[118] See Schliwski (2004), p. 5 § 8.

[119] In his *Commentary on Hippocrates' Aphorisms*, Maimonides, as Kottek (2009: 9) observes, criticizes Hippocrates for not contextualizing his statements and for the weakness of his logical reasoning. Given Maimonides' opinion that doctors should receive only a limited training in logic (see aph. 25.59: Bos 2017: p. 172 l. 16–p. 174 l. 5), the latter criticism is perhaps meant to highlight the epistemological deficiencies of medicine as a whole rather than merely Hippocrates'.

Conclusion: Medicine Disciplined

This book began with two texts, *Plat.Tim.* and *Com.Tim.*, that reveal Galen's efforts to discipline the *Timaeus* – that is, to divide its account of natural reality (*physiologia*) into bounded domains of knowledge – as part of his larger project to redefine and invest medicine with epistemic authority. As I have argued, Galen found in the dialogue a powerful instrument for establishing a new epistemic order, which denies medicine's inferiority to philosophy (contrary to prior hierarchical schemes), because the relations that entangle Plato's textual cosmos can be variously emphasized or cut to produce different topographies of knowledge. Galen's interpretation, moreover, had a deep and enduring impact through its reception in the medieval Islamicate world, which put Galen's innovations to even more innovative uses. As an example, Ḥunayn's use of the dialogue's analogy between the eye and macrocosm to legitimize his more expansive refiguring of ophthalmology has illustrated that the diverse spatial, causal, and comparative entanglements in the *Timaeus* accommodated even disciplinary constructions running counter to Galen's own vision of medicine. It has also emerged from the preceding chapters that, of the relations in the Timaean cosmos, Galen and his Islamicate readers viewed those interfaces between the body and the soul as being most fraught with potential. The issues from the *Timaeus* that Galen cited to contest philosophy's monopolistic claim to epistemic authority – provoking different responses in turn from Ḥunayn, al-Rāzī, Avicenna, and Maimonides – were mostly mind–body problems, where what is in question is the extent to which the soul and so-called mental processes (for example, rational thought and sensation) are separable from the corporeal realm.

The first chapter established that Galen saw the *Timaeus*' location of the soul's three parts in the brain, heart, and lower abdomen (or liver, according to him), as well as its linking of psychic and bodily disease, as being suggestive of a strong connection between the body and soul. Medieval Islamicate interpreters of Galen accused him of exploiting this connection to reduce the soul to a material entity in order to give medicine a role in psychological controversies and psychic well-being. These hermeneutically capacious passages of the *Timaeus*, which for Neoplatonic-inspired readers such as al-Rāzī seemed equally to support their dualistic psychologies, offered Galen a way to trouble the distribution of value based on the corporeal–incorporeal dichotomy, which privileged philosophers as the exclusive experts of the 'worthier' element of animate life, the soul. My analyses of Avicenna and Maimonides uncovered that Galen's most compelling case for granting medicine a share in psychological knowledge was his anatomical defence, built on theoretical study, experimentation, and contact with patients, of Plato's identification of the brain as the place of origin of sensation and other activities of the rational soul. Overwhelmingly concerned with dictating what doctors can and cannot investigate – in other words, with dictating doctors' proper epistemic behaviour – the two men's boundary policies, I asserted, worked to protect the credibility of their cardiocentric psycho-physiologies, and therefore their socio-cultural prestige as philosophers, from the threat posed by Galen. Ḥunayn and al-Rāzī, who were sympathetic to Galen's expansionist ambitions for medicine, also took a polemical approach to his interpretation of the *Timaeus*' tripartition of the soul, although the basis of their opposition differed from that of Avicenna and Maimonides. Both may have accepted that the brain governs the functions of the rational soul, but Ḥunayn then mobilized this information to undermine Galen's restrictive notion of ophthalmology, and al-Rāzī disputed whether it necessitates what he saw as a strong materialist hypothesis in *QAM*.

The Islamicate chapters appear to mark a philosophical divide that determined their actors' openness to or rejection of Galen's disciplinary project: Ḥunayn and al-Rāzī affiliated themselves with Plato (or, in the former's case, with definitive Platonic positions such as encephalocentrism) and pushed Galen's expansion of medicine further; whereas Avicenna and Maimonides expressed commitment to Aristotle and endeavoured to narrow down the field. The shift documented in the four chapters seems to give credence to what has been called the 'Aristotelian turn' that philosophy took in the fourth/tenth century.[1] Analysis of Avicenna's various formulations of his doctrine of pleasure, which have in common a Platonic emphasis on the involvement of perception in the experience,

1. See Rashed (2015), vi–vii, who argues that the increasing prominence of Aristotle in *kalām* (Islamic speculative theology) precipitated this Aristotelian turn in philosophy, and Das and Koetschet (2019), 384.

has shown, however, that this turn was by no means absolute. Further to this point, Maimonides' admission in the *Guide* that his cosmogony could be misinterpreted as Platonic signals an unease about his own doctrinal resemblance to the rival philosophical camp. The binary of support/opposition, which is often used to frame medieval attitudes towards past authorities, does not adequately capture how the four writers positioned themselves in relation to Galen as well as to both Plato and Aristotle. As noted, they are all adversarial in their attempts to promote their own disciplinary visions over Galen's but at the same time follow his discursive tactics in articulating those visions. The reception history in this book has offered a different approach to describing such dialogues between the classical and medieval worlds by regarding authorities such as Galen as setting patterns of knowledge that their successors need to negotiate.

In heading each chapter with autobiographical and biographical passages that evince their subjects' concern with their own disciplinary identities, I have tried to show that Galen, Ḥunayn, al-Rāzī, Avicenna, and Maimonides' pursuit of epistemic authority was bound up with their desire to institutionalize their personal expertise – that is, to inscribe it permanently into their epistemic landscapes.[2] These five figures' drawing and redrawing of the boundaries of medicine – and therefore of philosophy as well – to exclude or include certain subjects corresponds to what each knew and who they considered worthy of receiving that knowledge. Nowhere was this identification of the personal with the disciplinary more evident than in *Prop.Plac.*, where the *Timaeus* served as a point of reference for Galen to define the limits of his own knowledge and thus also define the topics 'necessary for' or 'useful to' medicine. Notwithstanding the reticence of Ḥunayn, al-Rāzī, Avicenna, and Maimonides about their own epistemic limitations, my examinations of the structural and critical elements of their compositions have revealed how they, like Galen, shaped the medical discipline to conform to their knowledge claims.

Of the four Islamicate actors in this book, Ḥunayn's authorial ego is the least conspicuous; nonetheless, my biographically inflected reading of *Ten Treatises on the Eye* has suggested that its constituent treatises produce an ophthalmology reflective of the knowledge frame of a translator of both medical and philosophical texts. *Ten Treatises on the Eye* has a counterpart in Maimonides' *Medical Aphorisms* in the sense

2. Cf. Shapin (1992), 355, who maintains, with regard to early modern and modern science, that actors' categories should be viewed as institutions.

that its compilatory work – selecting quotations from Galen and later doctors – also seeks to reassemble its field of knowledge, but in so doing it is much more explicit about the personal imprints that it receives from its author. In addition to stating at the start of the book that he has included what interests or would benefit him, Maimonides inserts his own Jewish and Aristotelian beliefs into the text, and therefore reframes the medicine that it purports to represent, by attacking Galen's Timaean positions on creation and the physiology of the soul. I mentioned in my chapters on Maimonides and Avicenna that the failure of the two to adhere to their own disciplinary prescriptions speaks to the authoritative status of Galen's pattern of medical knowledge: they were compelled to engage with him on 'philosophical' topics in 'medical' contexts because he had demonstrated persuasively that doctors could be credible contributors to these issues. I can now expand on this conclusion and propose that Maimonides and Avicenna's boundary work, or rules, aimed not to delineate a new medicine, which complies with the dominant hierarchical epistemologies, but to shut out Galen from the very disciplinary space that he himself created so they could overwrite it with their own expertise. With its progressive idea of knowledge, al-Rāzī's *Doubts about Galen* is more forward about its goal to supersede Galen. The theological concerns about Galen's thought with which al-Rāzī confronts his reader forces them to recognize the need for a medical expert who has the metaphysical grounding to offer an acceptable, less doubtable system of medicine.

Informed by philosophical and religious ideologies as well as the personal ambitions underlying them, the multiple iterations of medicine made visible in this book betray the individualistic nature of medicine, and science by extension, that its positivistic rhetoric – its assertions that it is founded on axiomatic and observable truths – cloaks. This conclusion about science's contingency is, as I pointed out in the Introduction, hardly novel in STS scholarship, but, on account of the field's modernist slant, pre-modern science tends to be left out of its histories of the constructedness of science. Besides redressing this scholarly lacuna in STS, I hope to have demonstrated the promise that a sensitivity to boundary work holds for the study of ancient and medieval medicine. This is especially true because a traditional focus of such study has been on the meaning of the epistemic labels (for example, *technē*, *epistēmē*, *ṣināʿa*, and *ʿilm*) that are applied to medicine rather than on the ever-shifting topography of the discipline. Even this established area of interest can acquire fresh significance if we approach the labels themselves as a performance of what Shapin calls 'boundary-speech', vocabularies that are developed to separate and privilege certain groups of knowers over others.[3] A history of pre-modern medicine that looks at the discursive uses to which knowledge categories are put would give a *longue durée* perspective on remappings of the field ongoing today.

For instance, the institutionalization of medical humanities programmes at the university level – and, more specifically, in medical schools – over the past twenty years or so has prompted calls for a reconceptualization of the field of medicine.[4] Meta-disciplinary reflections on the medical humanities seem to disagree about whether it is an autonomous unit of knowledge or something integral to medicine.[5] The consensus is, however, that the medical humanities are constitutive of the discipline of medicine because the training in history, creative writing, and the visual arts (among other subjects) serves the end of producing better doctors.[6] The medical humanities also do for medicine the intellectual work of theorizing, and thus reimagining, medicine's practices, spaces, participants, and objects (for example, the human body).[7] Moreover, the medical humanities seem to do the rhetorical work of safeguarding the epistemic authority of medicine by addressing the public's dissatisfaction with the 'dehumanization', or excessive biologism, of the discipline.[8]

Confronted with accusations from disciplinary insiders that the medical humanities are a pointless public-relations exercise that is 'parasitic' on their time, its defenders, such as Kirklin and Richardson, refer to medicine's status as an 'art' to legitimize this broadened map of medical knowledge: 'There is, of course, nothing new about the idea that the arts can play a valuable role in the education of health care professionals. The ancients conceived medicine as a fundamental branch of philosophy. To Hippocrates, medicine is an art.'[9] Leaving aside its generalizations, this narrative exploits medicine's ancient classification as a *technē* ('art'), which Kirklin and Richardson appear to understand in the modern sense of 'fine arts' (and perhaps as a synecdoche for the

3. Shapin (1992), 335.
4. Chiapperino and Boniolo (2014: 378) place the origin of the medical humanities in the 1960s but state that its initiatives have only recently gained momentum in universities and clinical research spaces.
5. On these conflicts about the disciplinary nature of the medical humanities, see Greco (2013).
6. See Gordon (2005); Evans and Macnaughton (2004); Shapiro et al. (2009); Chiapperino and Boniolo (2014). Cf. Rose (2014); Fitzgerald and Callard (2016).
7. See, e.g., Chiapperino and Boniolo (2014), 382.
8. Gordon (2005).
9. Kirklin and Richardson (2001), 1. Cf. Greco (2013), 229.

humanities), to historicize the medical humanities and, through this invocation of the distant past, justify their inclusion of a humanistic education in medicine.[10] From the appeal to classical authority, to the aim to 'charg[e] medicine with the power to (re)integrate the body, mind, and spirit', with the medical humanities, old lines are being drawn anew.[11]

10. Celsus is one ancient authority that does give medicine a philosophical origin. See p. 9n36 above.
11. Bolton (2008), 146.

References

Primary Sources

ʿAbd al-Ġanī, M. L. (ed.) 2005. *Kitāb al-Šukūk li-l-Rāzī ʿalā kalām fāḍil al-aṭibbāʾ Ǧālīnūs fī al-kutub allatī nusibat ilayh*. Cairo: Dār al-Kutub wal-Waṯāʾiq al-Qawmīya.

Abū Rayyān, M., ʿArab, M. M., and Mūsā, J. M. (eds.) 1978. *Masāʾil fī al-ṭibb li-l mutaʿallimīn*. Cairo: Dār al-Ǧāmiʿāt al-Miṣriyya.

Adamson, P. and Pormann, P. E. (trans.) 2012. *The philosophical works of al-Kindī*. Karachi: Oxford University Press.

ʿAlwān, H. B. (ed.) 1985. *Ṭabaqāt al-umam*. Beirut: Dār al-Ṭalīʿa.

Anawātī, G. and Zāyed, S. (eds.) 1960. *al-Šifāʾ al-Ilāhiyyāt 1*. Cairo: Organisation Général des Imprimeries Gouvernementales.

Avicenna 1877 (ed. anon.). *al-Qānūn fī l-ṭibb*. Cairo: Maṭbaʿat Būlāq.

1908 (ed. anon.). 'Fī Aqsām al-ʿulūm al-ʿaqliyya', in *Tisʿ rasāʾil fī l-ḥikma wa l-ṭabīʿiyyāt*. Cairo: Maṭbaʿa Hindiyya, 104–19.

al-Bābā, M. Z. (ed.) 1984. *Min muʾallafāt Ibn Sīnā al-ṭibbiyya: Kitāb Dafʿ al-maḍār al-kulliyya ʿan al-abdān al-insāniyya, al-Urǧūza fī l-ṭibb, Kitāb al-Adwiya al-qalbiyya*. Aleppo: Ǧāmiʿat Ḥalab, Maʿhad al-Turāṯ al-ʿIlmī al-ʿArabī.

Badawī, A. R. (ed.) 1955. *al-Aflāṭūniyya al-muḥdaṯa ʿinda l-ʿArab*. Cairo: Maktabat al-Nahḍa al-Miṣriyya.

(ed.) 1966. *Plotinus apud arabes: Theologia Aristotelis et fragmenta quae supersunt*. 2nd edn. Islamica 20. Cairo: Maktabat al-Nahḍa al-Miṣriyya.

(ed.) 1973. *al-Taʿlīqāt*. Cairo: al-Hayʾa al-Miṣriyya al-ʿĀmma li-l-Kitāb.

Bailey, C. (ed.) 1922. *Lucreti de rerum natura, libri sex*. 2nd edn. Oxford: Oxford University Press.

Baneth, D. H. (ed.) 1946. *Igrot ha-Rambam*. Jerusalem: Meḳitse Nirdamim.

Bar-Sela, A., Hoff, H. E., and Faris, E. (trans.) 1964. 'Two treatises on the regimen of health: "Fī Tadbīr al-ṣiḥḥah" and "Maqālah fī bayān baʿḍ al-aʿrāḍ wa-al-jawāb ʿanhā"', *Transactions of the American Philosophical Society* 54: 3–50.

Bergsträsser, G. (ed.) 1925. 'Ḥunain ibn Isḥāq über die syrischen und arabischen Galen-Übersetzungen', *Abhandlungen für die Kunde des Morgenlandes* 17: 1–53.

(ed.) 1932. 'Neue Materialien zu Ḥunain Ibn Isḥāq's Galen-Bibliographie', *Abhandlungen für die Kunde des Morgenlandes* 19: 1–108.

Bos, G. (ed. and trans.) 2002. *Maqālah fī al-rabw*. Graeco-Arabic Sciences and Philosophy Series. Provo: Brigham Young University Press.

(ed. and trans.) 2004. *Maimonides, Medical aphorisms: Treatises 1–5*. Provo: Brigham Young University Press.

(ed. and trans.) 2007. *Maimonides, Medical aphorisms: Treatises 6–9*. Provo: Brigham Young University Press.

(ed. and trans.) 2015. *Maimonides, Medical aphorisms: Treatises 16–21*. Provo: Brigham Young University Press.

(ed. and trans.) 2017. *Maimonides, Medical aphorisms: Treatises 22–25*. Provo: Brigham Young University Press.

Boudon-Millot, V. (ed. and trans.) 2002a. *Galien: Exhortation à l'étude de la médecine, Art médical*. Paris: Les Belles Lettres.

(ed. and trans.) 2007. *Galien: Introduction générale, Sur l'ordre de ses propres livres, Sur ses propres livres, Que l'excellent médecin est aussi philosophie*. Paris: Les Belles Lettres.

Boudon-Millot, V. and Pietrobelli, A. (ed. and trans.) 2005. 'Galien ressuscité: Édition *princeps* du texte grec du *De propriis placitis*', *Revue des études grecques* 118: 168–213.

Brock, A. J. (ed. and trans.) 1916. *Galen: On the natural faculties*. Cambridge, MA: Harvard University Press.

Bruns, I. (ed.) 1887. *De anima liber cum mantissa*. Berlin: Reimer.

Bryson, J. S. (ed.) 2001. 'The Kitāb al-Ḥāwī of Rāzī (ca. 900 AD), book one of the Ḥāwī on brain, nerve, and mental disorders: Studies in the transmission of medical texts from Greek into Arabic into Latin'. Ph.D. thesis. Yale University.

Burnet, J. (ed.) 1900. *Platonis opera*, vol. I: *Euthyphro, Apology, Crito, Phaedo, Cratylus, Theaetetus, Sophist, and Statesman*. Oxford: Clarendon Press.

(ed.) 1901. *Platonis opera*, vol. II: *Parmenides, Philebus, Symposium, Phaedrus, Alcibiades I, Alcibiades II, Hipparchus, and Amatores*. Oxford: Clarendon Press.

(ed.) 1902. *Platonis opera*, vol. IV: *Clitopho, Republic, Timaeus, and Critias*. Oxford: Clarendon Press.

(ed.) 1903. *Platonis opera*, vol. III: *Theages, Charmides, Laches, Lysis, Euthydemus, Protagoras, Gorgias, Meno, Hippias Maior, Hippias Minor, Io, and Menexenus*. Oxford: Clarendon Press.

(ed.) 1907. *Platonis opera*, vol. V: *Minos, Leges, Epinomis, Epistulae, Definitiones*. Oxford: Clarendon Press.

Busse, A. (ed.) 1900. *Eliae in Porphyrii isagogen et Aristotelis categorias commentaria*. Commentaria in Aristotelem Graeca 18.1. Berlin: Reimer.

(ed.) 1902. *Olympiodori prolegomena et in categorias commentarium*. Commentaria in Aristotelem Graeca 12.1. Berlin: Reimer.

(ed.) 1904. *Davidis prolegomena et In Porphyrii Isagogen commentarium*. Commentaria in Aristotelem Graeca 18.2. Berlin: Reimer.

Channing, J. (ed. and trans.) 1766. *Rhazes de variolis et morbillis, arabice et latine; cum aliis nonnullis eiusdem argumenti*. London: Guilielmus Bowyer.

Cheikho, L. (ed.) 1899. 'Fī l-ḍaw' wa ḥaqīqatihi', *al-Mashriq* 2: 1105–13.

(ed.) 1911. 'Risāla fī l-farq bayna l-rūḥ wal-nafs', *al-Mashriq* 14: 94–109.

Clarke, E., Dillon, J., and Hershbell, J. P. (trans.) 2003. *Iamblichus: De mysteriis.* Atlanta: Society of Biblical Literature.

Colson, F. H. and Whitaker, G. H. (ed. and trans.) 1939. *Philo*, vol. IV: *On the confusion of tongues. On the migration of Abraham. Who is the heir of divine things? On mating with the preliminary studies.* Cambridge, MA: Harvard University Press.

Cooperson, M. (trans.) 2001. 'The Autobiography of Ḥunayn ibn Isḥāq (809–73 or 877)', in K. E. Brustad (ed.), *Interpreting the self: Autobiography in the Arabic literary tradition.* Berkeley: University of California Press, 107–18.

Cornford, F. M. (trans.) 1937. *Plato's cosmology: The Timaeus of Plato.* London: Kegan Paul.

Craik, E. (ed. and trans.) 2006. *Two Hippocratic treatises: 'On sight' and 'On anatomy'.* Studies in Ancient Medicine 33. Leiden: Brill.

Davies, D. (trans.) 2013. 'Character traits', in Singer (ed.), *Galen: Psychological writings*, 135–201.

de Boer, W. (ed.) 1937. *Galeni De propriorum animi cuiuslibet affectuum dignotione et curatione; De animi cuiuslibet peccatorum dignotione et curatione; De atra bile.* Leipzig: Teubner.

de Goeje, M. J. (ed.) 1965. *Kitāb al-Tanbīh wa l-išrāf.* Beirut: Maktabat Ḫayyāṭ.

De Lacy, P. (ed. and trans.) 1996. *Galeni De elementis ex Hippocratis sententia.* Berlin: Akademie-Verlag.

(ed. and trans.) 2005. *Galeni De placitis Hippocratis et Platonis.* Berlin: Akademie-Verlag.

Dillon, J. (trans.) 1993. *Alcinous: The handbook of Platonism.* Oxford: Clarendon Press.

Dodds, E. R. (ed.) 1963. *Proclus: The elements of theology.* 2nd edn. Oxford: Clarendon Press.

Drossaart Lulofs, H. J. and Poortman, E. L. J. (ed. and trans.) 1989. *Nicolaus Damascenus. De plantis: Five translations.* Amsterdam: North Holland.

Dunlop, D. M., Akasoy, A., and Fidora, A. (trans.) 2005. *The Arabic version of the Nichomachean ethics.* Leiden: Brill.

Fakhry, M. (ed.) 1985. *Kitāb al-Naǧāt.* Beirut: Dār al-Afāq al-Ǧadīda.

Flügel, G. (ed.) 1871. *Kitāb al-Fihrist.* 2 vols. Leipzig: F. C. W. Vogel.

Forget, J. (ed.) 1892. *Ibn Sīnā: Le livre des théorèmes et des avertissements.* Leiden: Brill.

Fowler, R. C. (trans.) 2016. 'Albinus: Introduction to the book of Plato', in R. C. Fowler (ed.), *Imperial Plato: Albinus, Maximus, Apuleius.* Las Vegas: Parmenides Publishing, 33–58.

Furley, D. J. and Wilkie, J. S. (trans.) 1984. *Galen: On respiration and the arteries.* Princeton: Princeton University Press.

Gabrieli, F. (ed. and trans.) 1952. *Compendium legum Platonis.* Plato Arabus 3. London: Warburg Institute.

Garofalo, I. (ed.) 2000. *Galenus: Anatomicarum administrationum libri qui supersunt novem: earundem interpretatio arabica Hunaino Isaaci filio ascripta; libros V–IX continens.* Naples: Istituto universitario orientale.

Gärtner, F. (ed. and trans.) 2015. *Galeni De locis affectis I–II*. Berlin: De Gruyter.

Gill, C. (trans.) 2013. *Marcus Aurelius: Meditations, Book 1–6*. Oxford: Clarendon Press.

Gohlman, W. E. (ed. and trans.) 1974. *The life of Ibn Sina*. Studies in Islamic Philosophy and Science. Albany: SUNY Press.

Goichon, A. M. (trans.) 1951. *Livre des directives et remarques*. Paris: J. Vrin.

Goodman, L. E. (trans.) 1972. *Ibn Tufayl's Hayy ibn Yaqzān: A philosophical tale*. Library of Classical Arabic Literature 1. New York: Twayne Publishers.

Gummere, R. M. (ed. and trans.) 1925. *Seneca: Epistles*, vol. III: *Epistles 93–124*. Cambridge, MA: Harvard University Press.

Hameed, H. A. (ed.) 1982. *al-Qānūn fī l-ṭibb*. Vol. I. New Delhi: Jamia Hamdard.

(trans.) 1983. *Avicenna's tract on cardiac drugs and essays on Arab cardiotherapy*. Karachi: Hamdard Foundation Press.

Hankinson, R. J. (ed. and trans.) 1998a. *Galen on antecedent causes*. Cambridge Classical Texts and Commentaries 35. Cambridge: Cambridge University Press.

Helmreich, G. (ed.) 1907. *Galen De usu partium libri xvii*, vol. I: *Libros 1–8 continens*. Leipzig: Teubner.

(ed.) 1909. *Galen De usu partium libri xvii*, vol. II: *Libros 9–17 continens*. Leipzig: Teubner.

Henry, P. and Schwyzer, H. R. (eds.) 1951–73. *Plotini opera*. 3 vols. Leiden: Brill.

Hyamson, M. (ed. and trans.) 1962. *Mishneh Torah: The book of knowledge*. Jerusalem: Boys Town.

Iskandar, A. Z. (ed.) 1961. *Rhazes' k. al-murshid aw al-fuṣūl (The Guide or Aphorisms), with texts selected from his medical writings*. Mağallat Maʿhad al-Maḫṭūṭāt al-ʿArabiyya. Cairo: Dhulqi.

(ed. and trans.) 1988. *Galeni De optimo medico cognoscendo libelli versio Arabica*. Berlin: Akademie-Verlag.

Johnston, I. (trans.) 2006. *Galen: On diseases and symptoms*. Cambridge: Cambridge University Press.

Kendall, B. and Thomson, R. W. (ed. and trans.) 1983. *David the invincible philosopher: Definitions and divisions of philosophy*. University of Pennsylvania Armenian Texts and Studies 5. Chico: Scholars Press.

Koch, K. (ed.) 1923. *Galeni De sanitate tuenda*. Leipzig: Teubner.

Koetschet, P. (ed. and trans.) 2019. *Abū Bakr al-Rāzī, 'Doutes sur Galien'*. Scientia Graeco-Arabica 25. Berlin: De Gruyter.

Kraus, P. (ed.) 1936a. 'Raziana II', *Orientalia* 5: 35–56.

(ed.) 1936b. *Risāla li-l-Bīrūnī fī fihrist kutub Muḥammad b. Zakariyyāʾ al-Rāzī*. Paris: Imprimerie orientaliste.

(ed.) 1937. 'Kitāb al-aḫlāq li-Ğālīnūs', *Bulletin of the Faculty of Arts, Egyptian University* 5: 1–51.

(ed.) 1939. *Abi-Bakr Mohammadi Filii Zachariae Raghensis (Razis) Opera Philosophica Fragmentaque quae supersunt*. Cairo: University Fuʾād.

Kraus, P. and Walzer, R. (ed. and trans.) 1951. *Plato Arabus I: Galeni compendium Timaei Platonis*. London: Warburg Institute.

Kroner, H. (ed. and trans.) 1923. 'Fī tadbīr aṣ-ṣiḥḥat, Gesundheitsanleitung des Maimonides für den Sultan al-Malik al-Afḍal: Zum ersten Male im Urtexte herausgegeben, ins deutsche übertragen und kritisch erläutert' (part 1), *Janus* 27: 101–16, 285–300.

(ed. and trans.) 1924. 'Fī tadbīr aṣ-ṣiḥḥat, Gesundheitsanleitung des Maimonides für den Sultan al-Malik al-Afḍal: Zum ersten Male im Urtexte herausgegeben, ins deutsche übertragen und kritisch erläutert' (part 2), *Janus* 28: 61–74, 143–52, 199–217, 408–19, 455–72.

Kuhne Brabant, R. (ed. and trans.) 1982. 'El "Sirr sinaʿat al-tibb" de Abu Bakr Muhammad B. Zakariyaaʾ al-Razi', *al-Qanṭara: Revista de estudios árabes* 3.1–2: 347–414.

Lamb, W. R. M. (ed. and trans.) 1924. *Plato*, vol. II: *Laches, Protagoras, Meno, Euthydemus*. New York: Putnam.

Lami, A. and Garofalo, I. (ed. and trans.) 2012. *L'anima e il dolore: De indolentia-De propriis placitis. Testo greco a fronte*. Milan: Biblioteca universale Rizzoli.

Lamoreaux, J. C. (ed. and trans.) 2016. *Ḥunayn ibn Isḥāq on his Galen translations: A parallel English–Arabic text*. Provo: Brigham Young University Press.

Larrain, C. J. (ed.) 1991. 'Ein unbekanntes Exzerpt aus Galens Timaioskommentar', *ZPE* 85: 9–30.

(ed. and trans.) 1992. *Galens Kommentar zu Platons Timaios*. Stuttgart: Teubner.

Lightfoot, J. L. (ed. and trans.) 1999. *Parthenius of Nicaea: The poetical fragments and the Erotika pathemata*. Oxford: Oxford University Press.

Lippert. J. (ed.) 1903. *Tāʾrīḫ al-Ḥukamāʾ*. Leipzig: Dieterich.

Long, A. A. and Sedley, D. N. (ed. and trans.) 1987. *The Hellenistic philosophers*. 2 vols. Cambridge: Cambridge University Press.

Lopez Pereira, J. E. (ed. and trans.) 2009. *Crónica mozárabe de 754=Continuatio isidoriana hispana*. León: Centro de Estudios e Investigación San Isidoro.

Louis, P. (ed. and trans.) 1956. *Aristote: Les parties des animaux*. Paris: Les Belles Lettres.

Lucchetta, F. (ed.) 1969. *Epistola sulla vita futura*. Padua: Antenore.

Lyons, M. (ed. and trans.) 1969. *Galeni De partibus artis medicativae*. Berlin: Akademie-Verlag.

Mahdi, M. (trans.) 2001. *Alfarabi: Philosophy of Plato and Aristotle*. Ithaca: Cornell University Press.

Mann, J. E. (ed. and trans.) 2012. *Hippocrates: On the art of medicine*. Studies in Ancient Medicine 39. Leiden: Brill.

Marmura, M. E. (ed. and trans.) 2005. *The metaphysics of the healing: A parallel English–Arabic text*. Islamic Translations Series. Provo: Brigham Young University Press.

Marx, A. (ed.) 1935. 'Texts by and about Maimonides', *Jewish Quarterly Review* 25.4: 371–428.

May, M. T. (trans.) 1968. *Galen: On the usefulness of the parts of the body. (Περὶ χρείας μορίων.) (De usu partium.)* 2 vols. Cornell Publications in the History of Science. Ithaca: Cornell University Press.

McGinnis, J. and Reisman, D. C. (trans.) 2007. *Classical Arabic philosophy: An anthology of sources*. Indianapolis: Hackett Publishing Company.
Meyerhof, M. (ed. and trans.) 1928. *The book of the ten treatises on the eye, ascribed to Ḥunain ibn Isḥâq (809–877 A.D.): The earliest existing systematic text-book of ophthalmology*. Princeton University Arabic Collection. Cairo: Government Press.
Migne, J.-P. (ed.) 1860. *Patrologiae cursus completus: Patrologia Graeca*. Vol. LXIV. Paris: Migne.
Moraux, P. (ed. and trans.) 1965. *Aristote. Du ciel*. Paris: Les Belles Lettres.
Morewedge, P. (trans.) 1973. *The metaphysica of Avicenna (Ibn Sīnā): A critical translation-commentary and analysis of the fundamental arguments in Avicenna's Metaphysica in the Dāniš Nāma-i ʿalāʾī (The book of scientific knowledge)*. Persian Heritage Series 13. New York: Columbia University Press.
Mudry, P. (ed. and trans.) 1982. *La préface du De medicina de Celse*. Bibliotheca Helvetica Romana 19. Bern: Francke.
Mugler, C. (ed. and trans.) 1966. *Aristote: De la génération et de la corruption*. Paris: Les Belles Lettres.
Muḥaqqiq, M. (ed.) 2005. *Kitāb al-Šukūk ʿalā Ǧālīnūs*. Islamic Thought 1. Tehran: International Institute of Islamic Thought and Civilization.
Muntaṣir, A., Zāyid, S., and Ismāʿīl, A. (eds.) 1980. *al-Šifāʾ: al-Ṭabīʿiyyāt, t. 8, al-Ḥayawān*. Cairo: al-Hayʾa al-Miṣriyya al-ʿĀmma li-l-Kitāb.
Naṣr, S. H. and Muḥaqqiq, M. (eds.) 1995. *al-Asʾila wal-aǧwiba*. Kuala Lumpur: International Institute of Islamic Thought and Civilization.
Nickel, D. (ed. and trans.) 2001. *Galeni De foetuum formation*. Berlin: Akademie-Verlag.
Nutton, V. (ed. and trans.) 1979. *Galeni De praecognitione*, Berlin: Akademie-Verlag.
(ed. and trans.) 1999. *Galeni De propriis placitis*. Berlin: Akademie-Verlag.
Nutton, V. and Bos, G. (ed. and trans.) 2011. *Galen: On problematical movements*. Cambridge Classical Texts and Commentaries 47. Cambridge: Cambridge University Press.
Pines, S. (trans.) 1963. *The guide to the perplexed*. 2 vols. Chicago: University of Chicago Press.
Prüfer C. and Meyerhof, M. (trans.) 1911. 'Die aristotelische Lehre vom Licht bei Ḥunain b. Isḥâq', *Der Islam* 2: 117–28.
Rabe, H. (ed.) 1899. *Ioannes Philoponus: De aeternitate mundi contra Proclum*. Leipzig: Teubner.
Rackham, H. (ed. and trans.) 1931. *Cicero: De finibus bonorum et malorum*. Cambridge, MA: Harvard University Press.
(ed. and trans.) 1934. *Aristotle: The Nicomachean Ethics*. Cambridge, MA: Harvard University Press.
(ed. and trans.) 1951. *Cicero: De natura deorum, Academica*. Cambridge, MA: Harvard University Press.
Rahman, F. (trans.) 1952. *Avicenna's psychology*. London: Oxford University Press.
(ed.) 1959. *Avicenna's De anima (Arabic text); Being the psychological part of Kitāb al-Šifāʾ*. London: Oxford University Press.

Ramelli, I. (ed. and trans.) 2009. *Hierocles the Stoic: Elements of ethics, fragments and excerpts*. Atlanta: Society of Biblical Literature.

Rappe, S. (trans.) 2010. *Damascius' 'Problems and solutions regarding first principles'*. Oxford: Oxford University Press.

Rashed, M. (ed. and trans.) 2015. *al-Ḥasan ibn Mūsā al-Nawbaḫtī, Commentary on Aristotle 'De generatione et corruption'*. Scientia Graeco-Arabica 19. Berlin: De Gruyter.

al-Rāzī 1955–70 (ed. anon). *al-Kitāb al-Ḥāwī fī l-ṭibb*. Hyderabad: Maṭbaʿat Mağlis Dāʾirat al-Maʿārif al-ʿUṯmāniyya.

Rescher, N. and Marmura, M. (ed. and trans.) 1965. *The refutation by Alexander of Aphrodisias of Galen's treatise On the theory of motion*. Islamabad: Islamic Research Institute.

Riḍā, N. (ed.) 1965. *ʿUyūn al-anbāʾ fī ṭabaqāt al-aṭibbāʾ*. Beirut: Dār Maktabat al-Ḥayāt.

Rolfe, J. C. (ed. and trans.) 1952. *Attic Nights*, vol. III: *Books 14–20*. Cambridge, MA: Harvard University Press.

Ross, W. D. (ed.) 1924. *Aristotle's Metaphysics*. 2 vols. Oxford: Clarendon Press.

(ed.) 1955. *Aristotle: Parva naturalia*. Oxford: Clarendon Press.

(ed.) 1957. *Aristotelis Politica*. Oxford: Clarendon Press.

(ed.) 1961. *Aristotle: De anima*. Oxford: Clarendon Press.

(ed.) 1964. *Aristotelis Analytica priora et posteriora*. Oxford: Clarendon Press.

(ed.) 1965. *Aristotelis De arte poetica liber*. Oxford: Clarendon Press.

(ed.) 1966. *Aristotelis Physica*. Oxford: Clarendon Press.

Rowson, E. (ed. and trans.) 1988. *A Muslim philosopher on the soul and its fate: al-ʿĀmirī's Kitāb al-Amad ʿalā l-abad*. American Oriental Series 70. New Haven: American Oriental Society.

Runia, D. R. and Share, M. J. (ed. and trans.) 2008. *Proclus: Commentary on Plato's 'Timaeus' II*. Cambridge: Cambridge University Press.

Sachau, E. (ed.) 1887. *Kitāb al-Bīrūnī fī taḥqīq mā li-l-Hind min maqūla maqbūla fī l-ʿaql aw marḏūla*. London: Trübner & Co.

Sbath, P. and Meyerhof, M. (ed. and trans.) 1938. *Le livre des questions sur l'oeil de Honain ibn Ishaq*. Cairo: Imprimerie de l'Institut Français d'Archéologie Orientale.

Schiefsky, M. J. (ed. and trans.) 2005. *Hippocrates: On ancient medicine*. Studies in Ancient Medicine 28. Leiden: Brill.

Schliwski, C. (ed. and trans.) 2004. 'Moses Ben Maimon, Sharḥ fuṣūl Abuqrāṭ: Der Kommentar des Maimonides zu den Aphorismen des Hippokrates; Kritische Edition des arabischen Textes mit Einführung und Übersetzung'. Ph.D. thesis. University of Cologne.

Schöne, H. (ed.) 1911. *De partibus artis medicativae: Eine verschollene griechische Schrift in Übersetzung des 14. Jahrhunderts*. Greifswald: J. Abel.

Schröder, H. O. (ed.) 1934. *Galeni In Platonis Timaeum comentarii fragmenta*. Berlin: Teubner.

Scopelliti, P. and A. Chaouech. (ed. and trans.) 2006. *Liber Aneguemis*. Milan: Mimesis.

Singer, C. (trans.) 1956. *Galen: On anatomical procedures*. London: Oxford University Press for the Wellcome Historical Museum.
Singer, P. N. (trans.) 1991. *Galen: Selected works*. Oxford: Oxford University Press.
(trans.) 2013a. 'The capacities of the soul depend on the mixtures of the body', in Singer (ed.), *Galen: Psychological writings*, 374–424.
(ed.) 2013b. *Galen: Psychological writings: Avoiding distress; Character traits; The diagnosis and treatment of the affections and errors peculiar to each person's soul; The capacities of the soul depend on the mixtures of the body*. Cambridge: Cambridge University Press.
Sodano, A. R. (ed. and trans.) 1958. *Porfirio Lettera ad Anebo*. Naples: Arte Tip.
(ed.) 1964. *Porphyrii In Platonis Timaeum commentariorum fragmenta*. Naples: Istituto della Stampa.
Spies, O. (ed. and trans.) 1937. 'al-Kindī's treatise on the cause of the blue colour of the sky', *Journal of the Bombay Branch of the Royal Asiatic Society* 13: 7–19.
Swain, S. (ed. and trans.) 2013. *Themistius, Julian, and Greek political theory under Rome: Texts, translations, and studies of four key works*. Cambridge: Cambridge University Press.
Tarrant, H. (ed. and trans.) 2007. *Proclus: Commentary on Plato's 'Timaeus' I*. Cambridge: Cambridge University Press.
Tecusan, M. (ed. and trans.) 2004. *The fragments of the Methodists: Methodism outside Soranus*. Studies in Ancient Medicine 24. Leiden: Brill.
Telfer, W. (trans.) 1955. *Cyril of Jerusalem and Nemesius of Emesa*. Library of Christian Classics. Philadelphia: Westminster Press.
Theoharides, T. C. (trans.) 1971. 'Galen on marasmus', *Journal of the History of Medicine and Allied Sciences* 26: 369–90.
Thurn, I. (ed.) 2000. *Ioannis Malalae chronographia*. Berlin: De Gruyter.
Twersky, I. (trans.) 1972. *A Maimonides reader*. Library of Jewish Studies. Springfield, NJ: Behrman House.
van der Eijk, P. J. (trans.) 2014. *Philoponus: On Aristotle On the soul 1.1–2*. Ancient Commentators on Aristotle. London: Bloomsbury.
van der Eijk, P. J. and Sharples, R. W. (trans.) 2008. *Nemesius: On the nature of man*. Translated Texts for Historians 49. Liverpool: Liverpool University Press.
von Staden, H. (ed. and trans.) 1989. *Herophilus: The art of medicine in early Alexandria*. Cambridge: Cambridge University Press.
Wakīl, A. A. (ed.) 1968. *al-Milal wal-niḥal*. Cairo: Muʾassasat al-Ḥalabī.
Walzer, R. (ed. and trans.) 1985. *al-Fārābī on the perfect state*. Oxford: Oxford University Press.
Westerink, L. G. (ed.) 1956. *Olympiodorus: Commentary on the first Alcibiades of Plato*. Amsterdam: North Holland.
Wilberding, J. (trans.) 2011. *Porphyry to Gaurus on how embryos are ensouled and on what is in our power*. London: Bloomsbury.
Zeyl, D. J. (trans.) 2000. *Plato: Timaeus*. Indianapolis: Hackett Publishing Company.

Secondary Sources

Adamson, P. 2002. *The Arabic Plotinus: A philosophical study of the 'Theology of Aristotle'*. London: Duckworth.

2004a. 'Non-discursive thought in Avicenna's commentary on the *Theology of Aristotle*', in J. McGinnis (ed.), *Interpreting Avicenna: Science and philosophy in medieval Islam*. Leiden: Brill, 87–111.

2004b. 'Correcting Plotinus: Soul's relationship to body in Avicenna's commentary on the Theology of Aristotle', in P. Adamson, H. Baltussen, and M. W. F. Stone (eds.), *Philosophy, Science and Exegesis in Greek, Arabic and Latin Commentaries*. Vol. II. Bulletin of the Institute of Classical Studies, Supplement 47: 59–75.

(ed.) 2008. *In the age of al-Fārābī: Arabic philosophy in the fourth/tenth century*. Warburg Institute Colloquia 12. London: Warburg Institute.

2012. 'Avicenna and his commentators on human and divine self-intellection', in D. N. Hasse and A. Bertolacci (eds.), *The Arabic, Hebrew and Latin reception of Avicenna's 'Metaphysics'*. Scientia Graeco-Arabica 7. Boston: De Gruyter, 97–122.

(ed.) 2013. *Interpreting Avicenna: Critical essays*. Cambridge: Cambridge University Press.

2014. 'Galen on void', in Adamson et al. (eds.), *Philosophical Themes in Galen*: 197–211.

Adamson, P., Hansberger, R., and Wilberding, J. (eds.) 2014. *Philosophical Themes in Galen: Bulletin of the Institute of Classical Studies*, Supplement 114.

Adamson, P. and Pormann, P. E. (eds.) 2017. *Philosophy and medicine in the formative period of Islam*. Warburg Institute Colloquia 31. London: Warburg Institute.

Allen, J. V. 2011. 'Syllogism, demonstration, and definition in Aristotle's *Topics* and *Posterior analytics*', *Oxford Studies in Ancient Philosophy* 40: 63–90.

Allen, M. 2003. 'The Ficinian Timaeus and Renaissance science', in Reydams-Schils (ed.), *Plato's 'Timaeus' as cultural icon*, 238–50.

Alon, I. 1991. *Socrates in mediaeval Arabic literature*. Islamic Philosophy, Theology, and Science 10. Leiden: Brill.

Álvarez Millán, C. 2010. 'The case history in medieval Islamic medical literature: *Tajārib* and *Mujarrabāt* as source', *Medical History* 54.2: 195–214.

Anawātī, G. C. 1950. *Millénaire d'Avicenne: Essai de bibliographie avicennienne*. Cairo: Dar al-Maaref.

1956. 'Prolégomènes à une nouvelle édition du de causis arabe', *Mélanges Louis Massignon* 1: 73–110.

Anderson, G. 1993. *The Second Sophistic: A cultural phenomenon in the Roman Empire*. London: Routledge.

Aouad, M. 1989. 'La *Théologie d'Aristote* et autres textes du Plotinus Arabus', in R. Goulet (ed.), *Dictionnaire des philosophes antiques* Vol. I. Paris: CNRS, 541–90.

Appiah, K. A. 2012. 'Misunderstanding cultures: Islam and the West', *Philosophy and Social Criticism* 38.4–5: 425–33.

Arnaldez, R. 1978. 'Khalḳ', in *EI2*.

Arnzen, R. 1998. *Aristoteles' 'De Anima': Eine verlorene spätantike Paraphrase in arabischer und persischer Überlieferung; Arabischer Text nebst Kommentar, quellengeschichtlichen Studien und Glossaren*. Aristoteles Semitico-Latinus 9. Leiden: Brill.

2011. *Platonische Ideen in der arabischen Philosophie*. Berlin: De Gruyter.

2012. 'Plato's *Timaeus* in the Arabic tradition', in Celia and Ulacco (eds.), *Il Timeo*, 181–267.

2013. 'Proclus on Plato's *Timaeus* 89e3–90c7', *Arabic Sciences and Philosophy* 23: 1–45.

Balansard, A. 2001. *Technè dans les dialogues de Platon: L'empreinte de la sophistique*. International Plato Studies 14. Sankt Augustin: Academia Verlag.

Ballester, L. G. 1988. 'Soul and body, disease of the soul and disease of the body in Galen's medical thought', in Manuli and Vegetti (eds.), *Le opere psicologiche di Galeno*, 117–50.

Baltussen, H. 2000. *Theophrastus against the Presocratics and Plato: Peripatetic dialectic in the De sensibus*. Leiden: Brill.

Baneth, H. 1960–1. 'A doctor's library in Egypt at the time of Maimonides', *Tarbīṣ* 30: 171–85.

Barad, K. 2007. *Meeting the universe halfway: Quantum physics and the entanglement of matter and meaning*. Durham, NC: Duke University Press.

Bar-Asher, M. M. 1989a. 'Quelques aspects de l'éthique d'Abū-Bakr al-Rāzī et ses origins dans l'oeuvre de Galien (Premiere partie)', *Studia Islamica* 69: 5–38.

1989b. 'Quelques aspects de l'éthique d'Abū-Bakr al-Rāzī et ses origins dans l'oeuvre de Galien (Seconde partie)', *Studia Islamica* 70: 119–48.

Barker, A. D. 2003. 'Early Timaeus commentaries and Hellenistic musicology', in Sharples and Sheppard (eds.), *Ancient Approaches*, 73–87.

Barnes, J. 1969. 'Aristotle's theory of demonstration', *Phronesis* 14: 123–52.

Barnes, J., Jouanna, J., and Barras, V. (eds.) 2003. *Galien et la philosophie: Huit exposés suivis de discussions*. Geneva: Fondation Hardt.

Barney, R. and Brennan, T. (eds.) 2012. *Plato and the divided self*. Cambridge: Cambridge University Press.

Berman, L. V. 1974. 'Maimonides the disciple of Alfarabi', *Israel Oriental Studies* 4: 154–78.

Bertolacci, A. 2011. 'A community of translators: The Latin medieval versions of Avicenna's *Book of the Cure*', in J. N. Crossley and C. J. Mews. (eds.), *Communities of learning: Networks and the shaping of intellectual identity in Europe, 1100–1500*. Europa Sacra 9. Turnhout: Brepols, 37–54.

2013a. 'Averroes against Avicenna on human spontaneous generation: The starting-point of a lasting debate', in A. Akasoy and G. Giglioni (eds.), *Renaissance Averroism and its aftermath: Arabic philosophy in early modern Europe*. Dordrecht: Springer, 37–54.

2013b. 'Avicenna's Christian reception in Latin medieval culture', in Adamson (ed.), *Interpreting Avicenna*, 242–69.

Betegh, G. 2010. 'What makes a myth eikôs? Remarks inspired by Myles Burnyeat's EIKÔS MYTHOS', in Mohr and Sattler (eds.), *One book, the whole universe*, 213–24.

Biesterfeldt, H. H. 2000. 'Medieval Arabic encyclopedias of science and philosophy', in S. Harvey (ed.), *The medieval Hebrew encyclopedias of science and philosophy: Proceedings of the Bar Ilan University conference.* Amsterdam Studies in Jewish Thought 7. Dordrecht: Kluwer Academic Publishers, 77–98.

2002. 'Arabisch-islamische Enzyklopädien: Formen und Funktionen', in C. Meier (ed.), *Die Enzyklopädie im Wandel vom Hochmittelalter bis zur frühen Neuzeit, Akten des Kolloquiums des Projekts D im Sonderforschungsbereich 231 (29.11–1.12. 1996) hrsg.* Munich: Wilhelm Fink, 43–83.

Black, D. L., 2008. 'Avicenna on self-awareness and knowing that one knows', in S. Rahman, T. Street, and H. Tahiri (eds.), *The unity of science in the Arabic tradition.* Dordrecht: Springer, 63–87.

Blau, J. 1981. *The emergence and linguistic background of Judaeo-Arabic: A study of the origins of Middle Arabic.* Jerusalem: Ben-Zvi Institute.

Bolton, G. 2008. 'Boundaries of humanities: Writing medical humanities', *Arts and Humanities in Higher Education* 7.2: 131–48.

Bosworth, C. E. 2010. 'Bīrūnī, Abū Rayḥān, life', in Yarshater (ed.), *Encyclopaedia Iranica.*

Boudon-Millot, V. 2002b. 'La théorie galénique de la vision: Couleurs du corps et couleurs des humeurs', in L. Villard (ed.), *Couleurs et vision dans l'Antiquité classique.* Mont-Saint-Aignan: Publications de l'Université de Rouen, 65–75.

2003. 'Art, science et conjecture chez Galien', in Barnes et al. (eds.), *Galien et la philosophie*, 269–98.

2004. 'Illustrer les médecins grecs à la Renaissance: Les schémas d'optique galénique', in V. Boudon-Millot and G. Cobolet (eds.), *Lire les médecins grecs à la Renaissance: Aux origines de l'édition médicale.* Paris: de Boccard, 209–32.

2012. 'Vision and vision disorders: Galen's physiology of sight', in Horstmanshoff et al. (eds.), *Blood, sweat and tears*, 549–67.

Bouras-Vallianatos, P. and Zipser, B. (eds.) 2019. *Brill's companion to the reception of Galen.* Brill's Companions to Classical Reception 17. Leiden: Brill.

Bourdieu, P. 1993. *The field of cultural production: Essays on art and literature.* New York: Columbia University Press.

Bowersock, G. W. 1969. *Greek sophists in the Roman Empire.* Oxford: Clarendon Press.

Brentjes, S. 2012. 'The prisons of categories – "decline" and its company', in F. Opwis and D. Reisman (eds.), *Islamic philosophy, science, culture, and religion: Studies in honor of Dimitri Gutas.* Leiden: Brill, 133–56.

2014. 'Sanctioning knowledge', *al-Qanṭara: Revista de estudios árabes* 35: 277–309.

2018. *Teaching and learning the sciences in Islamicate societies (800–1700).* Studies on the Faculty of Arts 3. Turnhout: Brepols.

Brisson, L. 2012. 'Why is the *Timaeus* called an *eikôs muthos* and an *eikôs logos*?', in C. Collobert, P. Destrée, and F. Gonzalez (eds.), *Plato and myth: Studies on the use and status of Platonic myths.* Leiden: Brill, 369–92.

Brisson, L. and Meyerstein, F. W. (eds.) 1995. *Inventing the universe: Plato's 'Timaeus', the Big Bang, and the problem of scientific knowledge*. SUNY Series in Ancient Greek Philosophy. Albany: SUNY Press.

Broadie, S. 2012. *Nature and divinity in Plato's 'Timaeus'*. Cambridge: Cambridge University Press.

Burnett, C. 2012. 'Plato amongst the Arabic-Latin translators of the twelfth century', in Celia and Ulacco (eds.), *Il Timeo*, 269–306.

Burnyeat, M. 2005. 'Εἰκὼς μῦθος', *Rhizai: Journal for Ancient Philosophy* 2: 143–65.

Carone, G. 2005. 'Mind and body in late Plato', *Archiv für Geschichte der Philosophie* 87.3: 227–69.

Carpenter, A. 2010. 'Embodied intelligent (?) souls: Plants in Plato's *Timaeus*', *Phronesis* 55: 281–303.

Celia, F. and Ulacco, A. (eds.) 2012. *Il Timeo: Esegesi greche, arabe, latine*. Pisa: Pisa University Press.

Chang, H. 2008. 'Rationalizing medicine and the social ambitions of physicians in classical Greece', *Journal of the History of Medicine and Allied Sciences* 63.2: 217–44.

Chiapperino, L. and Boniolo, G. 2014. 'Rethinking medical humanities', *Journal of Medical Humanities* 35.4: 377–87.

Chiaradonna, R. 2009a. 'Galen and Middle Platonism', in Gill et al. (eds.), *Galen and the world of knowledge*, 243–60.

2009b. 'Le traité de Galien *Sur la démonstration* et sa postérité tardo-antique', in R. Chiaradonna and F. Trabattoni (eds.), *Physics and philosophy of nature in Greek Neoplatonism*. Leiden: Brill, 43–77.

Cohen, M. R. 2017. *Maimonides and the merchants: Jewish law and society in the medieval Islamic world*. Jewish Culture and Contexts. Philadelphia: University of Pennsylvania Press.

Connelly, C. 2016. 'New evidence for the source of al-Fārābī's philosophy of Plato', in J. Stover (ed.), *A new work by Apuleius: The lost third book of the 'De Platone'*. Oxford: Oxford University Press, 183–97.

Cooper, G. 2016. 'Ḥunayn ibn Isḥāq's Galen translations and Greco-Arabic philology: Some observations from the *Crises* (*De crisibus*) and the *Critical Days* (*De diebus decretoriis*)', *Oriens* 44: 1–43.

Cooperson, M. 1997. 'The purported autobiography of Ḥunayn ibn Isḥāq', *Edebiyât* 7.2: 235–49.

Craik, E. M. 2015. *The Hippocratic corpus: Content and context*. London: Routledge.

Cribiore, R. 2001. *Gymnastics of the mind: Greek education in Hellenistic and Roman Egypt*. Princeton: Princeton University Press.

Dalen, J. E., Ryan, K. J., and Alpert, J. S. 2017. 'Where have the generalists gone? They became specialists, then subspecialists', *American Journal of Medicine* 130.7: 766–8.

D'Ancona, C. (ed.) 2003a. *Plotino. La discesa dell'anima nei corpi (Enn. IV 8[6]). Plotiniana Arabica (pseudo-Teologia di Aristotele, capitoli 1 e 7; 'Detti del Sapiente Greco')*. Padua: Il Poligrafo.

2003b. 'The Timaeus' model for creation and providence: An example of continuity and adaptation in early Arabic philosophical literature', in Reydam-Schils (ed.), *Plato's 'Timaeus' as cultural icon*, 206–37.

2006. 'The topic of the "harmony between Plato and Aristotle": Some examples in early Arabic philosophy', in A. Speer and L. Wegener (eds.), *Wissen über Grenzen: Arabisches Wissen und lateinisches Mittelalter*. Berlin: De Gruyter, 379–405.

Das, A. R. 2014. 'Reevaluating the authenticity of the fragments from Galen's *On the medical statements in Plato's* Timaeus (Scorialensis Graec. Φ-III-11, ff. 123r–126v)', *ZPE* 192: 93–103.

2017a. 'Beyond the disciplines of medicine: Greek and Arabic thinkers on the nature of plant life', in Adamson and Pormann (eds.), *Philosophy and medicine*, 206–17.

2017b. 'The Hippocratism of ʿAlī ibn Riḍwān: Autodidacticism and the creation of a medical *isnād*', *Journal of Islamic Studies* 28.2: 155–77.

2019. 'Probable new fragments and a testimonium from Galen's commentary on Plato's *Timaeus*', *CQ* 69.1: 384–401.

Das, A. R. and Koetschet, P. 2019. 'Para-Plutarchan traditions in the medieval Islamicate world', in S. Xenophontos and K. Oikonomopoulou (eds.), *The Brill companion to the reception of Plutarch*. Boston: Brill, 373–86.

Davidson, H. 1979. 'Maimonides' secret position on creation', in I. Twersky (ed.), *Studies in Medieval Jewish History and Literature*. Vol. I. Cambridge: Cambridge University Press, 16–40.

1987. *Proofs for eternity, creation and the existence of God in medieval Islamic and Jewish Philosophy*. New York: Oxford University Press.

De Lacy, P. 1966. 'Galen and the Greek poets', *GRBS* 7: 259–66.

1979. 'Galen's concept of continuity', *GRBS* 20: 355–69.

1988. 'The third part of the soul', in Manuli and Vegetti (eds.), *Le opere psicologiche di Galeno*, 43–64.

Dench, E. 2017. 'Ethnicity, culture, and identity', in Richter and Johnson (eds.), *The Oxford handbook to the Second Sophistic*, 99–114.

De Rohden, P. and Dessau, H. 1897. *Prosopographia imperii romani, saec. I.II.III*. 3 vols. Berlin: Reimer.

Diamond, J. A. 2012. 'R. Abraham Isaac Kook and Maimonides: A contemporary mystic's embrace of a medieval rationalist', in J. A. Diamond and A. Hughes (eds.), *Encountering the medieval in modern Jewish thought*. Leiden: Brill, 101–28.

2014. *Maimonides and the shaping of the Jewish canon*. Cambridge: Cambridge University Press.

Dillon, J. 1996. *The Middle Platonists: 80 B.C. to A.D. 220*, rev. edn. Ithaca: Cornell University Press.

Dold-Samplonius, Y. 2007. 'Archimedes', in *EI3*.

Donini, P. 2008. 'Psychology', in Hankinson (ed.), *The Cambridge companion to Galen*, 184–209.

Dörrie, H. 1973. 'La doctrine de l'âme dans le néoplatonisme de Plotin à Proclus', *Revue de théologie et de philosophie* 2: 116–34.

Dörrie, H. and Baltes, M. 1993. *Der Platonismus im 2. und 3. Jahrhundert nach Christus: Text, Übersetzung, Kommentar*. Vol. III. Stuttgart-Bad Canstatt: Frommann-Holzboog.

2002. *Die philosophische Lehre des Platonismus*, vol. VI.1: *Von der 'Seele' als der Ursache aller sinnvollen Abläufe, Bausteine 151–168: Text, Übersetzung, Kommentar*. Stuttgart-Bad Cannstatt: Frommann-Holzboog.

Drossaart Lulofs, H. J. 1957. 'Aristotle's ΠΕΡΙ ΦΥΤΩΝ', *JHS* 77.1: 75–80.

Druart, T.-A. 2003. 'Philosophy in Islam', in A. S. McGrade (ed.), *The Cambridge companion to medieval philosophy*. Cambridge: Cambridge University Press, 97–120.

Dulieu, L. 1955. 'L'arabisme médical à Montpellier du XIIe au XIVe siècle', *Les cahiers de Tunisie* 3: 86–95.

Dunlop, D. M. 1959. 'The translations of al-Biṭrīq and Yaḥyā (Yuḥannā) b. al-Biṭrīq', *Journal of the Asiatic Society of Great Britain and Ireland* 3.4: 140–50.

Durling, R. J. 1988. 'The innate heat in Galen', *Medizinhistorisches Journal* 23.3: 210–12.

Eastwood, B. 1981. 'Galen on the elements for the olfactory sensation', *Rheinisches Museum für Philologie* 124: 268–90.

1982. 'The elements of vision: The micro-cosmology of Galenic visual theory according to Ḥunayn Ibn Isḥāq', *Transactions of the American Philosophical Society* 72: 1–59.

Ebrahimnejad, H. 2008. 'Jālinus', in Yarshater (ed.), *EIr*.

Eichholz, D. E. 1951. 'Galen and his environment', *Greece and Rome* 20: 60–71.

Ekroth. G. 2014. 'Animal sacrifice in antiquity', in G. L. Campbell (ed.), *The Oxford handbook of animals in classical thought and life*. Oxford: Oxford University Press, 324–54.

Emilsson, E. K. 1991. 'Plotinus on soul–body dualism', in S. Everson (ed.), *Psychology*. Cambridge: Cambridge University Press, 148–65.

Endress, G. 1991. 'La *Concordance entre Platon et Aristote*, l'Aristote arabe et l'émancipation de la philosophie en Islam medieval', in B. Mojsisch and O. Pluta (eds.), *Historia philosophiae medii aevi: Studien zur Geschichte der Philosophie des Mittelalters*. Amsterdam: B. R. Grüner, 237–57.

1997. 'The circle of al-Kindī: Early Arabic translations from the Greek and the rise of Islamic philosophy', in Endress and Kruk (eds.), *The ancient tradition in Christian and Islamic Hellenism*, 43–76.

Endress, G. and Kruk, R. (eds.) 1997. *The ancient tradition in Christian and Islamic Hellenism: Studies on the transmission of Greek philosophy and sciences dedicated to H. J. Drossaart Lulofs on his ninetieth birthday*. Leiden: Research School CNWS.

Engberg-Pedersen, T. 1990. *The Stoic theory of oikeiosis: Moral development and social interaction in early Stoic philosophy*. Aarhus: Aarhus University Press.

Eshleman, K. 2012. *The social world of intellectuals in the Roman Empire: Sophists, philosophers, and Christians*. Cambridge: Cambridge University Press.

Evans, H. M. and Macnaughton, J. 2004. 'Should medical humanities be a multidisciplinary or interdisciplinary study?', *Medical Humanities* 30.1: 1–4.

Fakhry, M. 1968. 'A tenth-century Arabic interpretation of Plato's cosmology', *Journal of the History of Philosophy* 6.1: 15–22.

Ferrari, F. 1998. 'Galeno interprete del *Timeo*', *Museum Helveticum* 55: 14–34.

Festugière, A. 1952. 'Le compendium Timaei de Galien', *Revue des études grecques* 62: 97–118.

Fischer, K.-D. 1980. 'Der früheste bezeugte Augenarzt des klassischen Altertums', *Gesnerus* 37: 324–25.

Fitzgerald, D. and Callard, F. 2016. 'Entangling the medical humanities', in A. Whitehead, A. Woods, S. Atkinson, J. Macnaughton, and J. Richards (eds.), *The Edinburgh companion to the critical medical humanities*. Edinburgh: Edinburgh University Press, 35–49.

Foucault, M. 1969. *L'archéologie du savoir*. Paris: Gallimard.

1975. *Surveiller et punir: Naissance de la prison*. Paris: Gallimard.

Fowler, R. 2017. 'Platonism', in Richter and Johnson (eds.), *The Oxford handbook to the Second Sophistic*, 563–80.

Frank, D. H. 1997. 'What is Jewish philosophy', in D. H. Frank and O. Leaman (eds.), *History of Jewish philosophy*. Routledge History of World Philosophies 2. London: Routledge, 1–8.

Freudenthal, G. and Zonta, M. 2013. 'The reception of Avicenna in Jewish cultures, East and West', in Adamson (ed.), *Interpreting Avicenna*, 214–41.

Friedman, M. A. 2007. 'Did Maimonides teach medicine? Sources and assumptions', in C. del Valle, S. G. Jalón, and J. P. Monferrer (eds.), *Maimónides y su época*. Madrid: Sociedad Estatal de Conmemoraciones Culturales, 365–80.

Gardner, S. and Grist, M. (eds.) 2015. *The transcendental turn*. Oxford: Oxford University Press.

Garofalo, I. 2002. 'Alcune questioni sulle fonti greche nel Continens di Razes', *Medicine nei Secoli* 14: 383–406.

Gersh, S. 1973. *Κίνησις ἀκίνητος: A study of spiritual motion in the philosophy of Proclus*. Leiden: Brill.

Gieryn, T. F. 1983. 'Boundary-work and the demarcation of science from non-science: Strains and interests in professional ideologies of scientists', *American Sociological Review* 48.6: 781–95.

1999. *Cultural boundaries of science: Credibility on the line*. Chicago: University of Chicago Press.

Gill, C. 2000. 'The body's fault? Plato's *Timaeus* on psychic illness', in M. R. Wright (ed.), *Reason and necessity in Plato's 'Timaeus'*. London: Duckworth, 59–84.

2006. *The structured self in Hellenistic and Roman thought*. Oxford: Oxford University Press.

2009. 'Galen and the Stoics: What each could learn from the other about embodied psychology', in D. Frede and R. Burkhard (eds.), *Body and soul in ancient philosophy*. Berlin: De Gruyter, 409–23.

2010. *Naturalistic psychology in Galen and Stoicism*. Oxford: Oxford University Press.

Gill, C., Whitmarsh, T., and Wilkins, J. (eds.) 2009. *Galen and the world of knowledge*. Cambridge: Cambridge University Press.

Girard, M. C. 1990. 'L'hellébore: Panacée ou placébo?', in P. Potter, G. Maloney, and J. Desautels (eds.), *La maladie et les maladies dans la collection hippocratique: Actes du VIe colloque international hippocratique (Québec, du 28 septembre au 3 octobre 1987)*. Quebec: Éditions du Sphinx, 393–405.

Gleason, M. 1995. *Making men: Sophists and self-presentation in Ancient Rome*. Princeton: Princeton University Press.

2009. 'Shock and awe: The performance dimension of Galen's anatomy demonstrations', in Gill et al. (eds.), *Galen and the world of knowledge*, 85–114.

Goitein, S. D. 1963. 'The medical profession in light of the Cairo Geniza documents', *Hebrew Union College Annual* 34: 177–94.

1980. 'Moses Maimonides, man of action: A revision of the master's biography in light of the Geniza documents', in G. Nahon and C. Touati (eds.), *Hommage à Georges Vajda: Études d'histoire et de pensée juives*. Louvain: Peeters, 155–67.

Goitein, S. D. and Friedman, M. 2007. *India traders of the Middle Ages*. Études sur le judaïsme médiéval 31. Leiden: Brill.

Goldstein, J. 1984. 'Foucault among the sociologists: The "disciplines" and the history of the professions', *History and Theory* 23.2: 170–92.

Goodman, L. E. 1971. 'The Epicurean ethic of Muḥammad ibn Zakariyā' ar-Rāzī', *Studia Islamica* 34: 5–26.

1975. 'Rāzī's myth of the fall of the soul: Its function in his philosophy', in G. Hourani (ed.), *Essays on Islamic Philosophy*. Albany: SUNY Press, 25–40.

1995. 'Abū Bakr Muḥammad ibn Zakarīyā' ar-Rāzī', in *EI2*.

2015. 'How Epicurean was Razi', *Studia graeco-arabica* 5: 247–80.

Gordon, J. 2005. 'Medical humanities: To cure sometimes, to relieve often, to comfort always', *Medical Journal of Australia* 182.1: 5–8.

Grafton, A., Most, G. W., and Settis, S. 2010. *The classical tradition*. Harvard University Press Reference Library. Cambridge, MA: Belknap Press of Harvard University Press.

Grant, B. 2016. *The aphorism and other short forms*. New York: Routledge.

Greco, M. 2013. 'Logics of interdisciplinarity: The case of the medical humanities', in A. Barry and G. Born (eds.), *Interdisciplinarity: Reconfigurations of the social and natural sciences*. London: Routledge, 226–46.

Gregory, A. 2003. 'Aristotle and some of his commentators on the *Timaeus*' receptacle', in Sharples and Sheppard (eds.), *Ancient Approaches*, 29–47.

Gross, A. 1996. *The rhetoric of science*. Cambridge, MA: Harvard University Press.

Gruen, E. S. 1990. 'Philosophy, rhetoric, and Roman anxieties', in E. S. Gruen (ed.), *Studies in Greek culture and Roman policy*. Cincinnati Classical Studies 7. Leiden: Brill, 158–92.

Gutas, D. 1975. *Greek wisdom literature in Arabic translation: A study of the Graeco-Arabic gnomologia*. American Oriental Series 60. New Haven: American Oriental Society.

1983. 'Paul the Persian on the classification of the parts of Aristotle's philosophy: A milestone between Alexandria and Baġdâd', *Der Islam* 60.2: 231–67.

1987–8. 'Avicenna's *maḏhab*: With an appendix on the question of his date of birth', *Quaderni di Studi Arabi* 5–6: 323–36.

1988. *Avicenna and the Aristotelian tradition.* Islamic Philosophy and Theology 4. Leiden: Brill.
1997. 'Galen's synopsis of Plato's Laws and Fārābī's Talkhīs', in Endress and Kruk (eds.), *The ancient tradition in Christian and Islamic Hellenism*, 101–19.
1998. *Greek thought, Arabic culture: The Graeco-Arabic translation movement in Baghdad and early 'Abbāsid society (2nd–4th/8th–10th c.).* London: Routledge.
2002. 'The study of Arabic philosophy in the twentieth century: An essay on the historiography of Arabic philosophy', *British Journal of Middle Eastern Studies* 29.1: 5–25.
2003. 'Medical theory and scientific method in the age of Avicenna', in D. C. Reisman (ed.), *Before and after Avicenna: Proceedings of the first conference of the Avicenna study group*. Leiden: Brill, 145–62.
2007. 'The text of the Arabic Plotinus: Prolegomena to a critical edition', in C. D'Ancona (ed.), *The libraries of the Neoplatonists: Proceedings of the meeting of the European Science Foundation Network 'Late antiquity and Arabic thought: Patterns in the constitution of European culture' held in Strasbourg, March 12 –14*. Leiden: Brill, 371–84.
2012. 'Platon: Tradition arabe', in R. Goulet (ed.), *Dictionnaire des philosophes antiques*. Vol. Va. Paris: CNRS Éditions, 845–63.
2014. *Avicenna and the Aristotelian tradition.* Leiden: Brill.
Gutman, O. 2003. *Pseudo-Avicenna: Liber celi et mundi.* Aristoteles Semitico-Latinus 14. Leiden: Brill.
Hankinson, R. J. 1988. 'Galen explains the elephant', *Canadian Journal of Philosophy* 14: 135–57.
1989. 'Galen and the best of all possible worlds', *CQ* 39: 206–27.
1992. 'Galen's philosophical eclecticism', *ANWR* II.36.5, 3505–22.
1998b. *Cause and explanation in ancient Greek thought.* Oxford: Oxford University Press.
(ed.) 2008. *The Cambridge companion to Galen.* Cambridge: Cambridge University Press.
2009. 'Medicine and the science of soul', *Canadian Bulletin of Medical History* 26.1: 129–54.
Hansberger, R. 2011. 'Plotinus Arabus rides again', *Arabic Sciences and Philosophy* 21.1: 57–84.
Hardwick, L. 2003. *Reception studies.* Oxford: Oxford University Press.
Harris, W. V. 2018. 'Pain and medicine in the classical world', in W. V. Harris (ed.), *Pain and pleasure in classical times.* Leiden: Brill, 55–82.
Harte, V. 2004. 'The *Philebus* on pleasure: The good, the bad and the false', *Proceedings of the Aristotelian Society* 104.2: 111–28.
Harvey, S. 2004. 'The impact of Philoponus' commentary on the *Physics* on Averroes' three commentaries on the *Physics*', in P. Adamson, H. Baltussen, and M. Stone (eds.), *Philosophy, Science and Exegesis in Greek, Arabic and Latin Commentaries.* Vol. II. *Bulletin of the Institute of Classical Studies*, Supplement 47: 89–105.

2018. 'The story of a twentieth-century Jewish scholar's discovery of Plato's political philosophy in tenth-century Islam: Leo Strauss' early interest in the Islamic *falāsifa*', in O. Fraisse (ed.), *Modern Jewish scholarship on Islam in context: Rationality, European borders, and the search for belonging*. Berlin: De Gruyter, 219–44.

Harvey, W. Z. 1991. 'Why Maimonides was not a Mutakallim', in J. L. Kraemer and L. V. Berman (eds.), *Perspectives on Maimonides: Philosophical and historical studies*. London: Littman Library of Jewish Civilization, 105–14.

Hasnawi, A. 1990. 'Fayḍ', in *Encyclopédie philosophique universelle*, vol. II: *Les Notions philosophiques: Dictionnaire, tome 1, publiée sous la direction d'A. Jacob*. Paris: Presses Universitaires de France, 966–72.

Hasse, D. N. 2000. *Avicenna's 'De anima' in the Latin West: The formation of a peripatetic philosophy of the soul 1160–1300*. Warburg Institute Studies and Texts 1. London: Warburg Institute.

Havrda, M. 2015. 'The purpose of Galen's treatise On Demonstration', *Early Science and Medicine* 20: 265–87.

2017. 'Body and cosmos in Galen's account of soul', *Phronesis* 62.1: 69–89.

Hein, C. 1985. *Definition und Einteilung der Philosophie*. Europäische Hochschulschriften. Reihe 20, Philosophie 177. Frankfurt: Lang.

Heinrichs, W. 1995. 'The classification of the sciences and the consolidation of philology in classical Islam', in J. W. Drijvers and A. A. McDonald (eds.), *Centres of learning: Learning and location in pre-modern Europe and the Near East*. Leiden: Brill, 119–40.

Hemelrijk, E. A. 1999. *Matrona docta: Educated women in the Roman elite from Cornelia to Julia Domna*. London: Routledge.

Hine, H. 2016. 'Philosophy and *philosophi*: From Cicero to Apuleius', in G. D. Williams and K. Volk (eds.), *Roman reflections: Studies in Latin philosophy*. New York: Oxford University Press, 13–29.

Hirschberg, J. 1908. *Geschichte der Augenheilkunde. 2. und 3. Buch (i.e.: 1–3. Abschnitt): Buch 1–3, Abschnitt 1–25: Geschichte der Augenheilkunde im Mittelalter und in der Neuzeit*. Leipzig: Engelmann.

Hirt Raj, M. 1987. 'Le statut social du médecin à Rome et dans les provinces occidentales sous le haut-empire', in *Archéologie et médecine: VIIèmes Rencontres internationals d'archéologie et d'histoire d'Antibes (23, 24, 25 octobre 1986)*. Juan-les-Pins: Association pour la Promotion et la Diffusion des Connaissances Archéologiques, 95–107.

Hodgson, M. G. S. 1974. *The venture of Islam: Conscience and history in a world civilization*. Vol. I. Chicago: University of Chicago Press.

Hoenig, C. 2018. *Plato's 'Timaeus' and the Latin tradition*. Cambridge Classical Studies. Cambridge: Cambridge University Press.

Holmes, B. 2010. *The symptom and the subject: The emergence of the body in ancient Greece*. Princeton: Princeton University Press.

2013. 'Disturbing connections: Sympathetic affections, mental disorder, and the elusive soul in Galen', in W. V. Harris (ed.), *Mental disorders in the classical world*. Leiden: Brill, 147–76.

2014. 'Galen on the chances of life', in V. Wohl (ed.), *Probabilities, hypotheticals, and counterfactuals in ancient Greek thought*. Cambridge: Cambridge University Press, 230–50.

2015. 'Galen on sympathy', in Schliesser (ed.), *Sympathy*, 61–9.

Hopkins, S. 2005. 'Languages of Maimonides', in Tamer (ed.), *The trias of Maimonides*, 85–106.

Horstmanshoff, M. 1990. 'The ancient physician: Craftsman or scientist?', *Journal of the History of Medicine and Allied Sciences* 45: 176–97.

Horstmanshoff, M., King, H., and Zittel, C. (eds.) 2012. *Blood, sweat, and tears: The changing concepts of physiology from antiquity into early modern Europe*. Leiden: Brill.

Ierodiakonou, K. 2014. 'On Galen's theory of vision', in Adamson et al. (eds.), *Philosophical Themes in Galen*: 235–47.

Inwood, B. 1985. *Ethics and human action in early Stoicism*. Oxford: Clarendon Press.

Isnardi Parente, M. 1966. *Techne: Momenti del pensiero greco da Platone a Epicuro*. Florence: La Nuova Italia.

Israelowich, I. 2015. *Patients and healers in the high Roman Empire*. Baltimore: Johns Hopkins University Press.

Ivry, A. L. 1986. 'Islamic and Greek influences on Maimonides' philosophy', in S. Pines and Y. Yovel (eds.), *Maimonides and philosophy*. Dordrecht: Springer, 139–56.

Jackson, R. P. J. 1996. 'Eye medicine in the Roman world', in *ANRW* II.37.3, 2228–51.

Jacobs, J. A. 2013. *In defense of disciplines: Interdisciplinarity and specialization in the research university*. Chicago: University of Chicago Press.

Jacquart, D. 1996. 'The influence of Arabic medicine in the medieval West', in R. Rashed and R. Morelon (eds.), *Encyclopedia of the history of Arabic science*. Vol. III. London: Routledge, 963–84.

2005. 'Gerard of Cremona (1187)', in A. Vauchez, M. Lapidge, R. B. Dobson (eds.), *Encyclopedia of the Middle Ages*. Oxford University Press (online).

Janssens, J. 1987. 'Ibn Sīnā's ideas of ultimate realities: Neoplatonism and the Qurʾān as problem solving paradigms in the Avicennian system', *Ultimate Reality and Meaning* 10.4: 252–71.

2007. 'The reception of Avicenna's *Physics* in the Latin Middle Ages', in A. Vrolijk, J. P. Hogendijk, and R. Kruk (eds.), *O ye gentleman: Arabic studies on science and literary culture in honour of Remke Kruk*. Islamic Philosophy, Theology, and Science 74. Leiden: Brill, 55–64.

2011. 'Ibn Sīnā (Avicenna), Latin translations of', in H. Lagerlund (ed.), *Encyclopedia of medieval philosophy: Philosophy between 500 and 1500*. Vol. I. Berlin: Springer, 522–7.

Johansen, T. K. 1997. *Aristotle on the sense-organs*. Cambridge: Cambridge University Press.

2004. *Plato's natural philosophy: A study of the 'Timaeus-Critias'*. Cambridge: Cambridge University Press.

Johnson, A. P. 2013. *Religion and identity in Porphyry of Tyre: The limits of Hellenism in late antiquity*. Cambridge: Cambridge University Press.

Johnson, W. A. 2010. *Readers and reading culture in the high Roman Empire: A study of elite communities*. Classical Culture and Society. Oxford: Oxford University Press.

Jouanna, J. 2009. 'Does Galen have a medical programme for intellectuals and the faculties of the intellect?', in Gill et al. (eds.), *Galen and the world of knowledge*, 190–205.

2012. *Greek medicine from Hippocrates to Galen: Selected papers*. Leiden: Brill.

Kahl, O. 2015. *The Sanskrit, Syriac and Persian sources in the 'Comprehensive book' of Rhazes*. Islamic Philosophy, Theology and Science 93. Leiden: Brill.

Kalderon, M. E. 2015. *Form without matter: Empedocles and Aristotle on color perception*. Oxford: Oxford University Press.

Karamanolis, G. E. 2006. *Plato and Aristotle in agreement? Platonists on Aristotle from Antiochus to Porphyry*. Oxford: Oxford University Press.

Kargar, D. 2012. 'Irānšahri', in Yarshater (ed.), *EIr*.

Kaukua, J. 2015. *Self-awareness in Islamic philosophy: Avicenna and beyond*. Cambridge: Cambridge University Press.

Kellner, M. 1987. 'Heresy and the nature of faith in medieval Jewish philosophy', *Jewish Quarterly Review* 77.4: 299–318.

Kennedy, E. S., 1970. 'al-Bīrūnī', in *Dictionary of Scientific Biography*. Vol. II. New York: Scribner, 147–58.

Kerferd, G. B. 1972. 'The search for personal identity in Stoic thought', *BJRL* 55: 177–96.

Kirklin, D. and Richardson, R. 2001. 'Introduction: Medical humanities and tomorrow's doctors', in D. Kirklin and R. Richardson (eds.), *Medical humanities: A practical introduction*. London: Royal College of Physicians, 1–6.

Klein, J. 1996. *Crossing boundaries: Knowledge, disciplinarities, and interdisciplinarities*. Charlottesville: University Press of Virginia.

Knuuttila, S. 2004. *Emotions in ancient and medieval philosophy*. Oxford: Clarendon Press.

Kobayashi, M. 1988. 'The social status of doctors in the early Roman Empire', in T. Yuge and M. Doi (eds.), *Forms of control and subordination in antiquity*. Leiden: Brill, 416–19.

Koetschet, P. 2015. 'Galien, al-Rāzī, et l'éternité du monde: Les fragments du traité *Sur la démonstration*, IV, dans *Les doutes sur Galien*', *Arabic Sciences and Philosophy* 25.2: 167–98.

2017. 'Abū Bakr al-Rāzī on vision', in Adamson and Pormann (eds.), *Philosophy and medicine*, 170–89.

Kohler, G. Y. 2012. *Reading Maimonides' philosophy in 19th century Germany: The guide to religious reform*. Amsterdam Studies in Jewish Philosophy 15. Dordrecht: Springer Netherlands.

König, J. 2009. 'Conventions of prefatory self-presentation in Galen's *On the Order of My Own Books*', in Gill et al. (eds.), *Galen and the world of knowledge*, 35–58.

König, J. and Whitmarsh, T. 2007. 'Ordering knowledge', in J. König and T. Whitmarsh (eds.), *Ordering knowledge in the Roman Empire*. Cambridge: Cambridge University Press, 3–39.

Korhonen, T. 1997. 'Self-concept and public image of philosophers and philosophical schools at the beginning of the Hellenistic age', in J. Frösén (ed.), *Early Hellenistic Athens: Symptoms of a change*. Papers and Monographs of the Finnish Institute at Athens 6. Helsinki: Foundation of the Finnish Institute at Athens, 33–101.

Kottek, S. 2009. 'Critical remarks on medical authorities: Maimonides' commentary on Hippocrates' *Aphorisms*', in C. Fraenkel (ed.), *Traditions of Maimonideanism*. IJS Studies in Judaica 7. Leiden: Brill, 3–15.

Kraemer, J. L. 1984. 'On Maimonides' messianic posture', *Studies in Medieval Jewish History and Literature* 2: 109–42.

2008. *Maimonides: The life and world of one of civilization's greatest minds*. New York: Random House.

Kraus, P. and Pines, S. 2012. 'al-Rāzī', in *EI*.

Kudlien, F. 1976. 'Medicine as a "liberal art" and the question of the physician's income', *Journal of the History of Medicine and Allied Sciences* 31.4: 448–59.

Kühn, C. G. 1828. *Opuscula academica medica et philologica: Collecta, aucta et emendate*. Vol. II. Leipzig: Voss.

Lami, A. 2010. 'Sul testo del *De propriis placitis* di Galeno', *Galenos* 4: 81–126.

Langermann, Y. T. 1992. 'Maimonides' repudiation of astrology', *Maimonidean Studies* 2: 123–58.

1993. 'Maimonides on the synochous fever', *Israel Oriental Studies* 13: 175–98.

Lassner, J. 1970. *The topography of Baghdad in the early Middle Ages: Text and studies*. Detroit: Wayne State University.

Latour, B. and Woolgar, S. 1986. *Laboratory life: The construction of scientific facts*. Princeton: Princeton University Press.

Leaman, O. 2003. 'Introduction to the study of Jewish philosophy', in D. H. Frank and O. Leaman (eds.), *The Cambridge companion to medieval Jewish philosophy*. Cambridge: Cambridge University Press, 3–15.

Le Coz, R. 2006. *Les chrétiens dans la médecine arabe*. Peuples et cultures de l'Orient chrétien. Paris: L'Harmattan.

Leggett, A. J. 2010. 'Plato's *Timaeus*: Some resonances in modern physics and cosmology', in Mohr and Sattler (eds.), *One book, the whole universe*, 31–6.

Lettinck, P. 1999. *Aristotle's Meteorology and its reception in the Arab world*. Leiden: Brill.

Levin, S. B. 2014. *Plato's rivalry with medicine: A struggle and its dissolution*. Oxford: Oxford University Press.

Lévy, C. 2003. 'Cicero and the *Timaeus*', in Reydams-Schils (ed.), *Plato's 'Timaeus' as cultural icon*, 95–110.

Lewis, B. 1993. *Islam in history: Ideas, people, and events in the Middle East*. Chicago: Open Court.

Lewis, O. 2017. *Praxagoras of Cos on arteries, pulse and pneuma: Fragments and interpretation*. Leiden: Brill.

Lieber, E. 1979. 'Galen: Physician as philosopher; Maimonides: Philosopher as physician', *Bulletin of the History of Medicine* 53: 268–85.
Linant de Bellefonds, Y., Cahen, C., and İnalcık, H. 2012. 'Ḳānūn', in *EI2*.
Lindberg, D. C. 1976. *Theories of vision from Alkindi to Kepler*. Chicago: University of Chicago Press.
Lloyd, G. E. R. 1987. 'Empirical research in Aristotle's Biology', in A. Gotthelf and J. Lennox (eds.), *Philosophical issues in Aristotle's biology*. Cambridge: Cambridge University Press, 53–63.
1988. 'Scholarship, authority and argument in Galen's *Quod animi mores*', in Manuli and Vegetti (eds.), *Le opere psicologiche di Galeno*, 11–42.
1991. 'The definition, status, and methods of the medical τέχνη in the fifth and fourth centuries', in A. C. Bowen (ed.), *Science and philosophy in classical Greece*. New York: Garland, 249–60.
1992. 'The theories and practices of demonstration in Aristotle', in J. Cleary and D. Shartin (eds.), *Proceedings of the Boston Area Colloquium in ancient philosophy*. Vol. VII. Lanham: University Press of America, 371–412.
1996. 'Theories and practices of demonstration in Galen', in M. Frede and G. Striker (eds.), *Rationality in Greek thought*. Oxford: Clarendon Press, 255–77.
2009. *Disciplines in the making: Cross-cultural perspectives on elites, learning, and innovation*. Oxford: Oxford University Press.
Löbl, R. 2003. *Techne: Untersuchung zur Bedeutung dieses Wortes in der Zeit von Homer bis Aristoteles. 2: Von den Sophisten bis zu Aristoteles*. Würzburg: Königshausen und Neumann.
Long, A. A. 1996. 'Hierocles on *oikeiosis* and self-perception', in A. A. Long (ed.), *Stoic Studies*. Cambridge: Cambridge University Press, 250–63.
L'Orange, H. P. 1953. *Studies on the iconography of cosmic kingship in the ancient world*. Instituttet for Sammenlignende Kulturforskning, Serie A 23. Oslo: H. Aschehoug.
Lorenz, H. 2012. 'The cognition of appetite in Plato's *Timaeus*', in Barney and Brennan (eds.), *Plato and the divided self*, 238–58.
Lorusso, V. 2005. 'Nuovi frammenti di Galeno (*In Hp. Epid. IV Comm. VIII*; *In Plat. Tim. Comm.*)', *ZPE* 152: 43–56.
Mahdavī, Y. 1954. *Bibliographie d'Ibn Sīnā*. Publications de l'Université de Tehran 206. Tehran: University of Tehran.
Mahdi, M. 1996. 'Remarks on al-Rāzī's Principles', *Bulletin d'études orientales* 48: 145–53.
Makdisi, G. 1981. *The rise of colleges: Institutions of learning in Islam and the West*. Edinburgh: Edinburgh University Press.
Manetti, D. and Roselli, A. 1994. 'Galeno commentatore di Ippocrate', in ANRW II.37.2, 1529–1635.
Manuli, P. and Vegetti, M. (eds.) 1988. *Le opere psicologiche di Galeno: Atti del terzo colloquio galenico internazionale, Pavia, 10–12 settembre 1986*. Naples: Bibliopolis.
Marmura, M. E. 1986. 'Avicenna's "flying man" in context', *The Monist* 69.3: 383–95.

1992. 'Quiddity and universality in Avicenna', in P. Morewedge (ed.), *Neoplatonism and Islamic thought*. Studies in Neoplatonism 5. Albany: SUNY Press, 77–87.

2006. 'Avicenna's critique of Platonists in book VII, chapter 2 of the *Metaphysics* of his *Healing*', in J. E. Montgomery (ed.), *Arabic theology, Arabic philosophy: From the many to the one: Essays in celebration of Richard M. Frank*. Leuven: Peeters, 355–70.

Martijn, M. 2010. *Proclus on nature: Philosophy of nature and its methods in Proclus' 'Commentary on Plato's Timaeus'*. Philosophia Antiqua 121. Leiden: Brill.

Martin, W. M. 2015. 'Stoic transcendentalism and the doctrine of *oikeiosis*', in Gardner and Grist (eds.), *The transcendental turn*, 342–68.

Martindale, C. 1993. *Redeeming the text: Latin poetry and the hermeneutics of reception*. Cambridge: Cambridge University Press.

Mattern, S. 2008. *Galen and the rhetoric of healing*. Baltimore: Johns Hopkins University Press.

2013. *The prince of medicine: Galen in the Roman Empire*. Oxford: Oxford University Press.

Mazor, A. 2007. 'Maimonides' conversion to Islam: New evidence', *Pe'amim* 110: 5–8.

McAuliffe, J. D. (ed.) 2001. *Encyclopaedia of the Qu'rān*. Leiden: Brill (online).

McGinnis, J. 2010. *Avicenna*. Great Medieval Thinkers.Oxford: Oxford University Press.

Mendell, H. 1998. 'Making sense of Aristotelian demonstration', *Oxford Studies in Ancient Philosophy* 16: 161–225.

Menn, S. 2002. 'Aristotle's definition of soul and the programme of the *De anima*', *Oxford Studies in Ancient Philosophy* 22: 83–139.

Messer-Davidow, E., Shumway, D. R., and Sylvan, D. J. 1993. 'Introduction: Disciplinary ways of knowing', in E. Messer-Davidow, D. R. Shumway, and D. J. Sylvan (eds.), *Knowledges: Historical and critical studies in disciplinarity*. Knowledge: Disciplinarity and Beyond. Charlottesville: University Press of Virginia, 1–24.

Meyer-Steineg, T. 1916. *Das medizinische System der Methodiker: Eine Vorstudie zu Caelius Aurelianus 'De morbis acutis et chronicis'*. Jenaer medizin-historische Beiträge. Jena: Fischer.

Micheau, F. 1997. 'Mécènes et médecins à Bagdad au IIIe/IXe siècle: Les commanditaires des traductions de Galien par Ḥunayn ibn Isḥāq', in D. Jacquart (ed.), *Les voies de la science grecque: Étude sur la transmission des textes de l'antiquité au dix-neuvième siècle*. Hautes études médiévales et modernes 78. Geneva: Droz, 147–79.

Mohr, R. D. 2010. 'Plato's cosmic manual: Introduction', in Mohr and Sattler (eds.), *One book, the whole universe*, 1–14.

Mohr, R. D. and Sattler, B. M. (eds.) 2010. *One book, the whole universe: Plato's 'Timaeus' today*. Las Vegas: Parmenides Publishing.

Moraux, P. 1977. 'Unbekannte Galen-Scholien', *ZPE* 27: 1–62.

Morgan, T. J. 1998. *Literate education in the Hellenistic and Roman worlds*. Cambridge: Cambridge University Press.

Morison, B. 2008. 'Logic', in Hankinson (ed.), *The Cambridge companion to Galen*, 66–115.

Moseley, G. 2018a. 'Found in translation: An Arabic *Phaedo* fragment (107d6–108c1) in Ruhāwī's *Adab al-ṭabīb* and the late antique transmission of Plato', *Mnemosyne* 71: 976–92.

2018b. 'Pl. *Leg.* 631c6–7: Textual gleanings from an Arabic fragment', *Mnemosyne* 71: 173–6.

2019. 'New witness to Plat. *Smp.* 191e and *Leg.* 7, 819d2–3', *Museum Helveticum* 76.1: 1–6.

Mourelatos, A. P. D. 2010. 'Epistemological section (29b–d) of the proem in Timaeus' speech: M. F. Burnyeat on eikôs mythos, and comparison with Xenophanes B34 and B35', in Mohr and Sattler (eds.), *One book, the whole universe*, 225–47.

Mudry, P. 1985. 'Médecins et spécialistes: Le problème de l'unité de la médecine à Rome au 1er siècle ap. J. C.', *Gesnerus* 42: 329–36.

Munk, S. 1842. 'Notice sur Joseph ben-Iehouda ou Aboul'hadjàdj Yousouf ben-Yahya al-Sabti al-Maghrebi, disciple de Maïmonide', *Journal asiatique* 3.14: 5–70.

Musallam, B. 1987. 'Avicenna: Medicine and biology', in Yarshater (ed.), *EIr*.

Naǧātī, M. U. 1985. *al-Idrāk al-ḥissī ʿinda Ibn Sīnā: baḥṯ fī ʿilm al-nafs ʿinda al-ʿArab*. Algiers: Dīwān al-Maṭbūʿāt al-Ǧāmiʿiyya.

Natali, C. 2007. 'Aristotle's conception of *dunamis* and *techne*', in S. Stern-Gillet and K. Corrigan (eds.), *Reading ancient texts: Essays in honour of Denis O'Brien*. Vol II. Leiden: Brill, 3–21.

Netton, I. R. 2002. *Muslim Neoplatonists: An introduction to the thought of the Brethren of Purity (Ikhwān al-Ṣafāʾ)*. London: Routledge.

Nicholls, M. 2011. 'Galen and libraries in the Περὶ ἀλυπίας', *JRS* 101: 123–42.

Nickel, D. 2002. 'On the authenticity of an "excerpt" from Galen's commentary on the *Timaeus*', in Nutton (ed.) *The Unknown Galen*: 73–8.

Niehoff, M. R. 2007. 'Did the *Timaeus* create a textual community?' *Greek, Roman and Byzantine Studies* 47: 161–91.

Nussbaum, M. 2001. *The fragility of goodness: Luck and ethics in Greek tragedy and philosophy*. Cambridge: Cambridge University Press.

2009. *The Therapy of desire: Theory and practice in Hellenistic ethics*. Princeton: Princeton University Press.

Nutton, V. 1972. 'Roman oculists', *Epigraphica* 34: 16–29.

1984. 'Galen in the eyes of his contemporaries', *Bulletin of the History of Medicine* 63: 305–14.

(ed.) 2002. *The Unknown Galen: Bulletin of the Institute of Classical Studies*, Supplement 77.

2004. *Ancient medicine*. Sciences of Antiquity. London: Routledge.

2009. 'Galen's library', in Gill et al. (eds.), *Galen and the world of knowledge*, 19–34.

O'Brien, D. 1984. *Plato: Weight and sensation; The two theories of the 'Timaeus'*. Philosophia Antiqua 41. Paris: Les Belles Lettres.
Overwien, O. 2012. 'The art of the translator, or: How did Ḥunayn ibn ʾIsḥāq and his school translate?' in Pormann (ed.), *Epidemics in context*, 151–69.
Owen, G. E. L. 1953. 'The place of the *Timaeus* in Plato's dialogues', *CQ* 47: 79–95.
Parker, H. 1997. 'Women physicians in Greece, Rome, and the Byzantine Empire', in L. Furst (ed.), *Women physicians and healers: Climbing a long hill*. Lexington: University Press of Kentucky, 131–50.
Pembroke, S. G. 1971. 'Oikeiosis', in A. A. Long (ed.), *Problems in Stoicism*. London: Athlone Press, 114–49.
Peters, F. E. 1968. *Aristoteles Arabus: The oriental translations and commentaries on the Aristotelian corpus*. Leiden: Brill.
Peterson, D. C. 2001. 'Creation', in McAuliffe (ed.), *Encyclopaedia of the Quʾrān*.
Pietrobelli, A. 2013. 'Galien agnostique: Un texte caviardé par la tradition', *REG* 126.1: 103–35.
Pigeaud, J. 1993. 'L'introduction du Méthodisme à Rome', in *ANRW* II.37.1, 565–99.
Pinault, J. R. 1992. *Hippocratic lives and legends*. Studies in Ancient Medicine 4. Leiden: Brill.
Pines, S. 1953. 'Rāzī critique de Galien', *Actes du septième congrès international d'Histoire des Sciences*. Paris: Académie International d'Histoire des Sciences, 480–7.
1954. 'La conception de la conscience de soi chez Avicenne et chez Abū al-Barakāt al-Baghdādī', *Archives d'histoire doctrinale et littéraire du moyen âge* 29: 21–56.
1997. *Studies in Islamic atomism*, trans. Y. T. Langermann. Jerusalem: Magnes Press.
Pingree, D. E. 2014. 'Plato's Hermetic Book of the Cow', *Transactions of the American Philosophical Society* 104.3: 463–75.
Pleket, H. W. 1995. 'The social status of physicians in the Greco-Roman world', *Clio Medica* 27: 27–34.
Polito, R. 2013. 'Asclepiades of Bithynia and Heraclides of Pontus: Medical Platonism?', in M. Schofield (ed.), *Aristotle, Plato, and Pythagoreanism in the first century BC: New directions for philosophy*. Cambridge: Cambridge University Press, 118–38.
Pormann, P. E. 2004. *The oriental tradition of Paul of Aegina's 'Pragmateia'*. Studies in Ancient Medicine 29. Leiden: Brill.
(ed.) 2012. *Epidemics in context: Greek commentaries on Hippocrates in the Arabic Tradition*. Scientia Graeco-Arabica 8. Boston: De Gruyter.
2013. 'Avicenna on medical practice, epistemology, and the physiology of the inner senses', in Adamson (ed.), *Interpreting Avicenna*, 91–108.
Pormann, P. E. and Joosse, N. P. 2012. 'Commentaries on the Hippocratic Aphorisms in the Arabic tradition: The example of melancholy', in Pormann (ed.), *Epidemics in context*, 211–50.

Pormann, P. E. and Savage-Smith, E. 2007. *Medieval Islamic medicine*. Edinburgh: Edinburgh University Press.

Porter, J. 2008. 'Reception studies: Future prospects', in L. Hardwick and C. Stray (eds.), *A companion to classical receptions*. Oxford: Blackwell, 469–81.

Prins, J. 2014. *Echoes of an invisible world: Marsilio Ficino and Francesco Patrizi on cosmic order and music theory*. Leiden: Brill.

Rapoport, Y. and Shahar, I. 2012. 'Irrigation in the medieval Islamic Fayyum: Local control in a large-scale hydraulic system', *Journal of the Economic and Social History of the Orient* 55.1: 1–31.

Rashed, M. 2000. 'Abū Bakr al-Rāzī et le kalām', *MIDEO* 24: 39–54.

2008. 'Abū Bakr al-Rāzī et la prophétie', *MIDEO* 27: 169–82.

2009. 'Le prologue perdu de l'abrégé de Timée de Galien dans un texte de magie noire', *Antiquorum Philosophia* 3: 89–100.

2011. 'Aristote à Rome au IIe siècle: Galien, *De indolentia* §§15–18', *Elenchos* 32: 55–77.

Reid, H. 2011. *Athletics and philosophy in the ancient world*. London: Routledge.

Reisman, D. C. 2013. 'The life and times of Avicenna: Patronage and learning in medieval Islam', in Adamson (ed.), *Interpreting Avicenna*, 7–27.

Repici, L. 2000. *Uomini capovolti: Le piante nel pensiero dei greci*. Rome: Laterza.

Reydams-Schils, G. J. (ed.) 2003. *Plato's 'Timaeus' as cultural icon*. Notre Dame, IN: University of Notre Dame Press.

Richter, D. S. and Johnson, W. A. (eds.). 2017. *The Oxford handbook to the Second Sophistic*. Oxford: Oxford University Press.

Robinson, J. 2003. 'Some remarks on the source of Maimonides' Plato in *Guide of the Perplexed* I.17', *Zutot, Perspectives on Jewish Culture* 3.1: 49–57.

Rocca, J. 2003. *Galen on the brain: Anatomical knowledge and physiological speculation in the second century AD*. Leiden: Brill.

2012. 'From doubt to certainty: Aspects of the conceptualisation and interpretation of Galen's natural pneuma', in Horstmanshoff et al. (eds.), *Blood, sweat, and tears*, 629–59.

Roochnik, D. L. 1996. *Of art and wisdom: Plato's understanding of techne*. University Park: Pennsylvania State University Press.

Rose, N. 2014. 'The human sciences in a biological age', *Theory, Culture, and Society* 30.1: 3–34.

Rosen, R. M. 2013. 'Galen on poetic testimony', in M. Asper (ed.), *Writing science: Medical and mathematical authorship in ancient Greece*. Berlin: De Gruyter, 177–90.

Rosenthal, F. 1954. 'Isḥāq b. Ḥunayn's Taʾrīḫ al-aṭibbāʾ', *Oriens* 7: 55–80.

1966. '"Life is short, the art is long": Arabic commentaries on the first Hippocratic aphorism', *Bulletin of the History of Medicine* 40.3: 226–45.

1978. 'The physician in medieval Muslim society', *Bulletin of the History of Medicine* 52.4: 475–91.

1992. *The classical heritage in Islam*. London: Routledge.

Roueché, M. 1999. 'Did medical students study philosophy in Alexandria?' *Bulletin of the Institute of Classical Studies of the University of London* 43: 153–69.
Samuelson, N. M. 1991. 'Maimonides' doctrine of creation', *Harvard Theological Review* 84.3: 249–71.
Savage-Smith, E. 1995. 'Attitudes toward dissection in medieval Islam', *Journal of the History of Medicine and Allied Sciences* 50.1: 67–110.
2002. 'Galen's lost ophthalmology and the Summaria Alexandrinorum', in Nutton (ed.), *The Unknown Galen*: 121–38.
2007. 'Anatomical illustration in Arabic manuscripts', in A. Contadini (ed.), *Arab painting: Text and image in illustrated Arabic manuscripts*. Leiden: Brill, 147–59.
Schacht, J. and Meyerhof, M. 1937. 'Maimonides against Galen, on philosophy and cosmogony', *Bulletin of the Faculty of Arts of the University of Cairo* 5: 53–88.
Schiefsky, M. J. 2007. 'Galen's teleology and functional explanation', *Oxford Studies in Ancient Philosophy* 33: 369–400.
Schliesser, E. (ed.) 2015. *Sympathy: A history*. Oxford Philosophical Concepts. Oxford: Oxford University Press.
Schwarb, G. 2017. 'Early kalām and the medical tradition', in Adamson and Pormann (eds.), *Philosophy and medicine*, 104–69.
Schwarz, M. 1992. 'Who were Maimonides' Mutakallimūn? Some remarks on *Guide of the Perplexed* part I, chapter 73', *Maimonidean Studies* 2: 159–209.
Sedley, D. 1982. 'Two conceptions of vacuum', *Phronesis* 27.2: 175–93.
2013. 'Cicero and the *Timaeus*', in M. Schofield (ed.), *Aristotle, Plato and Pythagoreanism in the first century BC: New directions for philosophy*. Cambridge: Cambridge University Press, 187–205.
Seeskin, K. 2005. *Maimonides: Origin of the world*. Cambridge: Cambridge University Press.
Septimus, B. 1975. 'Meir Abulafia and the Maimonidean controversy of the thirteenth century'. Ph.D. thesis. Harvard University.
Sezgin, F. 1970. *Medizin, Pharmazie, Zoologie, Tierheilkunde bis ca. 430 H.* Geschichte des arabischen Schrifttums 3. Leiden: Brill.
(ed.) 1986. *Augenheilkunde im Islam: Texte, Studien und Übersetzungen*. Vol. II. Frankfurt am Main: Institut für Geschichte der Arabisch-Islamischen Wissenschaften.
Shapin, S. 1992. 'Discipline and bounding: The history of the sociology of science as seen through the externalism–internalism debate', *History of Science* 30.4: 333–69.
Shapiro, J., Coulehan, J., Wear, D., and Montello, M. 2009. 'Medical humanities and their discontents: Definitions, critiques, and implications', *Academic Medicine* 84.2: 192–98.
Sharples, R. W. and Sheppard, A. D. R. (eds.) 2003. *Ancient Approaches to Plato's 'Timaeus': Bulletin of the Institute of Classical Studies*, Supplement 78.
Shatzmiller, M. 1994. *Labour in the medieval Islamic world*. Leiden: Brill.
Shihadeh, A. 2015. *Doubts on Avicenna: A study and edition of Sharaf al-Dīn al-Mas'ūdī's commentary on the Ishārāt*. Leiden: Brill.

Silk, M. S., Gildenhard, I., and Barrow, R. J. (eds.) 2014. *The classical tradition: Art, literature, thought*. Hoboken, NJ: Wiley Blackwell.

Silver, D. J. 1965. *Maimonidean criticism and the Maimonidean controversy, 1180–1240*. Leiden: Brill.

Simms, D. L. 1991. 'Galen on Archimedes: Burning mirror or burning pitch?', *Technology and Culture* 32: 91–6.

Singer, P. N. 2014. 'Galen and the philosophers: Philosophical engagement, shadowy contemporaries, Aristotelian transformations', in Adamson et al. (eds.), *Philosophical Themes in Galen*: 7–38.

2017. 'The essence of rage: Galen on emotional disturbances and their physical correlates', in R. Seaford, J. Wilkins, and M. Wright (eds.), *Selfhood and the soul: Essays on ancient thought and literature in honour of Christopher Gill*. Oxford: Oxford University Press, 161–96.

2018. 'Galen's pathological soul: Diagnosis and therapy in ethical medical texts and contexts', in C. Thumiger and P. Singer (eds.), *Mental illness in ancient medicine*. Leiden: Brill, 381–420.

Siraisi, N. G. 1987. *Avicenna in Renaissance Italy: The Canon and medical teaching in Italian universities after 1500*. Princeton: Princeton University Press.

Skemp, J. B. 1947. 'Plants in Plato's *Timaeus*', *CQ* 41: 53–60.

Smith, M. 2015. *From sight to light: The passage from ancient to modern physics*. Chicago: University of Chicago Press.

Somfai, A. 2002. 'The eleventh-century shift in the reception of Plato's *Timaeus* and Calcidius' *Commentary*', *Journal of the Warburg and Courtauld Institutes* 65: 1–21.

Stern, J. 2013. *The matter and form of Maimonides' 'Guide'*. Cambridge, MA: Harvard University Press.

Strauss, L. 1935. *Philosophie und Gesetz: Beiträge zum Verständnis Maimunis und seiner Vorläufer*. Berlin: Schocken.

1936. 'Quelques remarques sur la science politique de Maïmonide et de Fârâbî', *Revue des études juives* 100: 1–37.

1937. 'Der Ort der Vorsehungslehre nach der Ansicht Maimunis', *Monatsschrift für Geschichte und Wissenschaft des Judentums* 80.1: 93–105.

1952. *Persecution and the art of writing*. Chicago: University of Chicago Press.

Striker, G. 1995. 'Cicero and Greek philosophy', *Harvard Studies in Classical Philology* 97: 53–61.

1996. 'The role of oikeiosis in Stoic ethics', in G. Striker (ed.), *Essays on Hellenistic epistemology and ethics*. Cambridge: Cambridge University Press, 281–97.

Strohmaier, G. 1965. 'Ḥunain ibn Isḥāq und die Bilder', *Klio* 43–5:525–33.

1968. 'Die griechischen Götter in einer christlich-arabischen Übersetzung: Zum Traumbuch des Artemidor in der Version des Ḥunain ibn Isḥāḳ', in F. Altheim and R. Stiehl (eds.), *Die Araber in der Alten Welt*, vol. V.1: *Weitere Neufunde: Nordafrika bis zur Einwanderung der Wandalen. Ḏū Nuwās*. Berlin: De Gruyter, 127–62.

1998. 'Bekannte und unbekannte Zitate in den *Zweifeln an Galen* des Rhazes', in K. Fischer, D. Nickel., and P. Potter (eds.), *Text and tradition: Studies in ancient medicine and its transmission presented to Jutta Kollesch*. Studies in Ancient Medicine 18. Leiden: Brill, 263–87.

2012. 'Galen the Pagan and Ḥunayn the Christian: Specific transformations in the commentaries on *Airs, Waters, Places* and the *Epidemics*', in Pormann (ed.), *Epidemics in context*, 171–84.

Stroumsa, S. 1993. 'al-Fārābī and Maimonides on medicine as a science', *Arabic Sciences and Philosophy* 3.2: 235–49.

1999. *Freethinkers of medieval Islam: Ibn al-Rāwandī, Abū Bakr al-Rāzī, and their impact on Islamic thought*. Islamic Philosophy and Theology 35. Leiden: Brill.

2009. *Maimonides in his world*. Jews, Christians, and Muslims from the Ancient to the Modern World. Princeton: Princeton University Press.

Swain, S. 1996. *Hellenism and empire: Language, classicism, and power in the Greek world AD 50–250*. Oxford: Oxford University Press.

Tamer, G. (ed.) 2005. *The trias of Maimonides: Jewish, Arabic, and ancient culture of knowledge*. Studia Judaica 30. Berlin: De Gruyter.

Tarrant, H. A. S. 1993. *Thrasyllan Platonism*. Ithaca: Cornell University Press.

Taylor, C. A. 1996. *Defining science: A rhetoric of demarcation*. Madison: University of Wisconsin Press.

Taylor, C. C. W. 2008. 'Urmson on Aristotle on pleasure', in C. C. W. Taylor (ed.), *Pleasure, mind, and soul: Selected papers in ancient philosophy*. Oxford: Clarendon Press, 107–20.

Temkin, O. 1953. 'Greek medicine as science and craft', *Isis* 44.2: 213–25.

1973. *Galenism: Rise and decline of a medical philosophy*. Cornell Publications in the History of Science. Ithaca: Cornell University Press.

Tieleman, T. 1996. *Galen and Chrysippus on the soul: Argument and refutation in the 'De placitis' books II–III*. Leiden: Brill.

1998. 'Plotinus on the seat of the soul: Reverberations of Galen and Alexander in *Enn*. IV, 3 [27], 23', *Phronesis* 43.4: 306–25.

2003. *Chrysippus' 'On affections': Reconstruction and interpretation*. Leiden: Brill.

2005. 'Galen and Genesis', in G. Van Kooten (ed.), *The Creation of heaven and earth: Re-interpretations of Genesis 1 in the context of Judaism, ancient philosophy, Christianity, and modern physics*. Brill: Leiden, 125–45.

Tuozzo, T. M. 1996. 'The general account of pleasure in Plato's *Philebus*', *Journal of the History of Philosophy* 34.4: 495–513.

Ullmann, M. 1970. *Die Medizin im Islam*. Handbuch der Orientalistik I, Erg.-Bd. 6.1. Leiden: Brill.

2006. *Wörterbuch zu den griechisch–arabischen Übersetzungen des 9. Jahrhunderts. Supplement. Band 1: A–O*. Wiesbaden: Harrassowitz.

Urmson, J. O. 1967. 'Aristotle on pleasure', in J. M. E. Moravcsik (ed.), *Aristotle: A collection of critical essays*. Notre Dame, IN: University of Notre Dame Press, 335–41.

van Bladel, K. T. 2009. *The Arabic Hermes: From the pagan sage to prophet of science*. Oxford Studies in Late Antiquity. Oxford: Oxford University Press.

2011. 'The Bactrian background of the Barmakids', in A. Akasoy, C. Burnett, and R. Yoeli-Tlalim (eds.), *Islam and Tibet: Interactions along the musk routes*. London: Ashgate, 43–88.

van der Eijk, P. J. 2009. 'Aristotle! What a thing for you to say! Galen's engagement with Aristotle and Aristotelians', in Gill et al. (eds.), *Galen and the world of knowledge*, 261–81.

van Gelder, G. J. 2011. 'Canon and canonisation, in classical Arabic literature', in *EI3*.

van Riel, G. 2000. *Pleasure and the good life: Plato, Aristotle, and the Neoplatonists*. Philosophia Antiqua 85. Leiden and Boston: Brill.

Vegetti, M. 1994. 'L'immagine del medico e lo statuto epistemologico della medicina in Galeno', in *ANRW* II.37.2, 1672–1717.

Verrycken, K. 1997. 'Philoponus' interpretation of Plato's cosmogony', *Documenti e Studi sulla Tradizione Filosofica Medievale* 8: 269–318.

Vesel, Ž. 1986. *Les encyclopédies persanes: essai de typologie et de classification des sciences*. Bibliothèque iranienne 31. Paris: Recherche sur les civilisations.

Viguera Molins, M. J. 2014. 'Almohads', in *EI3*.

Vlastos, G. 1939. 'The disorderly motion in the *Timaios*', *CQ* 33.2: 71–83.

von Staden, H. 1995 'Anatomy as rhetoric: Galen on dissection and persuasion', *Journal of the History of Medicine and Allied Sciences* 50: 47–66.

1997. 'Galen and the "Second Sophistic"', in R. Sorabji (ed.), *Aristotle and after. Bulletin of the Institute of Classical Studies*, Supplement 68: 33–54.

2002. 'Division, dissection, and specialization: Galen's On the parts of the medical techne', in Nutton (ed.) *The Unknown Galen*: 19–45.

2007. '*Physis* and *technē* in Greek medicine', in B. Bensaude-Vincent and W. R. Newman (eds.), *The artificial and the natural: An evolving polarity*. Cambridge, MA: MIT Press, 21–49.

2009. 'Staging the past, staging oneself: Galen on Hellenistic exegetical traditions', in Gill et al. (eds.), *Galen and the world of knowledge*, 132–56.

Walker, P. E. 1992. 'The political implications of al-Rāzī's philosophy', in C. Butterworth (ed.), *The political aspects of Islamic philosophy*. Cambridge, MA: Harvard University Press, 61–94.

Weisser, U. 1983. 'Ibn Sīnā und die Medizin des arabisch-islamischen Mittelalters – Alte und neue Urteile und Vorurteile', *Medizinhistorisches Journal* 18.4: 283–305.

1991. 'Zur Rezeption der Methodus Medendi im Continens des Rhazes', in R. Durling and F. Kudlien (eds.), *Galen's method of healing*. Studies in Ancient Medicine 1. Leiden: Brill, 123–46.

White, M. J. 2006. 'Plato and mathematics', in H. Benson (ed.), *A companion to Plato*. Malden, MA: Blackwell Publishing, 228–43.

Whitmarsh, T. 2001. *Greek literature and the Roman Empire*. Oxford: Oxford University Press.

2005. *The Second Sophistic*. Oxford: Oxford University Press.

Wilberding, J. 2014. 'The secret of sentient vegetative life in Galen', in Adamson et al. (eds.), *Philosophical Themes in Galen*: 249–68.

Wilburn, J. 2013. 'Moral education and the spirited part of the soul in Plato's *Laws*', *Oxford Studies in Ancient Philosophy* 45: 63–102.
Wisnovsky, R. 2003. *Avicenna's metaphysics in context*. Ithaca: Cornell University Press.
2013. 'Avicenna's Islamic reception', in Adamson (ed.), *Interpreting Avicenna*, 190–213.
Wolfsdorf, D. 2013. *Pleasure in ancient Greek philosophy*. Cambridge: Cambridge University Press.
Xenophontos, S. 2016. *Ethical education in Plutarch: Moralising agents and contexts*. Beiträge zur Altertumskunde 349. Berlin: De Gruyter.
Yarshater, E. (ed.) 1996. *Encyclopaedia Iranica*. Encyclopaedia Iranica Foundation (online).
Zimmermann, F. 1976. 'al-Fārābī und die philosophische Kritik an Galen von Alexander zu Averroes', in A. Dietrich (ed.), *Akten des VII. Kongresses für Arabistik und Islamwissenschaft*. Abhandlungen der Akademie der Wissenschaften in Göttingen, Phil.-Hist. Kl., Dritte Folge 98. Göttingen: Vandenhoeck und Ruprecht, 401–14.
1986. 'The origins of the so-called *Theology of Aristotle*', in J. Kraye (ed.), *Warburg Institute surveys and texts XI: Pseudo-Aristotle in the Middle Ages*. London: Warburg Institute, 110–240.
Zipser, B. 2009. 'Deleted text in a manuscript: Galen *On the Eye* and the *Marc. Gr. 276*', *Galenos* 3: 107–12.
Zonta, M. 2005. 'Maimonides' knowledge of Avicenna: Some tentative conclusions about a debated question', in Tamer (ed.), *The trias of Maimonides*, 211–22.

Index Locorum

'Āmirī, al-
Kitāb al-Amad 'alā al-abad (ed. Rowson)
p. 74 ll. 15–18, 105
Andalusī, Ṣā'id al-
Kitāb Ṭabaqāt al-umam (ed. 'Alwān)
§ 7, p. 180, l. 2–p. 181, l. 6, 109
Aristotle
Analytica Priora
26a10–13, 10
64a40–b28, 10
De Anima
412a19–22, 153
415b23, 59
417a3–9, 75
418a27–419a25, 74
De Partibus Animalium
656a27–657a12, 84–5
De Sensu et Sensibilibus
437a19–440b26, 74
437b12–25, 75n24
438a18–19, 75n25
Ethica Nicomachea
1097a9, 10
1139b, 7n28
1140a, 7n27
1152b–1154b, 162
1172a20–1175b35, 82
Metaphysica
981b13–25, 7
1070a29, 10
Meteorologica
1.14 (351a10–353a25), 143
Poetica
1460b20, 10
Politica
1279a1, 10
1282a4–8, 9n35
Avicenna
al-As'ila wa l-aǧwiba (ed. Naṣr and Muḥaqqiq)
p. 13 ll. 10–13, 104
al-Ilāhiyyāt
9.7, 165–7
9.7.4, 166
9.7.14, 166, 167
9.7.15–16, 167
9.7.17–18, 166
al-Qānūn fī l-ṭibb
1.1.1.2, 144–8, 156
1.1.5.1, 148–52
1.1.6.1, 154–5
1.1.6.4, 155–6
1.2.1.14, 161n79
1.2.2.23, 157–9
De Anima
1.5, 164n97
2.2, 163
4.4, 160–1
5.8, 153
Fī Aqsām al-'ulūm al-'aqliyya (ed. in Avicenna 1908)
p. 101 l. 8–p. 111 l. 7, 162
Kitāb al-Išārāt wa l-tanbīhāt
2.8, 165–7
Kitāb al-Naǧāt
2.6.10, 164n97
2.6.15, 153
Maqāla fī Aḥkām al-adwiya al-qalbiyya (ed. al-Bābā)
p. 226 ll. 2–3, 161
p. 226 ll. 5–6, 161
p. 226 l. 10–p. 230, l. 5, 162–4
p. 226 ll. 11–15, 162–3
p. 228 l. 1, 163
p. 228 ll. 3–4, 163–4
p. 228 ll. 9–13, 164
p. 229 l. 4–p. 230, l. 5, 164
pp. 234–6, 161
Sīrat al-šayḫ al-ra'īs (ed. Gohlman)
p. 24 l. 6–p. 26, l. 2, 140

General Index

Afḍal, Malik al-, 182
Alexander of Aphrodisias, 17–18
Alexander of Damascus, 83
Almohad caliphate, 171
ʿĀmirī, al-, 105
anatomy
  Galen on, 43–7, 82–4
  Maimonides on, 182
  ocular, 74, 84, 90–5
Andalusī, Ṣāʿid al-, 109
appropriation, Stoic. *See* οἰκείωσις
Aristides, Aelius, 55
Aristotle
  Galen on, 42–4
  Islamicate receptions of, 23
  Maimonides on, 173–4, 177
  on medicine, 10
  on pleasure, 162
  on sensation, 84–5
  on *technē* and *epistēmē*, 7
  on vegetative sensation, 59
  on vision, 74–5, 85
Aristotle, works of
  De Anima (On the Soul), 23, 74–5
  De Sensu et Sensibilibus (On Sense and Sensibles), 74–5, 183
  Meteorology, 143
  Nicomachean Ethics, 162
  On Plants, 59
  On the Heavens, 23
artes liberales, 8
Avicenna, 26–7
  cardiocentrism of, 148–56
  on disciplinary boundaries, 142, 144–8
  education and career, 140–1
  hierarchy of the sciences, 146
  on perception, 162–4
  and Platonism, 143–4
  on pleasure, 143, 156–60, 162–8
  on pneumatic theory, 154–6, 161
  on al-Rāzī, 104
  on sensation, 154–5
  on the soul, 142–3, 152–3
Avicenna, works of
  Autobiography, 140–1
  Canon of Medicine, 141–3, 144–59
  Cardiac Drugs, 143, 159–65
  Cure, The, 141–3
  De Anima (of The Cure), 153, 156
  Metaphysics (of The Cure), 165–8
  On the Divisions of the Intellectual Sciences, 146, 165
  Pointers and Reminders, 143, 165–8
  Salvation, 153, 156

Baghdad, 93–5
Ben Maimon, Moshe. *See* Maimonides
Bīrūnī, Abū l-Rayḥān al-, 104, 141
  Book Confirming What Pertains to India, The, 40–1, 67–8
  List of al-Rāzī's Books, 112
Boethus, Flavius, 42, 83n61
Book of Laws, The, 39
boundary work, 12–13
  and disciplinary identities, 200–1
  the soul in, 198–9
boundary-speech, 201–2

canon, 144
Celsus, Cornelius, 76
Chrysippus, 42–4, 64–5
classical tradition, 28
cosmogony, 111, 124–8, 175–9
creation. *See* cosmogony
crystalline humour, 90–3

David of Armenia, 19–20
Dawla, Šams al-, 161
discipline, 11–12
dissection, 43–4, 194n112

Lightning Source UK Ltd.
Milton Keynes UK
UKHW020833190321
380619UK00004B/106

9 781108 499484